CURED!

The Insider's Handbook
for Health Care Reform

CURED!

The Insider's Handbook for Health Care Reform

Stephen S. S. Hyde

HOBNOBPUBLISHING

First printing 2009

ISBN: 978-0-9840556-0-9 (hardcover)
        978-0-9840556-1-6 (paperback)
LCCN: 2009928297

**ATTENTION CORPORATIONS, UNIVERSITIES, COLLEGES,
AND PROFESSIONAL ORGANIZATIONS:** Quantity discounts are available on bulk
purchases of this book for educational, gift purposes, or as premiums for
increasing publication subscriptions or renewals.
For information, please contact Hobnob Publishing at
(303) 641-0946 or www.hobnobpublishing.com.

To Loren, Evan, and Erin

Contents

Part I—THE PROBLEM

A Troubling Conclusion—Market Failure

Premium Rate Setting

Why Not Mandate Health Insurance?

Part II—GOVERNMENT ATTEMPTS TO FIX THE PROBLEM

Part III—The Cure

The Upside-Down Economics and Persistent Myths of American Health Care

The American health care system is a disaster. The purpose of this book is to describe how it came to be this way and to offer a way out. The punch line of this book is a deceptively simple proposition. We can resolve virtually all the problems of our massively dysfunctional health care system if we can figure out how to get America's consumers to demand and to act on the answers to two questions:

1. For my medical needs and personal circumstances, which health care providers, procedures, services, and products offer me the highest quality, most beneficial outcomes?

2. Of those high-quality treatment options, which ones cost the least?

Let me ask you to suspend any disbelief that consumers ever can, will, or even should ask these questions or act on the answers. The arguments that they can't, won't, or shouldn't are bogus. That's lesson number one from my nearly forty years of toiling in the fields of health care regulation and management.

If the two questions above seem somehow familiar, it's because they focus on the basic value proposition that all American consumers ask every day of their lives for virtually everything they buy—food, clothing, housing, transportation, recreation—everything, that is, except health care.

The problem lies in the failure of consumer markets to evolve in health care the way they have in other aspects of our lives. At the heart of this failure is a fundamental difference that separates health care from our other wants and needs—but it's probably not the one you think. It is this: Although high prices almost always connote optional luxury goods and services, they don't with health care. A quarter-million-dollar liver transplant can be just as necessary as a two-cent aspirin. There is nothing luxurious about it. Thus, for everyone to have the ability to consume the full range of necessary medical care, they must have insurance to pay for the expensive stuff. The primary market failure in health care is that markets have not emerged to offer such insurance to everyone. This is the crux of our problem.

We have failed to recognize and fix this market failure largely because its existence has been obscured by uncounted layers of myth and practice that almost all of us have accepted as the way things must be. Almost utterly ignored, or even rejected, is the reality that medical care is what economists refer to as an economic good that is subject to the dynamics of price-mediated supply and demand. It is not, as many believe, a public good or a basic human right. I wish it were. Because of this market failure, we now suffer under a system that would be more familiar to Lewis Carroll than Adam Smith.

We spend more and more money while excluding more and more people from care. Only in health care does excess supply create its own excess demand with no decrease in price. This phenomenon even has a name in economics—the Roemer Effect. Therefore, to lower costs, we have tried to restrict the supply of health care facilities and providers—a futile effort in defiance of basic economics.

Increasingly, the more innovative new providers (such as specialty hospitals) are, the more state and federal governments have suppressed them because of the threat they represent to existing, far less efficient players. And if competition is considered bad in health care, price competition is especially bad. Maybe that's why we let the federal government control prices on virtually all doctor and hospital services. Then, in an effective *coup de grâce* to any sort of microeconomic market solution, we have hidden even these artificial prices from consumers, lest they foolishly use them as a guide to actual value.

We face a dire shortage of primary care doctors, yet the government continues to set their reimbursement rates at the lowest levels, with insurers going along as willing co-conspirators. At the same time we legislatively restrict highly qualified nurse practitioners from practicing to the full extent of their well-documented capabilities.

Often, low-cost generic drug competition causes sales of a brand-name medication to suddenly drop by 97 percent. So does the maker of the brand-name drug drop the price to compete more effectively? No, because the perverse rules of health care economics dictate that the rational approach is actually to *raise* the price. The same drug companies sell their most expensive drugs to you for not one price but two: an extremely high one if you have insurance and free if you don't, thus providing perverse incentives for some sick people to actually drop their insurance coverage.

Why do we empower people to smoke, eat, and drink themselves to death by requiring those with healthy lifestyles to subsidize their self-destructive behaviors? And why are we increasingly making doctors accountable for preventing the diseases that predictably result from their patients' 24/7 lifestyles?

As medical costs rise, we force insurers to cover even more unnecessary services, thus driving insurance premiums even higher. We require insurers to cover normal consumer purchases, no matter how cheap—even though this adds overhead, profit, and parasitic billing and reimbursement expenses that can double the cost—while completely hiding prices from consumers.

We justify all this on the basis that people supposedly value and use only the health care they think they're getting for free, even when it drives insurance premiums beyond anything many of them can afford. Even worse, people without insurance, who can nonetheless pay their doctors upfront, are required to pay the highest prices while bureaucratic insurers that delay payments get to pay less than half as much. And many uninsured consumers who could pay—but simply refuse—often escape paying anything. This leaves the hospitals and doctors to pass these costs on to those with health insurance, thus further driving up their premiums.

Every day ordinary consumers buy and integrate complex choices of computers, automobiles, software, and communications technologies into their lives. But they can't be trusted to make their own choices about medical care. Instead, we let others—the government, employers, insurers, and doctors—tell them what medical care they can have and which providers they can use. Then consumers are told how much they have to pay for it all. If we had a similar system for buying cars, we'd have a revolt on our hands. Because none of this has worked well, many health reform advocates now propose to let the government force everyone to buy what they supposedly need—a uniform set of health insurance benefits that takes no account of individual needs, circumstances, means, or preferences.

Even though advertising is generally viewed as an essential, informative—if frequently annoying—component of our consumer economy, prescription drug advertising is increasingly castigated as harmful and in need of prohibition, as it is in Europe. In our everyday lives technological advances make virtually everything better and cheaper—except health care, where technology is blamed for driving costs higher. Maybe this helps explain why doctors have resisted electronic medical records, thus leaving health care as our sole remaining paper-documented industry.

We have witnessed no improvements in the office productivity of many doctors over the past forty years, yet the states persist with restrictive corporate-practice-of-medicine laws that prevent medical practices from adopting organizational, ownership, and management forms that have transformed the rest of American industry from the 1800s to this day.

Our private health insurance system is employer-based. That means people too sick to work can't get coverage. Small business is the great economic driver of the American economy. Yet we saddle it with excessive health care costs, regulations, and mandates while we exempt large employers. Then the big companies squander their privilege by hiring pharmacy benefit managers who make their employees pay higher prices than they could have gotten on their own with a modicum of savvy retail shopping.

This system is so upside down that workers actually complain when expensive prescription drugs become available over the counter at 70 percent lower prices. Why? Because they now have to pay *more* for them. What on earth is going on here, and why do so many of us accept this situation as normal?

Many reform proponents argue that richer people should pay more for their health insurance than poorer people. Yet they simultaneously support employer-based insurance that requires younger, lower-paid employees to subsidize their older, richer colleagues—or drop their own insurance altogether. When many young workers quite rationally do the latter, the reformers then blame them for supposedly believing they're invincible. These same reform advocates would fix the situation with the simple expedient of making it illegal not to buy health insurance—despite the fact that no one has *ever* been required to purchase anything as a condition of living in America—and that includes car insurance.

Everywhere else in our economy, profits are a sign of customer acceptance, efficient operations, and good management. In health care, they are seen by many pundits as evidence of rapacity, wasted resources, and denied care. Drug companies, whose products prevent disease, heal the sick, and reduce medical costs, are demonized as conniving price gougers because they rationally follow the rules of an irrational game not of their invention—not that they've done much to try to change such a lucrative game. Health insurers that keep their members out of bankruptcy are said to be the greedy, heartless bad guys who are in cahoots with an all-consuming black hole of medical providers, yet reformers would have us believe we're supposed to force everyone to buy from them anyway?

We celebrate when medical costs increase at *only* twice the prevailing inflation rate. Providers who harm patients are paid more than those who heal them. And if anyone tries to exclude sub-par doctors, we pass laws to require that they be treated and paid equally with the best ones. We claim to have "the best health care system in the world," even though your chance of being treated according to current medical standards is the same as getting heads on a coin toss. Doctors deride these professional standards as "cookbook medicine" that any well-trained nurse practitioner with a computer could achieve.

Many pundits support more federal debt and unfunded mandates to pay for more health care spending. Yet many of the same critics discourage consumer savings and investment that could support better individual health choices.

In this upended universe, we hear calls for yet more government control to improve, of all things, private sector efficiency. Better yet, say others, we should force business out of health care altogether and let the government run it all more responsively, compassionately, and cost-effectively—presumably as the government has done with banking and securities regulation, mortgage lending, the Congress, military weapons procurement, the FAA, the FDA, and the IRS. True, increased government control hasn't worked so far, but surely more of it will. Top-down, rules-based control is all the rage. Market capitalism has become the new pariah of health care.

Widespread acceptance of such inverted economic thinking by people who should know better has deeply affected public perceptions of health care's problems and how we should go about solving them. It has led to numerous beliefs that simply don't hold up to rational scrutiny. It is as if the ruling mantra in health care is "We hold these myths to be self-evident." And the myths come in all sizes and flavors. Here are some of the big ones:

- Insurance coverage for primary and preventive care saves money by preventing expensive diseases.

- Such insurance coverage is necessary because people won't buy preventive services on their own.
- Electronic medical records will reduce total health care spending.
- There are forty-six million Americans who can't find or can't afford health insurance.
- The uninsured are the biggest problem in health care. Solving it will lower total health care spending.
- Our health care system produces the worst life expectancy and infant mortality statistics in the developed world.
- Requiring everyone to buy health insurance is the only way to deal with free riders and to solve the problem of the uninsured.
- So many young people have no insurance because they think they're immortal and don't need it.
- Getting the uninsured youngsters to buy insurance will help pay the growing health care costs of the aging boomers.
- Insurance company profits are a big contributor to excessive health care costs.
- Letting Medicare negotiate drug prices will solve the problem of excessive pricing by Big Pharma.
- Uninsured people who use hospital emergency rooms are a big cause of cost-shifting to the rest of us.
- A large percentage of all health care spending occurs during the last year of patients' lives.
- We may spend a lot more for health care than other countries, but at least we have "the best health care system in the world."
- A national health board that sets medical practice standards will improve quality and lower costs.
- Paying more money to doctors who do the right thing will improve quality.
- Doctors have a natural, rightful monopoly on the practice of medicine.
- Health care is a public good.

- All licensed doctors are created equal and must be treated that way. (Question: What do you call a medical student who squeaks through graduation at the bottom of his class? Answer: Doctor.)
- Doctors are the key factor in preventing chronic diseases.
- Specialty hospitals unfairly harm community hospitals.
- Medicare, with its low administrative costs, is more efficient than private insurers.
- The free market can solve all our problems in health care.
- A consumer market-based system can never work because medical care is too technical and too complex for consumers ever to be able to navigate and purchase on their own.
- Employer-based health insurance is dominant because of a World War II tax ruling that excluded employees' health benefits from their income taxes.
- The dominance and success of employer-based health insurance makes it worth preserving and strengthening.
- Requiring employers to cover health insurance will improve workers' living standards.
- The lack of insurer motivation to promote long-term prevention is the result of frequent membership turnover.
- Community rating, in which everyone pays the same health insurance premium, is the fairest pricing method.
- Individual insurance is inherently inferior to employer-based group insurance.
- Consumer-driven health care and health savings accounts (HSAs) don't and won't work because consumers can't get good information on health care prices and quality.
- Consumer-driven health care is just another way of saying "the patient pays more" and is especially unfair to the poor and to people with chronic diseases.
- Health care quality and cost will improve if government, employers, providers, and insurers coordinate to focus on the patients.

In this book I will establish that each of these assumptions and assertions is either merely wrong or dead wrong—and that any attempt at serious reform founded on any combination of such beliefs is doomed.

Why do people believe these myths if they're not true? Liberal economist and Nobel laureate Paul Krugman's coinage of the "anti-Cassandra effect" may help explain it—if somewhat cynically. Cassandra was the beautiful young daughter of King Priam of Troy in Homer's *Iliad*. She was blessed by Apollo with the gift of prophecy but also cursed never to be believed by anyone. Krugman's anti-Cassandra effect holds that there are those "who have been wrong about everything—but are still, mysteriously, treated as men of wisdom"— an especially ironic bon mot, considering Krugman's own position favoring single-payer health insurance reform.[1]

Market economist Thomas Sowell takes a more analytical approach, pointing out that "fallacies are not simply crazy ideas. They are usually both plausible and logical—but with something missing. Their plausibility gains them political support. Only after that political support is strong enough to cause fallacious ideas to become government policies and programs are the missing or ignored factors likely to lead to 'unintended consequences,' a phrase often heard in the wake of economic or social policy disasters."[2]

Whether you prefer liberal Krugman's or conservative Sowell's explanation, each economist pretty well sums up the conventional state of health care—past and present. There is too much conventional thinking and too little objective scrutiny of its dynamics, defects, and potential solutions. It's a lot like Samuel Johnson's reference to second marriages as triumphs of hope over experience.

I propose we move to the fifty-thousand-foot level and look at the medical landscape as just another essential component of our national consumer economy but one that also presents a uniquely problematic market and regulatory failure. Such a perspective can suggest solutions that have thus far eluded those who see health care as something operating under a different set of economic principles.

It doesn't. The failure of the public and private sectors (and more than a few economists) to recognize this is at the root of virtually all the problems we now see in inadequate insurance, poor care quality, high costs, and a looming pandemic of preventable diseases. A more realistic view of health care can lead us to a uniquely American solution producing dramatically better quality, lower costs, and universal access to affordable health insurance.

From such an Olympian perch, it becomes apparent that the consumer markets reliably supplying us with high-quality affordable food, clothing, housing, and transportation just might be able to do the same thing with medical care. Let us take advantage of this view to seek clues for crafting a more effective bottom-up, appropriately regulated, consumer market-based approach that will replace the top-down, rules-based system that governs it now.

If we're going to address our needs in reforming health care, we must agree on two inconvenient truths. First, employers' and government's historic roles in health care have failed to deliver. Continuing or increasing those roles will only exacerbate and accelerate that failure. Second, unfettered market forces alone will never spontaneously create a market that will allow everyone to gain needed access to expensive medical care. Fixing health care will require a regulatory approach that renders unto government that which is rightly government's, and to markets that which is rightly markets'. It is my intent to show how we can do this and to resolve virtually all of the major problems in our health care financing and delivery system.

As for the myths, I used to believe a lot of them myself. If at times I appear preachy, please grant me the slack you would a former smoker who now proselytizes his newfound vision of abstinence. We mean well. And we have a valid point. We just need to be less pushy and more humble.

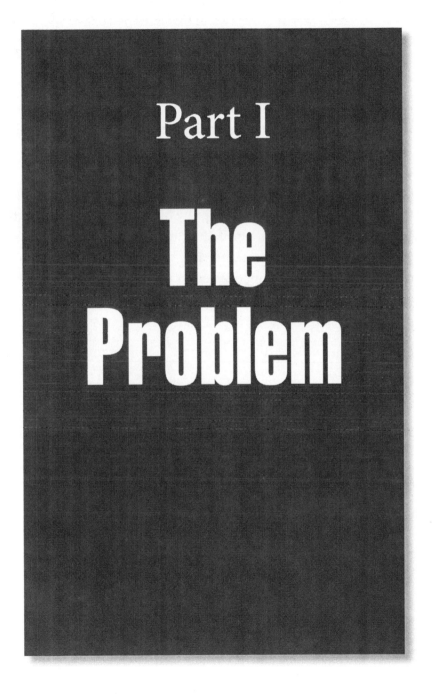

Part I

The Problem

PART I—THE PROBLEM

This book is organized into three parts. Part I is primarily focused on laying out and analyzing the problems of our unstable, unsustainable health care financing and delivery system—and especially why it has developed the way it has. The first chapter provides an outline of my proposed cure: The American Choice Health Plan. Part II covers past steps and missteps by the government to fill in the gaps presented by the market's failure to provide affordable health insurance to everyone who wants and needs it. Part III provides a look at two diametrically opposed cures for our sick system, the first a single-payer system and the second my prescription for The American Choice Health plan.

CHAPTER 1

The Fundamental Problem with American Health Care and a Proposal to Remedy It

The thesis of this book is simple. Our current health care mess is the result of a largely unrecognized but correctable market failure. This failure has prevented a viable consumer market from emerging to efficiently deliver the necessary, high-quality, and affordable medical care we all need. What we have instead is a balkanized system of private and government programs that lack a comprehensive focus on meeting the medical needs of America's consumers in an economically sustainable fashion.

Virtually all current proposals for health reform suffer from major—usually fatal—flaws that fail to address this market failure. Fixing the system will require what many will consider a radical approach, a fundamental realignment of the relationships among government, employers, insurers, health care providers, and consumers, effected in the following ways:

- *Government*: First, government must establish and enforce a regulatory environment in which comprehensive consumer health insurance and medical care markets can function; and second, government must provide financial and social safety nets for those who lack the ability to participate in these newly empowered markets. Among other things, this means getting government out of the health insurance business.

- *Employers*: We must change employers' role from providing their employees with little or no choice in health benefits to one of providing them the funds to purchase their own coverage from a plethora of private insurance offerings.

- *Insurers*: The insurers' role must revert to the fundamental function of providing financial protection against the unaffordable costs of medical care while becoming directly responsible to the people they insure rather than to government, employers, and providers.
- *Providers*: Each health care provider must become directly accountable to its consumers and patients rather than to government, insurers, and employers.
- *Consumers*: To gain the clout to demand all this accountability, consumers must control all the money for their own health insurance and medical care.

Once again, the effectiveness standard of such a regulated market solution would be the extent to which America's consumers demand and act on the answers to the two questions I raised in the introduction:

1. For my medical needs and personal circumstances, which health care providers, procedures, services, and products offer me the highest quality, most beneficial outcomes?

2. Of those high-quality treatment options, which ones are the least expensive?

Giving consumers the authority and responsibility to purchase their own health insurance and health services may sound deceptively simple, but doing so will correct virtually all of the current system's shortcomings. It will fix the inadequate access to health insurance, lack of affordability, inconsistent quality, under-funded government programs, and health care provider shortages. We are clearly a long way from such a solution now.

America is a market capitalist society in which the voluntary behavior of millions of buyers, interacting with millions of sellers, allocates limited economic resources to satisfy individual wants and needs. Despite manifold attempts to develop better systems over the centuries, none has ever topped market capitalism's status as the most effective known approach for creating and distributing economic wealth. Yet market capitalism has utterly failed to deliver an efficient and effective health care system, despite the fact that medical care is a scarce economic good that is subject to the same supply-and-demand dynamics as our other essential needs in life.

Why is that? Some claim it's a problem of excess profiteering by insurers, health care CEOs, and drug companies and thus too much rampant capitalism. Others see the culprit as too much government regulation and intervention and therefore too little market capitalism. Neither explanation properly characterizes the real issue, nor does it form the basis for a comprehensive solution. The real problem lies in a fundamental market failure that neither private nor public remedies have recognized or corrected.

Market Failure

The market failure is that—unlike in the cases of our other basic necessities of life—no naturally arising market mechanism will allow everyone to obtain the health insurance required to afford the full range of necessary medical treatments for expensive, life-threatening maladies. Let me explain.

There are essentially five fundamental human needs necessary to survive in modern society: food, clothing, housing, transportation, and medical care. (We might also include education, but that discussion is well beyond the scope of this book.) In our country we obtain the first four efficiently and affordably via essentially self-organizing markets operating under the rule of law—i.e., regulation. In meeting such needs, we find in each category a vast range of prices for different goods and services. In almost every case the high-priced products and services constitute luxuries that may add to our enjoyment of life but are hardly necessary. The basic necessities, on the other hand, are always cheaper and are affordable for almost everyone in any advanced economy like ours. Chicken is as nourishing as lobster, and clothes from Wal-Mart will keep a person as warm as those from Saks Fifth Avenue.

Health care is different. Expensive medical services are just as necessary as the inexpensive ones. With non-relevant exceptions, such as some elective procedures, they are rarely a luxury. Thus, while with food, clothing, shelter, and transportation we can distinguish between necessary and luxury goods on the basis of low and high prices, with medical care we cannot (see graph below). It is unique among life's necessities in not having a significant luxury component that correlates with price. If you need a liver transplant, no one would consider it a luxury in the commonly accepted sense of the word. None of my classmates at Harvard Business School ever told me they wanted to make a lot of money so they could enjoy a heart transplant when they got older, even though it's something few people can afford on their own.

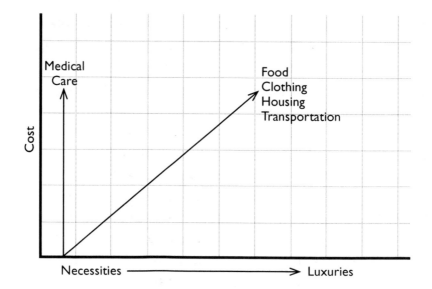

However expensive such medical services might be, few people feel they should have to forgo them in a prosperous economy. We tend to see them as unwelcome necessities foisted on us without regard to wealth or class, either as a result of bad luck or, increasingly, the long-term effects of bad behavior. Either way, access to them is not something most of us are willing to yield to the rich.

Because the need for expensive medical care strikes unpredictably and affects only a minority of the population at any given time, we have the fortunate opportunity to make it broadly affordable with insurance. By pooling financial resources from many individuals, we can pay the costs of those few who draw a losing number in life's medical sweepstakes. Economic history shows that insurance markets have spontaneously emerged to protect policyholders against financial losses in such diverse areas as ocean shipping, home ownership, personal disability, death, automobile accidents, credit defaults, beautiful legs, and many others.

Insurance markets allow a person to pay an affordable premium to an insurer that agrees to indemnify him against losses defined by the insurance contract. Insurance specialists, called actuaries, estimate the risks and costs and then set the premiums accordingly. Other specialists, called underwriters, make sure that each prospective client represents an acceptable risk that will not endanger the actuarial soundness of the overall risk pool.

This underwriting function is the point at which market failure in health insurance rears its nasty head because of the phenomenon of "adverse selection." If an insurer were to allow consumers the opportunity to buy insurance whenever they wanted it—as they can do in purchasing their other necessities—no rational person would do so until the benefits she would receive would equal or exceed the premiums she had to pay. Healthy people would wait until they were sick to buy health insurance, thus "adversely selecting" themselves into the insurance pool. Such a system can never be financially sustainable because the pool will always lack the necessary funds from the healthy majority to pay for the costs of the sick minority. No insurer would ever voluntarily enter such a market because—absent subsidy—it would inevitably go broke. A fire insurance company would not long survive if it sold home insurance to those whose houses were already on fire.

In health insurance, markets have dealt with the phenomenon of adverse selection via two market-generated mechanisms: employer-based group insurance and medically underwritten individual insurance. Therein lies the market failure. These insurance markets, by rationally protecting themselves from adverse selection, must systematically exclude large numbers of people altogether from buying their products—including the unemployed, the sick, the poor, the disabled, and the elderly. Over the decades this practice has led to increased governmental attempts to fill in these structural gaps with programs such as Medicare, Medicaid, and SCHIP.

Still, major gaps remain, with the result that—according to my calculations—fully fifteen million people are now excluded from affordable health insurance coverage in this country. That means fifteen million Americans are foreclosed from access to the full range of one of life's basic necessities. (Note: Fifteen million is only one-third of the frequently quoted number of forty-six million Americans who lack health insurance, a subject I will delve into later.) The market failure results from the fact that there is no known naturally arising market mechanism that will allow everyone to buy the insurance necessary to access the full range of medical treatments.

So we need to figure out how—via regulatory or other means— to correct this market failure and the adverse selection problem that causes it. We must allow everyone to purchase affordable, necessary health insurance. If we can do that, then insurance markets will no longer exclude anyone from coverage, allowing everyone the ability to afford a full range of necessary health services when and if they need them.

The health care market failure problem could have been identified and remedied by government regulatory action at any time within the past seven or eight decades, but that never happened. It's too bad, because relatively simple regulation could have obviated virtually all the problems we're now experiencing in our medical care financing and delivery system. Instead, what emerged was an employer-dominated insurance system, later augmented by numerous government interventions. As a result, consumers were effectively removed from any significant say about from whom they can buy insurance, what it will cover, how much they have to pay for it, which medical providers they can use, and whether they can keep their insurance when they lose their jobs or government support.

Equally dysfunctional is the substitution of corporate and government bureaucracy for the flexible, dynamic solutions that well-regulated markets are capable of producing automatically and far more effectively. As a result, the individuals who actually consume the medical services have lost the financial clout to demand the quantity, quality, and affordability they regularly expect when purchasing other necessities. This elimination of the normal consumer's role in medical care has been so thoroughgoing for so long that virtually everyone now sees it as the normal state of affairs. In fact, it is anomalous in the extreme when viewed in the context of the rest of our consumer economy.

Why the Market Failure Persists

Why hasn't this market failure been corrected so that we can all simply purchase medical services ourselves, along with the health insurance we need to protect ourselves from catastrophes? I suggest the reason lies in our common beliefs and fears. Here are five of them, which I discuss below:

1. We have faith in government solutions.

2. Medicine is different from our other basic needs.

3. We fear and distrust markets.

4. Don't we already have a market-based health care system?

5. Medical care is a public good, not an economic good.

Faith in Government Solutions

Health insurance came of age during the same period that Keynesian economics became popular in national economic circles. The Great Depression, along with heavily doctored evidence that the Soviet Union's collectivist economic model was as effective as market capitalism, shattered much of the American belief in the effectiveness of markets—what economists would call microeconomic solutions. The new conviction was that only top-down government action at what economists call the macroeconomic level could prevent destitution and "put a chicken in every pot." This belief was given further support during World War II, when the government took direct control over vast swaths of our industrial economy while heavily regulating the rest. The fact that we won the war gave even more credence to government's ability to manage our economy better than leaving it to the unplanned, chaotic whim of markets.

The government's focus on health care has tended to be directly interventionist in dealing with specific problems caused by market failure, which is reflected in the plethora of narrowly-targeted programs I describe in part II. The emphasis has not been on creating conditions to allow consumer insurance and medical care markets to function within reasonable regulatory confines. Of the numerous ad hoc attempts by employers and by federal and state governments to fix the problems caused by market failure, virtually all of them—though certainly benefiting particular interest groups—have made the overall system less effective, more expensive, and less sustainable.

So, instead of enabling a regulated health care market, our federal and state governments have cobbled together an increasingly inefficient bureaucratic patchwork of programs. These programs substitute for many of the functions that a market would perform automatically and far more responsively to the needs of its consumers. Employers, with their own bureaucratic management of group health insurance, have done no better.

There are many examples of distortional government interventions in health care—IRS policy, Medicare, Medicaid, the Hill-Burton

Act, certificate of need laws, medical practice acts, minimum benefit requirements, the HMO Act, SCHIP, state high-risk pools, guaranteed-issue requirements, any-willing-provider laws, corporate-practice-of-medicine prohibitions, COBRA, HIPAA, specialty hospital limitations, and many others. All are attempts to fix specific problems caused, one way or another, by market failure, and each has created unintended negative consequences that properly regulated markets could have prevented.

One of the most inadvertently destructive government actions has been the price regulation that has virtually eliminated the information and incentives that could have allowed providers and consumers to come together in the delivery of low-cost, effective medical care. A federal agency called CMS (Centers for Medicare and Medicaid Services) has for years quietly regulated, either directly or indirectly, the price for virtually every medical product and service in the United States, whether Medicare-related or not. So far, only prescription drugs have been excluded. Because doctors and hospitals are required to bill Medicare and Medicaid according to CMS rules, insurance companies have been forced to follow suit and base their own reimbursement systems on the CMS structure. It has become virtually impossible, even illegal, for doctors to charge their patients on any basis other than CMS's impossibly complex and arbitrary pricing system. Without clear prices, voluntarily arrived at between buyers and sellers, no market can exist for health care or anything else.

State and federal governments, by requiring insurers to cover even the most inexpensive consumer medical services, have further wrought havoc by misunderstanding the very principles of insurance. Not only does this result in hiding prices from consumers, but it also completely blurs the distinction between paying for normal consumer purchases and needing insurance as an instrument of protection only from unpredicted, unaffordable costs.

It's as though your car insurance also paid for oil changes and gasoline. You can telephone your local Lube Stop to find out exactly the price they'll charge for an oil change. But if you ask your doctor the price of a professional visit—not the copayment but the actual price the doctor is willing to accept for her services—she'll shrug and maybe send you to accounting. There, one of the myriad billing clerks will look at you as if you just arrived from Mars. If you persist, someone may dig out a fee schedule but then tell you it's irrelevant. Although the doctor will bill that amount to your insurer or other third-party payer, the doctor will almost always end up taking a much lower amount—based on what the government's Medicare agency says it is worth.

To learn the actual price, you'll first have to be seen by the doctor, then wait while she bills your insurance company or government program, then wait some more until she finds out how much it will pay, and then you may or may not finally receive a statement from the insurer telling you the allowable, negotiated rate owed to the doctor. Even then, it would not be the same price paid by another insurer. Dr. Benjamin Brewer, a family practitioner who writes a regular column for *The Wall Street Journal*, has observed, "Nobody I know would be willing to buy gas at an unknown price, only to find out the damage when the tab comes a month and a half later. But between the mind-numbing complexity of health-care charges and the reluctance of many in the health system to reveal their prices up front, you don't have much of a choice."[1] Because of government price controls there is no longer any such thing as a price that a doctor or a hospital holds out to the public in exchange for its services.

We have even eliminated the word *price* from our health care vocabulary, referring only to *cost*. We speak of the price of bread and the price of tires but the cost of prescription drugs. The inference is that some opaque back-office process in health care mysteriously determines an amount to be paid. Price is something that should be known upfront by both customer and seller. Cost is not.

Even the word *customer* has taken on a perverse meaning in health care. Ask drug manufacturers who their customers are. If you think they're the patients who consume the drug, then silly you. The customers are the doctors who prescribe the drugs without paying for them or even knowing their price—I mean *cost*.

A fundamental problem in American health care is that it has eliminated any necessity for the consumer to know or care about price. Price would allow—almost require—a prospective patient to judge the value of what he is being offered against the offerings of other providers. He could then commit his financial resources by choosing the best value—the best combination of quality, convenience, customer service, price, warranty, and net cost after insurance reimbursements. Price would give providers an objective way to differentiate their services from their competitors'. Yet the current system virtually forces consumers and providers to ignore price. In health care, the rigidity and complexity of government regulations and corporate rules have replaced the dynamic alacrity of market-determined prices to allocate and quickly reallocate resources to meet the real health care needs of Americans. Once again, markets cannot function without clear price signaling to both buyer and seller.

Medicine Is Different

Another factor weighing against a market solution in health care is the widespread belief that it is somehow different from our other necessities of life. There has long been an almost mystical belief that consumers needn't and shouldn't make medical purchase decisions. That's because only their doctors are supposed to know and follow the latest medical science to treat and cure them—even though most doctors don't. This belief has been encouraged by a medical profession that has long portrayed itself more as priesthood than occupation. At its worst, it has been resistant to change, protective of even its worst members, and highly successful in maintaining its monopoly on medical services—characteristics that have ill served many doctors and their patients. They both deserve better.

The common assumption is that ordinary people can't be relied on to make the kinds of decisions about buying health care that they make about virtually every other aspect of their lives. Instead, they must depend on the wizard behind the curtain—the doctors, employers, insurers, and bureaucracies—to decide what health care services they need and how much to pay for them. The medical industry is supposedly so different that technology is blamed for driving costs up, even though it has driven them down in virtually every other area of our lives.

Medical care can certainly be technical and complicated. We will never expect consumers to know on their own whether they need angioplasty versus a coronary bypass. But we also don't expect them to know how their cars, cable TVs, or computers work. With access to the right information, consumers could certainly make informed choices about which cardiologists and surgeons provide the best diagnoses, treatment recommendations, and outcomes at the lowest prices.

There is abundant evidence that, given adequate information—including price—consumers can do just as well buying health care products and services as they do making their other purchases. Just look at the consumer markets for Lasik eye surgery, cosmetic procedures, over-the-counter drugs, and high-deductible health insurance plans. Employer and government-dominated health insurance blocks consumers from access to information on medical options, quality, and price. Consumers are allowed neither the clout nor the incentives to demand it and use it.

Fear of Markets

Another reason for our lack of focus on market solutions is the widespread fear and distrust of markets. The late University of Pennsylvania economist Herbert S. Levine wrote, "While the entrepreneur is a positive force in the dynamic growth of society's well-being, he engenders social hostility because of the destructive aspect of [economist Joseph Schumpeter's concept of] 'creative destruction.'"[2] Creative destruction is the process by which innovative entrepreneurs create great value but at the cost of destroying older, less effective products and companies. Thus, as my friend Michael Rothschild has written, "Everyone wants the prosperity that markets yield, but no one wants to bear the risks implicit in market chaos. At bottom, this is why popular support for markets is so weak."[3]

It is common to fear what we don't understand, and the fact is that no one really understands *why* markets work—or periodically break down. Markets are human-based, complex adaptive systems that, by definition, defy comprehensive explication.[4]

Market-Based Health Care System

Many people mistakenly believe that our current health care system is already market-based, with insurance companies, drug manufacturers, doctors, and hospitals growing ever richer at the public's expense. In fact, we have never in modern times had a true market-based health care system. Today's private-sector players are merely playing by the rules of a horribly distorted game to maximize their own well-being—behaviors we normally applaud in a real market economy.

Medical Care As Public Good

A further complicating factor is that many policy advocates don't believe medical care should be viewed as an economic good at all but rather a public good. Some view medical care as more akin to a fundamental human right, like free speech or freedom of religion, rather than a limited resource subject to the laws of price-mediated supply and demand. They believe that health care is something best provided free of charge to people, not purchased by them. It is a belief held by a lot of influential and otherwise intelligent people, and it is not a new phenomenon. It was the theme of the extremely influential Flexner Report in 1910, in which educational theorist Abraham Flexner stated, "The medical profession is an organ differentiated by society for its highest purposes, not a business to be exploited."[5] This report set the tone for American medical training, practice, and regulation to this day. Related thinking in other industrialized countries has led them to adopt "socialized" health care systems that have removed most market roles altogether.

Mix all these ingredients into the health care batter, and you get a powerful combination of legislators, pundits, policy wonks, macroeconomists, presidential candidates, social theorists, and voters who think that government should ignore basic human economic behavior and bake in yet more government and corporate control. Their debates tend to focus on where and how much to increase that control—not on how to engage the time-tested ability of properly regulated markets, augmented by financial safety nets, to resolve these problems. Despite the repeated failures of government and employer interventions, these would-be reformers are now demanding even more government control and more employer mandates in the belief that this time we'll get a better outcome for everyone. We won't.

Many critics argue that we are a wealthy country that can afford to provide necessary care to all our citizens. I agree with them. But only to the extent that we can engage appropriately regulated market capitalism to do what it does best—allow self-interested individuals to choose how to allocate their own limited resources to purchase high-quality, affordable health care, including insurance for the expensive stuff that they can't otherwise afford. Then, with the addition of comprehensive social and financial safety nets for those otherwise unable to participate, we can ensure needed care for everyone—effectively and efficiently and far more humanely than under our current system and at probably half the cost.

But if we continue to default to top-down, rules-based control, we will ensure that we will *never* be wealthy enough as a society to meet everyone's medical needs *and* continue to improve our living standards. The inherent inefficiencies will eventually swamp whatever amounts of societal wealth we will ever be willing to allocate to medical care. We will increasingly be forced either to forgo other needs or to allow government to ration us into substandard medical care—perhaps to the point where future Harvard Business School students may indeed hope someday to have enough money to afford a heart transplant that some government functionary rules medically nonessential for someone of their advanced age.

The Goals of Health Reform

The first step to effective reform is to lay out a set of goals that we want health care reform to achieve. Although people may disagree on detail or philosophy, I think most would agree with, or at least reluctantly accede to, the following major objectives:

1. *Universal insurance availability*: Everyone in America should have access to affordable health insurance, regardless of individual health status or history.

2. *Sustainable value and affordability*: Whatever we do with health care reform, we must include mechanisms that will get spending under control while encouraging innovation and improving quality, all on a sustainable basis.

3. *Free-rider prevention*: Any insurance plan that allows anyone and everyone to enroll must also prevent them from gaming the system. They can't delay making insurance purchases until they become ill and then receive more in benefits than they pay in premiums.

4. *Voluntary participation*: Many advocates of universal insurance believe that it is either necessary or desirable to require everyone to purchase health insurance. It is neither, for reasons I will explain in chapter 4.

5. *Financial protection*: Health insurance should protect people against the unaffordable costs of necessary medical treatments.

6. *Choice of insurance, providers, and treatments*: People want choice. They're used to it elsewhere in their lives because it is functional. Choice acknowledges that different people have different needs, different priorities, and different financial means to meet those needs and priorities.

7. *Portability*: People should be able to keep their own health insurance policies, regardless of who they work for and whether they are unemployed, retired, eligible for government-sponsored coverage, or just taking long sabbaticals.

8. *Personal responsibility for prevention:* Health reform should include incentives for people to manage their own health risks, like obesity, smoking, alcohol abuse, blood pressure, cholesterol, blood sugar, and other individually controllable risk factors.

I'll discuss these goals in more detail in chapter 9, but now I must comment on their underlying focus on consumer control. Many people will tell you that the current medical system's focus is already on the patient. But seeing people as patients rather than as consumers or customers is actually part of the problem. The word *patient* is derived from the Latin *patiens* meaning "one who endures," a definition that could hardly be more appropriate for today's medical consumers. Viewing people this way puts them into a subordinate role to providers—and to insurers, governments, and employers. Yes, the patient is the focus of the current system—and many of the proposed ones—but more like an animal in a zoo is the focus of spectators, patrons, handlers, veterinarians, administrators, and fundraisers. A captive panda may indeed be the point of all these resources, but it hardly has a say in how it is treated. Consumers are too often viewed in a similar paternalistic way by our health care system. It assumes that it knows better than they what they need, what they can have, and how much they have to pay. We need a health care system that provides the information and the clout that allows people to make their own choices about what they consume and from whom. They should not be dependent on the benevolent intentions of others.

Those are the goals I propose for health care reform. Now let's see how we can create a workable consumer market to achieve them. I propose a concept I call the American Choice Health Plan. Its purpose is to engage regulated market forces to the maximum practicable extent as the most cost-effective means to funnel scarce health care resources to everyone who needs them. The following discussion provides a summary overview of American Choice, with chapters 9–12 going into considerably more detail.

The American Choice Health Plan

There are three essential reforms in American Choice. The first is to convert virtually all government and employer health insurance from the current defined-benefit group structure to a defined-contribution individual structure. Second, tax reform will extend to individuals the same favorable tax treatment currently available in health benefits provided by employers and government agencies. Third, insurance reform will allow a market for universally available, affordable, fully portable, individual health insurance to emerge on a self-sustaining, long-term basis.

Under American Choice, the government's ongoing role will change to one in which it will do two things—and refrain from doing a third.

- *Regulation*: First, the plan will establish and enforce a set of boundary rules, including tax reform, that will allow a private insurance market to emerge permitting all American residents to purchase health insurance to cover otherwise unaffordable, necessary medical care. This includes modifying or abolishing all current government and corporate programs and regulations that are in conflict with this approach.

- *Safety Nets*: Second, the government, augmented by private charitable organizations, will provide essential social and financial safety nets to protect the minority who can't otherwise participate in such a market on their own. Thus, government would continue to fund health benefits for the elderly, the poor, and the disabled—the traditional constituents of government-funded health care programs—but on a defined-contribution basis in the form of restricted cash payments. These would allow each individual to purchase his or her own health insurance in the same insurance market as everyone else.

- *Laissez-faire*: The third requirement is probably the most difficult. Government, having created a regulatory framework within which the market can finally function, must then be *lais-*

sez-faire—that is, it must leave consumers, insurers, and medical providers alone to make all the pricing, production, and purchasing decisions among themselves. Here the government can help most with, as Thoreau put it, the alacrity with which it would get out of the way. That would then allow Adam Smith's invisible hand to do its magic.

The government's legitimate roles would be those of rule maker, fair referee, enforcer, and safety net of last resort—not insurer or regulator of prices or benefits.

If there is a fundamental problem with this approach, it is not technical, actuarial, or financial—it is political. Although we know markets work in practice, too many influential politicians and policy wonks don't believe they work in theory—at least not for health care. The difficult task will be to transcend that way of thinking.

How the American Choice Health Plan Works

All employers and government agencies, such as Medicare and the state Medicaid programs, will get out of the insurance and benefits administration business entirely. That means no more setting benefits, premiums, or provider reimbursement rates—or choosing and paying medical providers. Instead, they will directly fund their constituents to enable them to purchase their own individual health insurance policies from private insurers and to buy their own health care services from their own choices of health care providers.

Tax equity will be achieved by allowing consumers to establish what I call health funding accounts (HFAs) that will receive these funding contributions on a tax-exempt basis and to which they may contribute their own funds, particularly when self-employed. HFAs are conceptually similar to today's Health Savings Accounts (HSAs) but are more comprehensive in scope. HFAs will allow individuals to receive the same tax treatment now given to employer health plans and will become the central funding mechanism for all of an individual's health insurance and health care purchases.

Reform of the insurance market will allow everyone to have access to many choices of private insurers, benefit options, and prices. Insurer participation will be voluntary, but participants will be subject to American Choice's regulatory regime, which will not allow any participating insurer to turn anyone away or discriminate on the basis of health status, history, or genetic predisposition. Consumer participation will also be voluntary, but a choice not to participate will carry with it substantial short-term and long-term financial and health risks that must be borne by the individual.

Private insurers participating in American Choice will be free to offer whatever kind of coverage at whatever premium levels in whatever markets they wish. The benefits, however, will have to meet minimum requirements for continuous creditable coverage. In essence, that means no qualified insurer may offer cut-rate, low-ball benefit plans that deny coverage for unaffordable, medically necessary services.

Each consumer, regardless of health status or history, will be eligible to purchase any health plan she chooses, making her own judgments as to the mix of benefits, premiums, terms, insurer reputation, and allowable providers, all depending on her own financial resources and HFA balances. After choosing her initial plan, she will then be able to change to any other qualified plan once each year, during open enrollment periods. Based on the experience of Medicare Part D, the Federal Employees Health Benefit Program (FEHBP), and countries such as Switzerland, France, and Germany, each American consumer will most likely be able to choose from as many as several hundred different private plans each year, which will ensure all individuals have access to plans that would best meet their particular needs and circumstances. FEHBP, for example, offers 269 different health plans across the country. Even tiny Switzerland's health care system offers ninety different private health plans to its citizens.

Consumers will be able to elect to purchase insurance that covers only high-cost health care, letting them pay directly for doctor visits, lab and X-ray tests, and most prescription drugs with their HFA funds. Or they might choose to purchase integrated insurance and primary care prepayment coverage, such as the Kaiser Foundation Health Plans offer. It will be up to each person to decide.

Any HFA balance left over at the end of a coverage year will roll over and be the consumer's to invest and use for future health care premiums and costs. Any shortfall will have to be made up with other personal funds, borrowings, or contributions from other people or organizations.

All premium rates will be set under what I call BAGLE (Behavior, Age, Gender, Location, and Employment/Extracurricular) rating principles that I describe in detail in chapter 11. These recognize the differing health risks and costs inherent in age, gender, residence, and chosen occupations and behaviors. Insurers will be allowed to provide premium discounts and benefit incentives to members who meet prevention standards, for example by: maintaining healthy body weight, not smoking, avoiding alcohol abuse, and maintaining healthy levels of cholesterol, blood sugar, and blood pressure.

In a free society like ours, it is important for participation in American Choice to be voluntary. The United States has never required anyone to buy anything as a condition of residency (the car insurance argument doesn't apply, as I will later explain). At the same time, it is crucial that consumers not be allowed to wait to buy insurance until they are sick without paying the costs of their own adverse selection. Many health reform proponents want to mandate coverage for all consumers in the belief that these two policy goals of voluntary insurance purchasing and prevention of free riders are mutually exclusive. They are not. We can deal with the adverse selection risk by imposing limited open enrollment periods, allowing insurers to charge penalties for late participation, permitting providers to withhold unpaid care in all but emergency situations, and imposing individual financial responsibility—including the risk of personal bankruptcy—for nonparticipation. Making American Choice voluntary recognizes that there are indeed people who will not want to buy health insurance because of religious, wealth, personal belief, constitutional, or other valid reasons.

American Choice could be a federalist as well as a federal program, in that the individual states might be allowed to experiment with different approaches within the same parameters. In any event, each state will retain regulatory authority over the financial soundness of insurers domiciled there, a role for which they have ample capability and experience. To guard against state legislative overreach in a federalist system, though, it would be important to allow interstate purchasing of health insurance.

Even with such a federalist system, it is essential that the federal government set the ground rules to allow American Choice to function. That would include necessary changes to ERISA, Medicare, Medicaid, SCHIP, TRICARE, veterans' benefits, tax laws, and continuous creditable coverage requirements and the preemption of state and federal laws that conflict with American Choice. Without federal action in most or all of these areas, effective comprehensive health care reform at the state level is all but impossible.

In a nutshell, that is the American Choice Health Plan. A more comprehensive explanation will follow in chapters 9–12.

The Benefits

You may have noticed that American Choice is really just insurance reform. You may be wondering: how will it deal with all the provider problems—such as price, cost, availability, accessibility, and quality?

Actually, it won't, at least not directly. A new, self-evolving medical delivery market would. If we reform the financing system properly, Adam Smith's invisible hand will lead the medical care delivery system to reform itself. I realize that, to many people, the vaunted dexterity of the great economist's ghostly extremity may seem somewhat palsied of late. Therefore, let me emphasize that American Choice is *not* a program of deregulation and derogation of health care to a free-for-all market system. It is a system of reregulation of health care along lines that correct deep flaws in the allocation of authority, responsibility, and accountability among the various players within our current system. I will go into considerably greater detail on these issues as the book progresses.

Under American Choice, the health care delivery system will have no choice but to provide clear pricing, improved access, higher quality, lower cost, modern information technology, and better customer service. In other words, health care providers and insurers will have to focus on and compete for the business of individual consumers, who will now control all the money. Consumers will no longer be viewed as objects of benevolent paternalism but as *customers*, without whose patronage providers and insurers will be unable to survive and thrive.

Once again, I ask you to suspend disbelief that a consumer-dominated medical system can or will work. I will discuss that later. What would American Choice accomplish? Here are some, but hardly all, of the major benefits:

1. *Universal health insurance availability*: Affordable insurance coverage will become available to everyone living in the United States. No one could be excluded from coverage because of health, employment, or financial status.

2. *Sustainable safety nets*: American Choice will rationalize government and private safety net programs to ensure adequate, high-quality health care for the poor, the working poor, the elderly, the disabled, and America's veterans. American Choice will enhance privacy, dignity, and affordability—all on a long-term, economically sustainable basis.

3. *High quality*: Consumers will have the clout to demand quality. Providers will have to demonstrate that they provide it. No longer will doctors and hospitals be able to get away with providing the accepted standard of care only half the time.

4. *Lower cost*: Over the course of five to fifteen years, American Choice can reduce health care costs by 50 percent or more. These savings will result from reductions in preventable diseases, poor quality care, inappropriate and excessive care, excessive prices, bad providers, parasitic billing and collection systems, unwise regulation, sloppy management, state-enforced provider monopolies, unneeded benefit mandates, adverse selection, and provider shortages. I analyze and discuss the cost issue in chapter 12.

5. *Consumer insurance choice*: Consumers will have a wide choice of health plans and the freedom to change to different plans annually if their current ones don't meet their needs.

6. *Consumer control of the money*: For the first time, consumers will control all the health care money. This will give them the clout to demand and receive the information and accountability they need from insurers and providers on quality, price, and customer service.

7. *Portability*: Everyone's insurance will be portable and no longer tied to an employer or government program. With appropriate financial safety nets, no one will involuntarily lose necessary insurance coverage.

8. *Consumer freedom to choose—or not*: No one will be required to purchase health insurance. At the same time, consumers will not be able to game the system to its detriment.

9. *Individual responsibility for preventable diseases*: BAGLE premium rating will require individual responsibility for control of preventable health risks, thus rewarding healthy behaviors and ending the current subsidization of unhealthy ones.

10. *Employer benefits*: The failed employer-based insurance system will end. Employees will get better insurance and better health care and have money left over. Employers will have no more say in the health care their employees consume than in the cars they

drive. Employers will instead focus on their core business strategies. They will no longer be forced to divert an ever-increasing portion of their efforts and resources to a health care system over which they have no effective control.

Unlike health reform proposals that merely tinker with the current dysfunctional system, the American Choice Health Plan completely restructures the system in a way consistent with America's social and economic values. It is a uniquely American solution to the health care crisis. The late presidential advisor and Presidential Medal of Freedom winner John W. Gardner's comment is apropos: "What we have before us are some breathtaking opportunities disguised as insoluble problems."

CHAPTER 2

Health Care Delivery:
The Key Problems and Issues

You've seen the statistics on health care costs. Total national spending in 2007 was $2.3 trillion—$7,600 per person. Employment-based health insurance premiums increased by 100% between 2000 and 2007, with average family premiums rising to $12,106 a year. The average employee share of premium costs has increased by 83% from $1,800 to $3,300. In 2000 most health insurance plans carried no deductible, and the ones that did averaged only $250. By 2008 deductibles had become the rule and averaged $1,000 per person. By comparison, the overall economy's prices increased over the same period at a relatively placid 24%. Worker income rose only 21%.[1]

Since 1970 health care spending has increased at an average rate of 9.9% annually while the Consumer Price Index (CPI) inflation rate has averaged 4.6%. In 2007 health spending accounted for 16% of Gross Domestic Product (GDP), up from 13.9% in 2001. This contrasts with Switzerland's 10.9%, Germany's 10.7%, Canada's 9.7%, and France's 9.5%. Even so, people in those other countries don't appear to be dropping dead in the streets from lack of health care. Some, however, are waiting in line for government-rationed health care.[2]

The Cost and Affordability Problem

Let's look at health care costs another way—from the consumer level. For all the *Sturm und Drang* about spending, they constituted only 5.7% of our personal expenditures in 2006.[3] So why all the angst over a relatively small personal expense that's only slightly more than we spend on entertainment—and far less than on housing, transportation, or food?

For one thing, health care products and services are probably close to the bottom on any scale of consumer enjoyment. No sane person gets pleasure from going to the doctor, taking (legal) drugs, or being hospitalized. It stands to reason that, however necessary health care may be, we believe we have better—or at least more enjoyable—uses for our money.

For another thing, we keep hearing that health care costs have been increasing at a much faster rate than almost anything else for as long as we can remember—even faster than college tuition, which has risen at only twice the general inflation rate.[4] Thus, we've become tired of its inexorable crowding out of more pleasurable activities and purchases. We want it to stop. The economically challenged even want "somebody else" to pay for it. Alas, Pogo, we have seen the enemy, and he is, indeed, us.

But average consumer spending on health care tells only part of the story. It masks the genuine financial and emotional pain of the millions of Americans who cannot get it on any basis and so face the risk of financial and personal catastrophe. The commonly cited figure of forty-six million uninsured Americans greatly exaggerates the magnitude of this problem. But it does not diminish the impact on the many people who actually do suffer and, in some cases, die from its lack.

We get a more complete understanding of our distress over health costs when we consider the fact that the consumer portion of spending grossly understates total health care expenditures. Consumer spending doesn't include what employers and government pay *on behalf of* U.S. consumers for insurance premiums and direct health care expenditures. When we add these figures to what consumers pay, we find health care taking up 20.6% of all personal consumption spending.[5]

This expenditure of nearly three-fourths of health care dollars by employers and governments—and not by the health care consumers themselves—is the portion that is largely hidden from consumers. It is at the root of our problem with health care costs at both the individual (micro) and societal (macro) levels.

It is important to understand that employer health care payments are actually unrecognized employee income. And that government payments are recycled consumer taxes and government borrowings. One way or another, it's all *our* money. We just don't get to control most of it.

In a 2004 article in *Health Affairs*, Princeton economist Uwe Reinhardt and two colleagues made an interesting argument. Their analysis concluded that, at a macroeconomic level, the United States can afford to continue high health care inflation for many years to come. That's because the expected growth in total GDP will still generate enough extra to advance our non-health-care standard of living:

> Although [projected] health spending in the amount of $3.36 trillion in 2013 may seem alarming, the nonhealth GDP projected to be available to Americans in that year would still be $5.6 trillion larger than it was in 2003. This implies that in 2003 U.S. dollars, Americans are projected to have 16.4 percent more nonhealth GDP per capita in 2013 than they had in 2003. While nonhealth GDP's share of total GDP is projected to fall over the decade (from 85.1 percent in 2003 to 81.6 percent in 2013), in absolute real dollars Americans are projected to have more of everything, besides health care.[6]

This isn't exactly the "don't worry, be happy" conclusion it may appear to be. The authors acknowledge that what might work at the national level doesn't necessarily work at the individual consumer level. Health costs will continue to displace wage increases, and they will eliminate them altogether for more and more workers at ever higher incomes.

The authors lay out a 2003 scenario of a firm that pays each of its workers total yearly compensation of $35,000. That includes $8,800 (25.1%) in health insurance and various other amounts for payroll taxes and other fringe benefits. They assume 1.5% annual productivity growth and 2.5% inflation, which is reflected in 4% annual compensation growth. They also assume 10% annual health insurance inflation. By the tenth year (2012), a worker will be earning total compensation of nearly $50,000, of which almost $21,000 (42%) will be required for health insurance premiums.

Despite insurance costs taking a progressively bigger bite out of total compensation each year, the worker will still see annual increases in his take-home pay—albeit by progressively lower percentages—at least through the tenth year. It's the eleventh year—2013—when health insurance cost increases will exceed total compensation increases. This will force employers to make a choice from three bad options. First, they can begin cutting workers' take-home pay by amounts that increase every year. Second, they can try to absorb the cost increases but lose money as a firm. Third, they can reduce or drop health benefits altogether.

Workers of all collar colors are notoriously reticent to accept reductions in their take-home pay. And employers are resistant to losing money and ultimately not being able to hire any employees at all. That is why we don't have to wait until 2013 to see employers—particularly small ones—dropping health insurance. Only 45% of small employers (with between three and two hundred employees) offered it in 2007, down from 57% in 2000. Overall, only 60% of all employers offered health benefits in 2007, compared with 69% in 2000.[7]

These firms, faced with the realities embodied in Prof. Reinhardt's scenario, are rationally deciding they're better off just paying out to their employees the money they previously spent on their behalf for health benefits. Some may even be trying to keep the suddenly reduced health insurance payments for themselves, but that is at best a short-term and ultimately self-destructive business strategy in any competitive labor market. Either way, this scenario forces workers to figure out how to buy insurance on their own in the individual market—or not. Except in states that mandate guaranteed-issue insurance to everyone who applies—without regard to medical condition—such individual insurance is frequently affordable. That's mostly true for the young and healthy, however, and it requires after-tax consumer dollars in any event. Older workers may have difficulty affording it, and those with serious medical conditions probably won't be able to get it at any price. (I will discuss all these issues later in more detail.)

In attempting to fix this problem, both federal and some state governments have imposed (Massachusetts in 1988, Washington in 1993) or proposed (President Obama) that employers be required to contribute a minimum percentage of employee compensation toward health benefits.[8]

Prof. Reinhardt's employer scenario points out the economic reality that any employer payment for an employee's benefit—whether in direct compensation or health care benefits—comes out of the same total compensation pool available to retain employees. If you arbitrarily increase one component, you necessarily decrease the amount of money available for the others. Viewed in that light—which is economically uncontroversial—laws requiring employers to spend on health insurance are really an enforced diversion of worker compensation for a government favored use. In this case the use is to support an inefficient, inflationary health care system that provides standard-of-quality care only half the time. The burden is placed squarely on the shoulders of the individual employees under the guise of employer responsibility.

Such employer mandates, therefore, do nothing to increase total worker compensation, which is determined by the competitive reality of the labor marketplace. Instead, mandates just redistribute more of the compensation from take-home pay to government-required health benefits, which leaves employees with less money in their pay envelopes. Workers also have to pay for the increasing insurance premiums not paid directly by the employer. For the government to expect such mandated quasi-taxes to achieve any significant value is reminiscent of Winston Churchill's observation, "We contend that for a nation to try to tax itself into prosperity is like a man standing in a bucket and trying to lift himself up by the handle." To be fair, employer mandates do provide two benefits for employees. First, they ensure that at least a part of employee compensation—the part used to pay insurance premiums—will be sheltered from taxes. Second, they provide access to health insurance to all employees at group rates. The former helps correct a deep flaw in federal tax policy. The latter relieves the effects of the market's failure to offer insurance to everyone. But, as proposed, mandates would not apply to small employers, part-time workers, and temporary workers. And by definition, they do nothing to extend insurance to the self-employed or to people without jobs.

It is critical to understand that mandates also do nothing to control health care inflation. That is primarily an artifact of forces unaffected by the number of uninsured. In fact, any increase in demand resulting from fewer uninsureds could actually worsen inflation.

There is something that mandates do reduce—the percentage of premiums paid by employers. That's because percentage-based employer contributions increase only at the same rate as overall compensation increases (4% in Prof. Reinhardt's example). Meanwhile, insurance premiums will continue to rise at two or three times that rate (10% in the example). This leaves the employee to pay *all* of the difference from increased payroll deductions. In the Reinhardt example, the employee's deductions will actually increase by 12% each year—higher even than the 10% health care inflation rate. Why is it higher? The phenomenon is what finance people call leverage—positive for the employer, negative for the employee.

Employer mandates initially appear to be a state-imposed burden on employers for the benefit of employees. In reality, they provide state-sponsored employer relief. They remove the employer's concern about health care inflation. No longer will their contributions be tied to increases in health insurance premiums. They will rise, instead, only with overall compensation increases. Employer mandates are a shell game that employees will lose every time. The math is simple for anyone with a calculator, something apparently in short supply in some state legislatures.

Prof. Reinhardt's example still holds. Without a reduction in the rate of medical inflation, workers will increasingly be unable to afford health insurance—mandates or no.

How Much Should We Spend?

We complain, quite legitimately, about the cost of medical care and how it consumes increasing portions of our personal and national treasure. We also view our expenditures vis-à-vis other countries and find ourselves suffering by comparison there, as well. This all begs the question of how much *should* we spend on medical care.

One way to look at it is that we consumers should have a right to expect that we get our money's worth, perhaps in the form of more QALYs (quality-adjusted life years) for the amount we spend. By that measure, we should be living longer, healthier lives and having the disposable income to enjoy them. Put another way, we should be getting real value for our money.

We cannot afford continuing high levels of medical inflation into the indefinite future. Even if we could, it makes sense to accept such a dynamic only as long as we're getting our money's worth—either subjectively as better, happier lives, or objectively as more QALYs. I will leave the happiness issue for the moment to philosophers, theologians, and Abraham Maslow. But let's take a closer look at the QALY issue.

How much is a QALY worth in money terms and who should determine its value to the person receiving it? One country with a nationalized health care system, the U.K., has an agency called NICE (National Institute for Health and Clinical Effectiveness) that says (perhaps not so nicely) that an incremental QALY is worth no more than about £30,000 (a little less than $45,000 in early 2009 exchange rates). That is its effective cutoff point for determining whether a patient will get a needed treatment.[9]

In rationing medical care by price, NICE has created a two-tier medical system based on personal wealth. A sixty-five-year-old man faced, for example, with the need for a liver transplant may be denied the operation by the National Health Service. That leaves him with two possible outcomes. Either he can afford to pay for it with his own money or he dies. The same goes for a number of drugs that haven't been found to add six months to a life for £10,000 or less. These include Revlimid for multiple myeloma, Kineret for rheumatoid arthritis, and Avonex for multiple sclerosis. These drugs are all normally paid for by insurance in the United States.[10]

A key factor to recognize is that the more QALYs you buy, the more each incremental one will cost, assuming you rationally buy the cheapest ones first. This creates an upwardly accelerating cost curve with marginal costs approaching infinity, especially as you age. That means the cost of an additional QALY is quite low when it results from the use of generic cholesterol-reducing statin drugs by populations at high risk for coronary heart disease, but the cost of a QALY resulting from a heart-lung transplant on a ninety-five-year-old patient is extremely high.

The evidence from the U.K., Canada, and other countries suggests that we put a significantly higher value on that last additional QALY in the United States than other nations do. Arguably, the heroic attempts often made to extend the life of an eighty-five-year-old patient in a persistent vegetative state indicates that we may actually place an infinite value on incremental QALYs. In such cases we're willing to spend a lot of money without any hope of improving anything other than a person's total number of artificially induced heartbeats. The obvious problem with accepting an infinite marginal QALY price is that we don't have infinite resources to pay for it.

The great science-fiction writer Robert A. Heinlein's first published short story, "Life-Line" (1939), told of a man named Professor Pinero who invented a machine that would predict the exact moment of any person's death with 100% accuracy. Although many of Heinlein's speculative musings later came to pass (e.g., waterbeds, rail guns, travel to the moon), this one, thankfully, did not. Such a device would cause no end of mischief, which could well include its use to save a lot of money on health care by simply denying it to people about to die. Medicare reported that it spent nearly 30% of its 2006 $408 billion budget on its beneficiaries in their final year of life.[11] That works out to about $122 billion per year in end-of-life care, or about 5% of total national health care expenditures. That's a tidy sum but not the bank-breaking amount circulated by urban legends and the occasional pundit. One can pick nits and say that Medicare's coverage for the elderly and disabled doesn't include all deaths. But that doesn't change the basic point that end-of-life care, though expensive, is not taking up the lion's share of our national health care expenditures.

In any event, I doubt we're ready for a Pineroesque system that would tell patients, "We regret to inform you that we're pretty sure you're in the last year of your life. So, beyond relieving your pain, we're not going to spend any more money on your care." Arguably, our British cousins are essentially doing this when they deny organ transplants for the elderly or withhold certain cancer therapies from everyone.

Fortunately, we have humane and entirely voluntary alternatives at the disposal of people who want to make their own preparations for shuffling off this mortal coil with their dignity intact. Living wills and hospice care have allowed an increasing number of patients and their families to make such decisions. They can thus avoid being plugged into machines that give them extended LY's but no QA's.

There is a lot of room for improvement in how America's hospitals and doctors deal with end-of-life treatment. The amount now spent varies tremendously depending solely on which hospital you—literally—end up in. The wondrous *Dartmouth Atlas of Health Care* reports the costs of care at different hospitals for elderly patients with multiple medical problems during their last two years of life.

Manhattan's New York University Medical Center costs an average of $105,000. Similar services at UCLA's Medical Center cost $94,000. Contrast that with the Mayo Clinic's world-renowned teaching hospital in Minnesota, which costs only $53,432.[12] A 2008 study by Dartmouth College researchers revealed that Medicare could have saved $50 billion over a five-year period if all hospitals had provided dying patients with the same level of care as those in the most efficient facilities.[13]

What could account for such large differentials among such well-regarded institutions? One factor is how well patients—and their families—are informed about their options and then listened to with respect to how they want to live their final days. Ideally, such fully-informed wishes would always trump doctor and institutional proclivities toward extraordinary efforts. Alas, they don't. Incidentally or not, heroic medical measures almost invariably result in greater doctor and hospital revenues.

All this still begs the question of how much we should collectively spend on health care at *any* stage of life. And more important, who should decide? Many pundits, politicians, doctors, and even economists seem to believe this should be answered via our democratic political process. They believe it should fall on our elected and civil service officials to make these expenditure decisions for us—as they now do for America's veterans, elderly, disabled, and poor, and as the U.K.'s NICE does for everyone. That, in my view, can be a terrible, dehumanizing approach that runs counter to almost everything we stand for as a country. It removes the individual from decisions that only that person can intelligently, fairly, and ethically make.

Fortunately, we have in this country a parallel decision-making process by which the national will on health care expenditures can be more rationally and ethically decided. It is via the expression of *individual* will through an even more democratic process than the political one—transparent, regulated markets. In the case of health care spending decisions, such markets would allow each person to make his own decisions about how much he is willing to spend on health insurance and health care and what those services should include. Through this democratic market process—with the inclusion of a substantial safety net component—the collective will would be made known. It would be the grand total of all voluntary individual expenditures for health care goods and services—just as it is with our equally essential needs of food, clothing, housing, and transportation. In other words, total health expenditures should be an *output* amount determined by individual priorities and decisions. They should not be an *input* amount established by politicians and bureaucrats—no matter how well-intentioned, intelligent, and well-informed these overlords may be. Such a market-based approach would be the moral high ground in health care and much more in keeping with American values and freedoms than any other system, existing or proposed.

Thus, I pose the question: Which do you trust more, our collective will expressed through individual choice or the quality of the sausage extruded through the tail-end of the political meat grinder? My fear is that the current national mood may actually favor the latter. Yet my roseate optimism whispers that—despite whatever detours we may take—sooner or later we will be willing to try even a regulated market-based solution. Sooner would be better.

The Quality Problem

Politicians like to tell us that we enjoy the best medical care in the world. If that's true, then have pity on the rest of the world. Medical practice is a combination of art and science. For too many American doctors, there is too much art and not enough science. This discrepancy shows up most obviously in wide statistical variations concerning how medicine is practiced in different parts of the country.

This variability kills people. In a 2003 *Managed Care* magazine article, "9 Ways to Reduce Unwarranted Variation," Martin Sipkoff reported that more than a thousand patients a week are needlessly dying because their doctors don't use evidence-based treatments.[14]

That's the equivalent of two full 747s flying into a mountain every week. In her book *Overtreated*, Shannon Brownlee estimates the number at thirty thousand deaths a year, which is only one 747 per week. "We're literally dying, waiting for the practice of medicine to catch up with medical knowledge," said Margaret O'Kane, president of the National Committee for Quality Assurance.[15] These deaths are not caused by medical mistakes but by doctors who are consciously providing or withholding care as they think appropriate. That care is just not in accordance with current medical standards. If you want to include medical mistakes in the death count, then you need to add another two hundred 747s per year (100,000 deaths) from medication errors alone and another 390 jumbo jets (195,000 deaths) for medical error-caused deaths in hospitals. Even the problem of surgeons operating on the wrong organ or the wrong patient is expected to occur once every year in every three-hundred–bed hospital in the United States.[16] That translates into about three thousand such "never events" every year. They're called that not because they never happen but because they *should* never happen.

Since Boeing tells us that only about fourteen hundred 747s were ever built, we're either going to have to fix the quality problem or find a new metaphor. Whether unwanted variation is by intent or mistake, it is horrendously tragic, inefficient, and costly. "Practice variation is one of the greatest problems we face in controlling costs," says Dwayne Davis, MD, medical director of Geisinger Health Care. For example, comparable Medicare patients in Miami cost almost two-and-a-half times as much to treat as those in Minneapolis. That means Medicare will pay $50,000 more in lifetime treatment for a sixty-five-year-old in Miami than in Minneapolis.[17] Why? It's not that the quality of care is any better in Miami. Arguably, it's worse. That's because so many more people there suffer high-tech hospital ICU deaths from the "need" to fully employ the larger number of doctors and hospital beds.

The problem isn't just in Miami. In Pennsylvania the 1999 rates of mastectomy for breast cancer showed variations as much as threefold for female Medicare beneficiaries across different regions *of the same state.* The frequency of one type of prostate removal procedure varied almost as much for Medicare men. For both conditions, less radical treatment options of equal medical value are available. But it is the doctor who decides which approach to follow. Too often, this happens without informing the patient and letting her or him in on the decision.

Across the U.S. cardiac bypass surgery rates showed an almost fourfold variation. The lowest was in Albuquerque and the highest in Redding, California. The difference wasn't attributed to any variation in illness rates or severity. The highest utilization occurred where the most cardiac catheterization labs were. As in Miami and virtually everywhere else, the supply of resources has created its own demand, regardless of objective patient need.

The quality of doctors varies as well, even for those with a lot of experience. In 2006 *The New England Journal of Medicine* reported a study of twelve highly experienced board-certified gastroenterologists. It found that some of the doctors were ten times better than others at finding precancerous polyps during colonoscopy procedures. The amount of time spent examining the colon explained much of the difference. Different doctors took between three and seventeen minutes per procedure.[18] In some practices thirty seconds was not unheard of. Insurers pay the same for the procedure regardless of the amount of time it takes. Americans get four million colonoscopies per year to detect and prevent colon cancer. Most patients will want to know how well their own doctors do this procedure, but few doctors keep track of their outcomes. Thus, there's really no way to find out.[19]

There are some medical treatments for which the medical evidence is so clear-cut that 100% of eligible patients should always receive them. Yet the use of beta-blocker drugs for heart attack patients varies from 5% to 92% in different parts of the country. Mammograms for Medicare females vary from 21% to 77%.[20] Obviously, nowhere do we see the 100% that we should.

It will surprise many people to know that doctors so frequently fail to do the right things. Numerous studies indicate that your overall likelihood of getting the current standard of care from an American doctor is approximately 50 percent.[21] That estimate is probably on the optimistic side. Such statistics are based on voluntary reports of doctors and health care organizations. It would not be a stretch to assume those who didn't report weren't doing as well.

Children are at even higher risk than adults. More than a fifth of the cases of hospitalized children with adverse drug reactions are preventable.[22] Children are also likely to receive the standard of medical care only 46% of the time. Adults aren't that much better off at 55%.[23] Virtually every medical specialty organization—the American Academy of Family Practitioners, the American Society of Clinical Oncology, the American College of Obstetricians and Gynecologists—has published its own recommended practice guidelines for its members to follow in treating patients for a wide variety of symptoms and conditions. Compliance with these guidelines has improved in some areas and specialties. Yet many doctors see these tools as insulting to them. They deride them as "cookbook medicine." That sounds a lot like an airline pilot refusing to use the preflight checklist because it's "cookbook flying."

Medical researchers began to look seriously at how the best doctors diagnosed and treated diseases in the 1970s. By the early 1990s medical entrepreneurs had incorporated their findings into easy-to-use computer programs. They allowed any doctor to access high-level expertise in her own practice as an aid to providing exemplary care. One such program, Symptom Analyst Plus, ran on a personal computer and sold for $295 in 1992. It allowed a doctor or nurse practitioner to perform consistent differential diagnoses of any combination of 537 signs, symptoms, and laboratory tests for 337 diseases and disorders. The possible diagnoses were displayed by rank according to their levels of support. Each diagnosis could then be compared with its disease reference in the program's database, which also displayed all the characteristics of that disease.[24]

By 1992 there were more than eighty such software programs commercially available. Almost all were offered only to doctors. They covered a broad range of medical disciplines, including backache, infectious disease, psychiatry, heart disease, coronary artery disease, sports medicine, pediatrics, emergency medicine, dermatology, dentistry, diabetes, general medicine, geriatrics, hypertension, medical history, allergy, endocrinology, enterology, hematology, laryngology, nephrology, neurology, obstetrics and gynecology, ophthalmology, otology, proctology, pulmonology, rheumatology, urology, anesthesia, and blood chemistry. Together, these computer applications represented a vast storehouse of readily usable expertise based on what was considered to be the best of the best in medical practice.[25] At the time, these computerized practice guidelines were the future of health care. Unfortunately, they still are, and under our current system they always will be. The companies that developed these medical practice applications are long gone, victims of a market that utterly failed to materialize. Doctors stayed away in droves. Essentially, their message was, "Why did I go through the rigors of eight years of medical school, internship, and residency training only to buy a $300 computer program that can do a better, more consistent job than I can? My patients would think I'm incompetent or that my nurse could do just as good a job. Egad, come to think of it, for many of the patients I see, she could!"

So today not much has changed, except that practice guidelines now tend to be in less-accessible printed form rather than in computer applications, which has further reduced the likelihood they will ever be used by doctors in their practices.

Estimates vary concerning the potential economic impact of widespread practice guideline use. Experts believe guidelines could eliminate a third of current medical spending. That would work out to about $700 billion—and scores of thousands of prevented deaths—per year.[26]

How Scientific *Is* Modern Medicine?

Voltaire once wrote, "The art of medicine consists in amusing the patient while nature cures the disease." We like to believe modern medicine has surmounted the woeful ignorance of the past and delivered us into a new age of medical enlightenment. It really hasn't. The awkward truth is that there is no scientific basis for most of what doctors do. The Institute of Medicine has estimated that there is strong scientific evidence for only 4% of the tests and treatments doctors use. More than 50% of them are backed by either very weak or no evidence at all.[27] Yet we all smile smugly at historical accounts of doctors bleeding their patients or dosing them with mercury or sulfuric acid for various maladies.

We can only shake our heads in puzzlement at more recent stories. For example, medical students were once taught not to use beta-blocker drugs for heart failure because, in theory, they don't work—but in practice they do. Even worse, most drugs that are prescribed don't work for most patients.[28]

One case of neglect by the medical establishment is particularly glaring. Doctors ignored for years the discovery that most stomach ulcers are caused by easily treated bacterial infections rather than an excess of stomach acid. The two Australian doctors who made this revolutionary discovery in the 1980s were met with criticism, disdain, and the refusal to publish their findings. The medical profession stuck with dogma that required the use of ineffective and expensive acid-suppression drugs, often followed by traumatic surgery.

Antibiotic treatment is now, finally, the standard of care. The Australian doctors, Barry Marshall and Robin Warren, were awarded the Nobel Prize for Medicine in 2005. How many tens of thousands of ulcer patients suffered and died because doctors ignored the evidence and continued their outdated treatments? What other breakthroughs have been made and are being ignored because they fail to fit the dominant paradigm?

Patients' medical records are rife with evidence of doctors ignoring scientific evidence in favor of their own flawed judgments.

In a 2004 editorial in the British medical journal *BMJ*, Australian medical professor Dr. Jenny Doust explored why doctors do things that don't work. She concluded there are multiple causes. Among the more interesting are: (1) undue reliance on clinical experience that is clouded when patients get well *despite* treatment (the "Voltaire Effect"); (2) a need to do something, even if it's wrong; (3) a failure to question the way things have always been done; (4) a reliance on explanatory disease models that are wrong; and (5) a need to maintain the ritual and mystique around medical practice.[29]

None of these is consistent with the popular image of the doctor as a lab-coated scientist utilizing the latest discoveries to cure patients. Honest doctors will tell you they see these contrary behaviors all the time. *Really* honest doctors will tell you they do them all the time. They will tell you they routinely order blood tests before surgery without any scientific evidence of benefit and that the results of such tests rarely change outcomes or even treatment. They will tell you that they have continued to prescribe drugs inappropriately despite prominent black box warnings on their labels.[30]

The problem isn't just that doctors do things for which there is contrary scientific evidence. For most medical treatments, there is no scientific evidence at all—pro or con. This problem is compounded when doctors fall into patterns of treatment that congeal into resistance to change. That can cause them to ignore scientific evidence when it does become available.

Most efforts to push for more evidence-based medicine come from government, employer groups, and some insurers. That makes sense since they're paying for the care—whether it works or not. Consumers, despite their well-established ability to avoid buying cars known to have exploding gas tanks or toys tainted with lead, are pretty much left out of the medical quality equation. They don't pay the bills, so they lack the clout necessary to demand information on the quality of medical procedures they receive or on the doctors who provide them.

Efforts to establish what scientifically works and what doesn't are sporadic. And the knowledge produced by these efforts is often slow to become an integral part of the medical delivery system. Thus, we have a system that: (1) doesn't systematically work to improve care based on outcomes research; (2) does a terrible job of adopting new standards once they've been developed; and (3) does an even worse job of providing the information that does exist to patients who choose the providers of their care.

What is missing is a mechanism to force effective change. The congressional budget office director in 2008 estimated we could save up to $700 billion in health spending—one-third of the total—just from identifying and eliminating treatments *that fail* to produce the best medical outcomes.[31]

Such findings have created serious interest in the government taking a bigger role in establishing medical comparative effectiveness standards. This has resulted in $1.1 billion of new funding in 2009 for comparative effectiveness studies to be conducted by the Agency for Healthcare Research and Quality, the National Institutes of Health, and the Department of Health and Human Services.[32] The program appears to focus on the laudable goal of providing better information for doctors and patients to use in making treatment decisions. Other influential health reform advocates, including former Senator Tom Daschle, would go considerably further, however, and establish a federal health board with broad power over federal and private insurance coverage decisions. With Federal Reserve Board-like independence, it would be responsible for "recommending coverage of those drugs and procedures backed by solid evidence. It would exert influence by ranking services and therapies by their health and cost impacts." It would include regional boards with the power to "concentrate on fulfilling national priorities" and to ensure "an adequate supply of certain services or linking payment to performance." Daschle also suggests "using the UK's NICE as a model." The board would employ a panel of a dozen or so experts who would be "chosen based on their stature, knowledge, and experience, ensuring that the decisions they make have credibility across the health-care spectrum."[33]

Concepts like the federal health board, although superficially appealing, raise several major concerns about how such an institution would operate and evolve:

1. *The Bottleneck Problem*: As a single, top-down arbiter of what is cost-effective and therefore what will or won't be covered by insurance, a federal health board could quickly become a bureaucratic bottleneck that inherently retards the adoption of new technologies. The idea of giving authority over literally scores of thousands of diagnoses, tests, drugs, and procedures to a single government agency led by a cadre of philosopher-kings is troubling. The pace and breadth of technological change makes this approach unworkable by a dozen such organizations.

2. *Linear Control of a Nonlinear System*: A bureaucracy with the power to implement "national priorities" such as the federal health board would necessarily involve the use of top-down rules for governing health care as though it were a machine. The board would decide which parts of the machine to improve and to approve in order to make it run more smoothly and efficiently. Health care, however, is not a machine. It is a complex adaptive system—much more akin to a constantly evolving ecosystem than an automobile.[34] Its inherent complexity and unpredictability can only be optimally addressed by the equally complex solutions that emerge from a rational, regulated marketplace in which millions of individual consumers and providers are allowed and empowered to seek their own best results according to their own needs and priorities.

3. *The Value Contradiction*: The concept of a federal health board does not seem to address the problem of health care pricing. That leaves open the question of how Daschle's proposed health board could really determine the value of health care services. Remember, value equals quality divided by price. Even if the health

board could identify everything that works and doesn't—the quality part—it still couldn't determine the intrinsic value of any of it. That's because it would have no market pricing upon which to base any value analyses. There are only the Resource Based Relative Value System and other mechanistic pricing automata produced and enforced by CMS. Such arbitrary standards are inherently incapable of supporting meaningful value calculations.

4. *Too Many Reasonable Men*: George Bernard Shaw memorably observed, "The reasonable man adapts himself to the world; the unreasonable one persists in trying to adapt the world to himself. Therefore all progress depends on the unreasonable man." One has to wonder what are the odds that a federal health board of medical leaders would include the kind of unreasonable, questioning, innovative iconoclasts necessary to truly challenge and advance the state of the medical art? It seems more likely that such a board would constitute a microcosm of the current medical establishment itself, complete with its attendant biases, dogmas, and reluctance to challenge or change conventional thinking. Under such a regime, one wonders if we would have, even yet, achieved widespread antibiotic treatment for ulcers.

5. *NICE Rationing*: Another concern about the proposed agency is the risk that it would become the primary means by which the government would ultimately ration medical care. One of the agencies Sen. Daschle points to as a model for his health board is the U.K.'s National Institute for Health and Clinical Effectiveness (with the ironic acronym NICE). NICE has decided that no new medical innovations will be paid for unless they can be shown to improve patients' lives for less than $45,000 per quality-adjusted life year, or QALY. This rule has effectively eliminated expensive procedures such as organ transplants for the elderly and certain well-established cancer therapies for anyone. Our British cousins have long since suppressed any notion of a medical services market. In doing so, they have eliminated any means of limiting

costs, short of rationing them based on government spending constraints. Senator Daschle's admiration for NICE is troubling although not so much as it was when he was briefly designated to become the Director of the White House Office of Health Care Reform. Nonetheless, his ideas continue to receive widespread interest from many would-be health reformers.

6. *A Roundabout Route to Change Doctor Behavior*: Another major weakness of the health board concept is that it seeks to force doctors to change their practice behavior on the basis of what it decides insurance will or won't cover. That's an awfully roundabout, inefficient route for getting doctors to change how they practice medicine. We did a lot of that top-down command-and-control stuff with HMOs and managed care. We were partially successful. But the doctors were at least as smart as we were. They became expert at gaming the system to get around any of our rules they considered arbitrary. A more efficient and direct route to change doctor behavior would be for their patients to demand evidence-based medicine, patronize doctors who practice it, and withhold their business from those who don't. There is no current mechanism that gives patients the information or the clout to do this. Patients don't control the money necessary to demand even the information on provider quality, much less compliance with medical standards. Nor are they allowed to choose providers who don't happen to be in their insurers' discount networks. This can all be fixed.

7. *The Mirage of Political Independence*: Cato Institute scholar Michael Cannon has challenged the myth of political independence for existing institutions such as the Fed and the SEC. Although nominally independent, they are indeed subject to significant fear of and suasion by the Congress. More specifically, he has pointed out how previous government efforts at comparative medical effectiveness research came to naught for the Office of Technology Assessment, the National Center for Health Care

Technology, and the Council on Health Care Technology. All of these agencies were disbanded after rendering findings that offended various components of the health care industry. Cannon's verdict: "If a government agency produces unwelcome research, those groups will spend vast sums on lobbying campaigns and political contributions to discredit or defund the agency."[35]

Insurers—whether Medicare, insurance companies, or employers—have a valid interest in promoting prevention and assuring payment for effective treatments. But they don't have the patient's vested interest in getting the most effective health care. Insurers' interests are financial. There is no way to make them effective proxies for patients when it comes to wanting, needing, and demanding excellent medical care. Patients are interested in improving their lives. They want to get the most appropriate medical treatments at the lowest cost to themselves. Patients have a lot more skin in the game than insurers ever will. That's why consumers need to be in a position to demand access to the best, most appropriate medical care available. That, and only that, will incentivize medical providers to compete for patients by actively seeking and adopting innovative care solutions. Top-down directives from government agencies and think tanks will never accomplish that. Doctors will game their way around such bureaucratic rulemaking in their sleep.

Thirty years from now, if we're fortunate, we'll remember our current era as the dark age of medical practice when Voltaire's aphorism still held true. But in the era of Google, eBay, iTunes, and YouTube, the idea of a central bureaucracy that establishes value standards for consumer health care is just so twentieth century.

The Chronic Disease Problem

According to the U.S. Centers for Disease Control and Prevention (CDC), chronic diseases afflict more than ninety million Americans and account for more than 75% of total medical costs. A hundred years ago, most illnesses and deaths were due to acute medical conditions. Now, the CDC says that "chronic diseases—such as cardiovascular disease (primarily heart disease and stroke), cancer, and diabetes—are among the most prevalent, costly, and *preventable* of all health problems" (my emphasis).

A 2006 mortality study by Harvard researchers identified six risk factors that lead to the diseases and injuries that make the largest contribution to mortality, and thus morbidity, disparities throughout the United States:[36]

1. Alcohol abuse

2. Tobacco smoking

3. Being overweight and obese

4. Elevated blood pressure

5. Elevated serum lipids (e.g., cholesterol)

6. Excess blood glucose

All of these risk factors share two characteristics: They are individually controllable and objectively measurable. Crucially, none of them is controllable by doctors or hospitals for anything longer than brief timeframes. That's a real problem because, collectively, these risks represent a rogues' gallery of chronic disease causes. Unmanaged, they progress to acute diseases, most notably cancer, heart disease, kidney failure, liver failure, blindness, pulmonary disease, limb loss, and stroke—and 75% of health care costs.

Our current medical care system simply does not work well for chronic problems. Its focus on episodic care does not and cannot meet the continuous needs of chronic disease patients. Our medical system was designed for acute conditions, such as infections, earaches, gunshot wounds, broken arms, automobile accidents, heart attacks, strokes, many cancers, and battered spouses. These are short-term conditions that respond to episodic care such as a doctor's office visit or a hospital stay in which antibiotic therapy, intensive medical treatment, surgery, or chemotherapy are provided.

The far more prevalent chronic diseases require day-to-day and even hour-to-hour awareness and attention by a completely different primary care giver—the patient herself. A study released in 2007 by the Milken Institute estimated we could save $190 billion a year in medical costs with lifestyle improvements and modest treatment advances for six diseases—cancer, diabetes, hypertension, stroke, heart disease, and pulmonary conditions. Since chronic diseases account for a total of $1.5 trillion in annual expenditures, this savings estimate would seem to be, as the authors themselves suggest, conservative.

Despite the critical need to improve patient responsibility for prevention and self-care, insurers and government payers are increasingly focused on incentivizing doctors to follow some of the simplest and most straightforward procedural guidelines for evaluating and treating their chronic disease patients. Such pay for performance (P4P) plans seek to reward doctors who, for example, prescribe antihypertensive medications for their patients with high blood pressure and check the hemoglobin A1c (a blood sugar measure) for their diabetes patients.

These programs may produce some patient benefit but miss the larger point. The primary effort necessary for effective chronic disease control has to be by the patient. If that is missing, nothing a doctor can do will be sufficient. This point was unintentionally captured in an article on P4P that stated, "Linking doctors' pay to how well they follow treatment guidelines can improve quality of care but not health outcomes."[37] Read that again. The writer has paraphrased the old saw, "The operation was a success, but the patient died." In doing so, he captured the essential problem in P4P—rewarding the wrong person to do the right things.

Take a look at this typical patient profile from an article on the Massachusetts Group Insurance Commission website:

> The patient had been diagnosed with hyperlipidemia, or high cholesterol. The doctor prescribed a statin, a lipid lowering drug. After taking the drug for a while, the patient's choles-

terol level came down. He stopped taking his medication. The patient later began to experience shortness of breath when exercising and some pressure in his chest. Subsequently, he experienced chest pain and had to have open-heart surgery.[38]

The patient was former President Bill Clinton.

It would be great if every doctor remembered to check hemoglobin A1c and to prescribe the correct drugs for all their diabetes patients during every visit. But if the patient isn't religiously checking his blood sugar levels every several hours, taking his medications, adjusting his insulin, exercising, and rigorously controlling his diet, then the doctor's actions will be like the chief engineer on the *Titanic* reporting the waterline level, post-iceberg.

Doctors need to prescribe statin drugs for cholesterol control, but until patients actually purchase the drugs (20% don't)[39] and take them every day for the rest of their lives (less than half do),[40] prescriptions won't do any good for preventing cardiovascular disease. Doctors can tell a patient that his body mass index of 30 (indicating obesity) is unlikely to permit a long and healthy life, but that is meaningless for preventing diabetes, cardiovascular disease, and cancer unless the patient is willing to engage in new habits to lose weight and exercise.

In today's system these efforts by doctors may be necessary to improve quality of care. But that's all about improvement in what the doctor does rather than how well the patient is doing. In other words, P4P is measuring quality of inputs instead of outcomes. Doctor support of chronic disease is certainly useful, even necessary. It is far from sufficient.

We know that educating patients on how such conditions will eventually make them sick or dead simply doesn't work for many Americans. The immediate pleasure of that bag of potato chips or the slice of German chocolate cake too often overcomes any concern about the long-term consequences. For whatever reason, fears of future personal agony and early death have not been sufficient to lead tens of millions of at-risk Americans to engage in healthy day-to-day personal behavior. We need something else.

A key challenge is to get people, first, to focus on preventing their own diseases and, second, to access the health care delivery system to provide necessary medical and other support. That's a tall order, especially since so many people now are going about their lives completely oblivious to their asymptomatic high blood pressure, unhealthy blood sugar, and ticking-time-bomb LDL cholesterol. Currently, an estimated 35% of workers with hypertension, 41% of those with high cholesterol, and 41% with diabetes have not been diagnosed.[41] Because these conditions can go for years without showing any symptoms, the people who have them think they're healthy. And many don't go to doctors to discover the truth. Likewise, doctors are accustomed to patients coming into their offices with specific complaints. They are trained to focus on those. The unspoken often remains undiagnosed. Thus, it's not just an issue of convincing people to manage their conditions. It's also one of motivating them *and* their health care providers to measure the conditions in the first place. And for those who are aware of these conditions, how do we then motivate them to do something about them?

Between doctors who refuse to follow accepted standards of care and patients who fail to prevent and manage their own chronic diseases, we have a major problem of responsibility and accountability in our health care system. Any attempt to reform health care that fails to resolve these issues will fail.

The Prevention Problem

The mantra of many health reform advocates is that improving access to preventive medical services will save a lot of money. The original argument for the financial value of medical prevention is often attributed to the co-founder of the Kaiser Foundation Health Plans, Dr. Sidney Garfield. He proposed to achieve prevention and its attendant savings through the mechanism of the periodic multi-phasic patient exam. These exams would separate the sick from the well. The sick would be treated. The healthy would be directed into separate health facilities for health education and counsel by allied health professionals.

Dr. Garfield's concept was originally embedded in Kaiser's genetic code, along with the concepts of prepayment and hospital utilization controls. Yet in an outcome more Lamarckian than Darwinian, even Kaiser now recognizes that Dr. Garfield, brilliant as he was in many of his innovations, went off in a wrong direction on the issue of early detection and prevention.[42]

It turns out that savings from prevention virtually always fall short of its costs. I realize that this statement runs directly counter to just about everything we hear and read about the value of prevention in the mainstream media and from the halls of Washington, so further discussion is necessary. There are primarily two reasons why prevention is not cost effective. First, individual health risk assessments have a terrible track record of predicting a person's future use of health services. Among other problems, there are too many false positives. Second, the cost of detecting and preventing nascent diseases almost always exceeds the cost of treating the relatively few such diseases that would have emerged—often much later—without such action. From a strictly medical cost-benefit standpoint—and that's what we're discussing here—medical prevention is a loser. From an individual quality-of-life standpoint, that's a different matter, but not one that insurance companies are equipped to deliver—or even to care about from a strictly actuarial and financial standpoint.

A 1995 review of prevention literature reported by the National Center for Policy Analysis concluded:

> Study after study has shown that preventive medicine adds to overall health care costs. The reason is fairly straightforward: Testing everyone costs a great deal of money, and the diseases being screened for are fairly rare. At best, the tests benefit only a few. And the savings generated by early detec-

tion of these few instances of disease are far outweighed by the costs of testing large numbers of people.[43]

The review added that preventive medical care showed savings only from prenatal care for poor women, tests for congenital disorders in newborns, and most childhood immunizations. Otherwise, flu and pneumonia vaccines, screening for various cancers (i.e., prostate, cervical, and colon), and periodic physical exams cost more than they saved.[44] This is not to say that such activities aren't beneficial from the standpoint of individual peace of mind, but the argument that improved access to preventive medical services will save money is, with very limited exceptions, untrue.

The definitive source of information on prevention cost-effectiveness can be found at the Tufts Medical Center's website for its Cost-Effectiveness Analysis (CEA) Registry. It is a comprehensive collection of virtually every known peer-reviewed article on health care cost-effectiveness analyses. A recent analysis of Registry data in *The New England Journal of Medicine* found that, indeed, "although some preventive measures do save money, the vast majority reviewed in the health economics literature do not."[45] Similarly, the journal *Health Affairs* concluded in 2009,

> Over the four decades since cost-effectiveness analysis was first applied to health and medicine, hundreds of studies have shown that prevention usually adds to medical costs instead of reducing them. Medications for hypertension and elevated cholesterol, diet and exercise to prevent diabetes, and screening and early treatment for cancer all add more to medical costs than they save.[46]

The goal of medical prevention is worthy, but providing blanket first-dollar insurance coverage for preventive services—except for the poor—was really never a good idea. It drives excess utilization and cost without concomitant reductions in the cost of prevented diseases. A landmark RAND study of health care costs and utilization demonstrated that requiring significantly higher patient payments for out-of-pocket costs had no adverse impact on patient health, except for the poorest populations.[47]

If anything, nearly free access to prescription drugs and medical care may have contributed to consumers feeling that they could actually increase their self-destructive behavior and then ask doctors for pills to fix any problems that resulted.

It is interesting that America's march toward epidemic obesity rather closely matched the upward trend in prevention coverage by managed care during much of the past forty years. According to the National Center for Health Statistics, the number of overweight and obese American adults ballooned from 47% in 1976–80 to about 67% in 2003–04, with the obesity rate more than doubling from 15% to 32%.[48] During that same period, HMO and managed-care enrollment, along with their coverage of preventive services, exploded from 8 million to 70 million members.[49] These statistics actually understate the prevalence of prevention coverage, since most insurers ended up providing it as well.

I'm not saying there is a cause-and-effect relationship here, just an interesting and suggestive coincidence that may be worth exploring further. Whether or not free preventive services have created a moral hazard, they certainly have not achieved an outbreak of healthy living.

Doctors and Prevention

A related flaw in the prevention argument is the idea that doctors can play a major role in preventing the diseases that are killing us. If that were true then, again, the virtual ubiquity of cheap primary and preventive care available under the managed-care system would have made us healthier. Instead, we got the opposite—an epidemic with no signs of abating.

Physician-provided health care is a misnomer. The medical profession is not and never has been focused on maintaining health but rather on curing sickness and correcting malfunctioning body states. It is in the nature of how the profession was established well over a century ago. Doctor education, training, practice, *and payment* are almost wholly focused on diagnosing and treating medical problems, not preventing them.

Of course, doctors have a valid role in prevention. But most of it involves prescribing drugs and informing their patients of the particular health risks they face beyond the obvious smoking, obesity, and drinking too much. According to Dr. Douglas Campos-Outcalt, associate chairman of the University of Arizona's department of family and community medicine, "Ninety percent of the things you [the doctors] need to know to make positive lifestyle changes you can get from a minimum battery of tests and taking a good medical and family history."[50] And that, in the grand scheme of things, is very inexpensive and within the financial means of the vast majority of Americans without resorting to insurance that can double its cost.

Public Health

A more fundamental fact is that public health efforts—not medical care—have delivered most of the great advances in prevention. Starting in the early twentieth century, public health efforts were responsible for the vast elimination of communicable, infectious, and deficiency diseases by the introduction of clean drinking water, public sanitation, vitamins, and antiviral vaccines.

In more recent years, public health, not organized medicine, has delivered notable accomplishments in prevention:

- *Smoking Cessation*: Anti-smoking public health campaigns have reduced the rate of youth and teen smoking in New York State by 45% between 2000 and 2006.[51]

- *Heart Disease and Stroke*: A major public health effort begun in 1999 to prevent heart disease and stroke—led by the American Heart Association/American Stroke Association, the Association of State and Territorial Health Officials, and the CDC—has been credited with helping reduce death rates in 2005 from coronary heart disease by 25.8% and from stroke by 24.4%.

- *HIV/AIDS*: Other public health prevention efforts have led to an 88% HIV/AIDS transmission rate reduction since 1984, with diagnoses dropping from 41,207 in 2001 to 38,685 in 2004.[52]

There is now scientific evidence that obesity and thinness as well as smoking cessation are socially contagious and thus worthy targets for future public health efforts.[53] There is much room for improvement in numerous causes of preventable diseases, particularly tobacco, alcohol, and illicit drug use, diet and activity patterns, violence, motor vehicle use, and sexual behavior.[54] Public health efforts continue to be a significant source of preventive success. Medical intervention has, without doubt, been a valued contributor to these and other prevention efforts, particularly the introduction of pharmaceutical statins and beta-blockers for cardiovascular health, but it has largely been in a support role backing up higher-leverage public health and individual efforts.

At bottom, true prevention now depends far more on the daily behavior of the affected individuals than it does on anything that doctors can do during an office visit. During the early twentieth century many people suffered and died from the scourges of deficiency diseases like rickets and pellagra, and from many communicable and infectious diseases. By the 1970s people in the United States were suffering and dying far more from cancer, cardiac and circulatory diseases, diabetes, stroke, and breathing disorders than from now virtually extinct traditional maladies. About all that doctors have been able to do to prevent these maladies has been to prescribe long-term maintenance medications and to make frequently ineffective recommendations for changes in patient behavior around diet, alcohol consumption, exercise, and smoking. Although a combination of public health, individual efforts, medical intervention, and especially new drugs has helped reduce mortality rates from heart attack and stroke by significant amounts, doctors have never done prevention very well on any kind of consistent, outcomes-supported basis.[55] And patients too often don't follow their advice anyway. Most chronic diseases are readily preventable—but not by doctors.

Chronic disease prevention depends on continual personal efforts to exercise; to eat, sleep, and drink responsibly; to avoid dangerous habits; and, when necessary, to take maintenance medications. Public health efforts can significantly assist in all this. Doctors can too, but they are not the main caregivers to these people—the people themselves are. Again, the current medical delivery model was designed a century ago to provide episodic treatment for acute conditions, and it hasn't changed. From the standpoint of prevention and chronic disease treatment, it is an outdated paradigm that fails to provide continual support for chronic medical conditions that burden their victims every hour of their lives and that cause 75% of today's health care expenditures.

Resolving the problem of these preventable diseases will require two major changes. The first is a change in individual behavior to avoid and control risk factors that lead to disease. The second is for both public health and new forms of health care delivery systems to emerge that will provide timely support dovetailing with their patients' lives.

There are other flaws in the argument that preventive services should be covered by insurance. The idea that people will not spend their own money on preventive care is—except for the poor—not supported by the evidence. Consumers now spend more than $50 billion a year just on alternative medications and treatments. If there's one thing that consumerism has taught us, it is that most people make mostly rational lifestyle and purchase decisions most of the time—but only when they have individual incentives and accountability (including a lack of moral hazard) *and* information on price, quality, and availability of their purchase options—almost none of which are available in our current health care financing and delivery system.

Instead, medical care is a black box in which we hide all the information and eliminate the consumer's ability to make rational decisions. The problem with primary and preventive care is that virtually no one knows how much (or how little) it actually costs, what the costs are of forgoing it, how effective it is, and where to find the best, most convenient value and customer service.

The Fallacy of Lifetime Medical Costs

Another aspect of prevention is illuminated by the following quiz (I warn you, it's a trick question):

Quiz

Who among the following people will incur the highest health care costs during his lifetime?

a) The Smoker: a twenty-year-old smoker

b) The Stout Guy: a twenty-year-old obese man

c) The Healthy Guy: a twenty-year-old non-smoker with normal weight.

The answer is (c). The healthy guy will cost the most (the smoker, the least). This is because the healthy guy will live considerably longer and will thus incur more diseases later in life—diseases unrelated to smoking or obesity that the smoker and the stout guy won't be burdened with (being dead and all). This was the conclusion of a recent study by Dutch researchers comparing the medical costs attributable to obesity, smoking, and healthy living.[56]

Does this mean we have the idea of prevention all wrong and we should actually encourage smoking and obesity in order to lower health care costs? And while we're at it, why not forbid seatbelts, have the police give tickets to people driving sober, and outlaw childhood immunizations and backup parachutes for skydivers?

To put this into perspective, let me ask a second question: Which of those three people will buy the most clothes in a lifetime? Or drive the most miles? Or eat the largest number of meals? Or enjoy more time with his grandchildren? The answer is also (c), the healthy guy who lives longest. Health care is a consumable that is no different from these others. The longer you live, the more you consume. By itself, it's a value-neutral proposition.

Looking a little deeper, however, the same study also shows that the stout guy will incur the highest health care costs *each year* until age fifty-six, after which the smoker's cost-per-year will be higher. Then, after they are both dead, the healthy guy's medical costs will eventually catch up and exceed their total costs.

A rational analyst will read the Dutch study and quickly realize that relative lifetime cost is not the correct metric for judging the financial benefits of prevention. Cost-effectiveness is. So the real question is: To what extent do the economic gains from the healthy guy's longer, more productive life overwhelm his increased medical costs in later life *on a net present value basis?*[57]

If his healthy life enables him to produce more, earn more, and save more than his higher medical costs in the far future, all on a discounted-value basis, then he—and the entire economy—is better off than if he had died earlier after suffering the debilitating, productivity-robbing effects of maladies caused by smoking and obesity. I'm not aware that these benefits have yet been measured, but then this discussion is merely about the economics of medical care, not the full range of benefits that accrue to the individual who enjoys good health. I will discuss that next.

Who Benefits from Cost-Benefit?

One way to look at the issue of cost-effectiveness is through the lens of Abraham Maslow's five-level hierarchy of individual needs.[58] This view reveals that insurers and employers have valid but very limited interests in the health of their constituent members and employees.

- *Insurers:* In Maslovian terms, insurers are concerned about profitably supporting a member's fundamental need for "Homeostasis." That is, the ability of a person's physiological and psychological systems to maintain their internal stability—a state we often refer to as health (on Maslow's lowest, most basic level of human need).

Insurers, as purely economic entities, are motivated to pay for only those preventive measures that generate cost-effective homeostatic results for their members. Thus, they have no economic interest in paying, for example, for general population screening for diabetes. The cost of detecting a few previously undiagnosed cases will overwhelm any savings that will result from medical interventions that might prevent a person's condition from worsening. (Please note that this is a completely different issue than that of turnover rates in an insurer's membership reducing the company's incentive for investing in long-term prevention.)

The only early illness detection and prevention services that make sense for insurers are those that provide short-term payback. Unfortunately, there are very few of these, as noted above. Therefore, it makes little sense to force insurers to bear responsibility for most costs of prevention since it fundamentally runs counter to their economic interests.

- *Employers*: Moving beyond insurers, we find that employers have a greater financial stake in the health of their employees. That's because a worker's productivity is directly affected by his health status. The employer is concerned not only with the employee's basic need for (and cost of) Homeostasis, but also with what Maslow called his Safety need (Maslow's second most basic human need)—specifically security of body, employment, and resources. It is an economic interest, however, not a benevolent one. All those things are necessary for a worker to perform productively for the employer.

  Thus, an insurer might not deem it economically worthwhile to subsidize weight loss programs on the basis of a net reduction in health claims. But an employer might find it to be cost-effective if it additionally improves a worker's attendance, job performance, safety record, attitude, and overall productivity—issues of little or no concern or benefit to insurers.

Even so, the employer's interest is confined only to the lowest two levels of Maslow's five levels of human needs.

- *Individuals*: It is the individual who has the most to gain from prevention. Those gains are not only economic, but also the non-economic ones that come from achieving ever higher Maslovian needs of Love and Belonging, Esteem (of self and others), and Self-actualization. These are in the predominantly non-economic realms of what makes us happy from a life well-lived. Employers and insurers have virtually no reliable interest in helping us achieve these goals.

  Only the individual, along with her family and friends, cares about enjoying a long, healthy, fulfilled life. She, therefore, is the one with the most to gain from investing in her own health. She alone is in the best position to judge such investments against other priorities in seeking happiness.

Making insurers and employers responsible for promoting an individual's health is targeting the wrong change agents. It should be the individual, who not only has the most to gain or lose but is in the best position to decide what her priorities should be to meet all of her needs, wherever they may fit into Maslow's universe.

The Free-Rider Problem

But what about individuals who are irresponsible about their health and are able to transfer the medical costs of that irresponsibility to their co-insured neighbors who do pursue healthy lives? An obese, alcohol-abusing smoker may indeed be setting his own priorities, but he's also creating what economists call negative externalities that he's forcing others to pay for—the excess medical costs that arise from his self-destructive pursuits.

All this suggests a solution. Why don't we give everyone a choice of not producing the negative externalities in the first place (by avoiding known health hazards) or of paying the predictable costs of their failure to do so? We could charge higher insurance premiums to people who smoke, people who are overweight, people who abuse alcohol or drugs, and people with unmanaged hypertension, high cholesterol, or high blood sugar. The additional charge would be calculated to cover the higher medical costs over a person's lifetime. Individuals would not be assessed on the basis of health status or history—only on reasonably controllable health risks. To be fair (and effective), all such health-risk indicators would have to be objectively measurable and individually controllable. Ensuring that could involve a straightforward regulatory role that I will discuss later.

One can argue that higher premiums won't make everyone live healthy lives. Probably nothing will do that. We will still have people who make choices that leave them fat, drunk, and smoking. But there will probably be a lot fewer of them, and they'll be paying the long-term costs of their own behavior as they age. They will also always have the option of changing their behaviors and spending less on insurance as a result.

In other words, we can achieve the financial and the higher-level benefits that prevention offers us by placing the authority, the responsibility, and the accountability squarely where it belongs—with each individual.

CHAPTER 3

Consumer Roles
and Rights

It should be abundantly clear by now that I am proposing to place the focus of effective, comprehensive health reform on America's citizens, or as I prefer to call them in this context, its consumers. It is they who must be enabled with the authority, the responsibility, and the personal accountability to engage with health insurers and health care providers from a position of power and authority, just as they do in procuring their other essential needs for food, clothing, housing, and transportation. Since this position runs counter to so much of the current thinking about health care and how it should be provided, I would like to address it more directly.

The Role of Consumers

I hear a lot of arguments against the idea of a consumer market in medical care. They primarily fall into five categories:

1. *The Inability-of-the-Poor-to-Cope Argument*: A consumer-based medical market won't work because the poor won't be able to function within it.

2. *The Above-the-Consumer's-Pay-Grade Argument*: Medical care is too complex and technical for mere consumers to understand; thus, they could never make intelligent decisions about how to get what they need.

3. *The Lack-of-Consumer-Information Argument*: Even if consumers were to ask the key questions about quality and price, they can't get the answers.

4. *The Emergency Argument*: How can I make a rational decision about who to buy medical services from when I'm being loaded into an ambulance far from home?

5. *The Medical-Care-Is-Special Argument*: Medical care is too essential a social need to be bought and sold like a mere commodity.

On inspection, none of these arguments holds up.

The Inability-of-the-Poor-to-Cope Argument

In conversations with many skeptics, I have gotten one objection to my American Choice Health Plan more than any other: "There's just no way the poor would be able to navigate your consumer market for health insurance and medical care." The implication is that this supposed fact for a part of the population somehow makes it true for the entire population. The issue of the poor is an important one that I will discuss in more detail later. But it is not dispositive of the overall question of fixing a broken health care system. That's because the argument suffers from something that logicians and economists call the fallacy of composition. The fallacy of composition arises from the inference that something true for the part must also be true for the whole. Here's an example of a fallacy of composition from NationMaster.com's online encyclopedia:[1]

1. Atoms are not visible to the naked eye.

2. Humans are made up of atoms.

3. Therefore, humans are not visible to the naked eye.

The argument about the poor suffers from the fallacy of composition at two levels. First, it assumes that because some poor people may lack the skills, intelligence, and ability to participate in a transparent medical market, then all of them do. This is clearly fallacious since we know that many members of the group we call "the poor" are actually highly mobile economically, socially, and educationally. Many who were in the lowest quintile of income at some time in their lives can, twenty years later, be found in the highest quintile, having been able to navigate a complex economy (I'm one of them). Second, even if the argument held for all the poor, it doesn't follow that the non-poor who make up 80–85% of the population would not be able to function in and benefit from a health care marketplace, or that special accommodations couldn't additionally meet the needs of the poor.

The real issue is not whether the problems of the poor would or should prevent such a market from remedying the problems of our health care financing and delivery system. It is how we should extend the inherent benefits of such a market to those who lack the financial means, skills, or ability to obtain them on their own. Framing the question this way helps suggest practical answers, perhaps in terms of additional economic and social safety nets to help make this happen. We don't forbid a marketplace in groceries because the poor can't afford them. We provide food stamps that allow them to participate like everyone else.

The Above-the-Consumer's-Pay-Grade Argument

Medical care can be technical, complex, scientific, nuanced, and ambiguous to an extent that defies decipherment by anyone lacking a high degree of specialty training. But so are PCs, iPods, Buicks, and Microsoft Vista. What makes these items rationally consumable by we mere mortals is our ability to access intermediate levels of information that tell us what we need to know to make rational, informed purchase decisions. There is nothing inherent in the art, science, or practice of medicine that would prevent the creation and dissemination of such information. It's just that under the current system there has been neither the demand by consumers nor the motivation by providers for it to be produced. If we could create the demand and the motivation, the information would flow. We would then be able to evaluate doctors, hospitals, and treatment regimens according to quality ratings, price levels, customer service rankings, warranty pledges, and other readily comprehensible measures of what we need to support sound value-based decisions.

The Lack-of-Consumer-Information Argument

This is the argument I get most often from those who have been long embedded professionally in our existing health care system. They've been inside this Alice-in-Wonderland construction for so long they can't imagine how it might look under a more rational design that resembles the rest of our economy.

It's a case of not seeing the forest for the trees or, as I like to think of it, of looking at the medical landscape from too low an altitude. Only by taking in the whole picture from a higher level can it become apparent where the system is broken and what other parts of the economic environment offer analogous solutions. If all you can see is a nonsensically complicated, government-dominated billing-and-collection system for doctors and hospitals, it can be hard to imagine it going away. It can be harder still to foresee it being replaced by market-based pricing. But then consumers would be the arbiters of value, not third parties possessed of their own inherently different priorities. Payment mechanisms could then function with the speed, cost, and simplicity of credit card transactions.

Again, there is nothing inherent in insurance or medicine that precludes dissemination of information that would allow most consumers to make mostly rational decisions most of the time. That's all any market requires to perform better than any other known system of economic organization.

The Emergency Argument

This is another version of the fallacy of composition. It suggests that the American Choice Health Plan won't work because rational consumer decisions won't be possible during medical emergencies, even though they are an infrequent occurrence for most people.

But even the limited case doesn't hold water. There is nothing to prevent the creation of emergency triage systems to direct ambulance drivers to the medical facilities best equipped to handle particular types of cases. If you collapsed with pain in your chest and left arm, and the ambulance med tech's EKG suspects or confirms a heart attack, then it is hardly a technological stretch to divert the driver to the best available facility for dealing with heart attacks.

If such a system had been in place when Bill Clinton suffered chest pains in 2004, he might have been rushed to five-star-rated Lenox Hill Hospital in Midtown Manhattan instead of the uptown three-star-rated New York Presbyterian Hospital—Columbia, where he actually received his quadruple bypass.[2] Fortunately, he seems to have come out okay although statistically his chances would seem to have been better at another hospital.

Just because many ambulances will now take you to the closest hospital or the one on the current rotation list or the one with which the ambulance company has a contract doesn't mean it needs to stay that way.

The Medical-Care-Is-Special Argument

This is the argument I address more fully below in the section "Is Health Care a Right?" At a conference on health reform in 2008, I was confronted by a fellow speaker who told me that health care was too important to be bought and sold. He said it should be provided free of charge by the government under a single-payer system. His argument was that medical care is a public good.

It's not. It's an economic good, just like food, clothing, housing, transportation, and recreation. As such, it is most efficiently, fairly, and effectively provided via regulated markets, not by governments. Government certainly has valid roles—as regulator and as safety net of last resort.

Actually, there are consumer health care markets. We've lived so long with the myth that patients can't or won't make their own health care decisions that it is necessary to present evidence that they indeed can and will. They are already doing it for a wide array of health care products and services that health insurance largely doesn't cover. These range from complex medical procedures performed by competing doctors, such as Lasik vision correction and bariatric weight loss surgery, to the market for FDA-approved over-the-counter medications, which is larger in unit volume than the market for prescription drugs. There is also a large and growing market for insurance plans that focus more responsibility on consumers.

Here are some examples:

Online Consumer Information

As noted at the beginning of this book, getting consumers to ask and act on the answers to two questions will fix virtually all the major problems in our health care financing and deliver system. Succinctly, (1) Who are the best providers?, and of those, (2) Which offer the lowest prices?

Only two things are needed for consumers to actually do this: motivation and information. Their motivation is slowly emerging as health insurance deductibles have increased from less than $250 in 2000 to more than $1,000 in 2008. And health plans with deductibles as high as $11,600, including HSA and HRA savings arrangements, have grown rapidly and now account for more than 20% of all insurance coverage for Americans under age sixty-five. This is a profound shift that is placing increasing purchasing responsibility directly on consumers and providing strong incentives for them to seek care with high quality and low price.[3]

Increased consumer financial responsibility is creating consumer demand for accurate, easily obtainable information on health service availability, quality, and, of course, price. Until recently, this information has been all but impossible to find. But, at least on the availability and quality front, that is changing rapidly.

Attempting to gain market share in meeting this demand, private companies like HealthGrades are providing online doctor and hospital quality ratings. Websites from UnitedHealth, Microsoft, Google, Revolution Health (25 million unique visitors per month), WebMD (18 million users per month), Consumer Reports, the Mayo Clinic, and other health information portals are competing by providing online consumer health records, health service pricing guides, and the latest information on medical treatments. According to comScore

Inc., a marketing research firm, health websites attracted 77 million visitors in 2008, up 14% from 2007.[4]

Laura Landro, who writes a consumer health column in *The Wall Street Journal*, listed some of the best and most improved sites:[5]

- *Consumermedsafety.org* allows consumers to report and seek information about medication safety, including the ability to receive automatic alerts by the FDA. Visitors to the site can list all their current medications and receive information on their safety ratings, possible side effects, and interactions.

- *WhyNotTheBest.org* allows both providers and consumers to compare the quality of their local and other hospitals, using Medicare data on 4,500 such institutions.

- *HazMap* (hazmap.nlm.nih.gov) is a federal site that provides visitors with information about exposure to chemicals and biologic substances and their known relationships to various diseases. Consumers can check by substance, disease, or symptoms. Also maintained by the government, the ToxTown site at www.toxtown.nlm.nih.gov provides consumer information on toxic chemicals and other environmental health risks.

- *EverydayHealth.com*, now part of Revolution Health, offers a seemingly encyclopedic range of health information, personal health calculators, site-links, and customized consumer websites.

- *WebMD.com* has further expanded its similarly extensive consumer site to include diet and nutrition.

- *HealthCentral.com* is a network of sites covering a wide variety of conditions and diseases, including a symptom checker.

- *Google Health* (google.com/health) and Microsoft Health Vault (healthvault.com) both offer a number of health-management tools and online personal health record capabilities.

Amid this growing universe of widely used information, there is one glaring lack: Consumer pricing information for commonly used health services is difficult or impossible to obtain. The barriers preventing it are a combination of provider pricing that has nothing to do with actual reimbursement expectations; insurer payments that ignore provider prices; and the eight-hundred-pound gorilla that drives these practices, the Center for Medicare and Medicaid Service's (CMS) chokehold on health care pricing and reimbursement systems.

A number of insurers do offer websites that estimate consumer costs for a range of providers and conditions, but these are based on historical data and confidential provider contracts, not actual provider prices.

One bright spot, however, is a website called DestinationRx (www.drx.com) that will give you current retail prices for virtually any drug and allow you to choose the pharmacy that currently offers the lowest price.

Unfortunately, there is little on the horizon to suggest the lack of medical service pricing will change anytime soon. Until it does, we will have to rely on crude proxies for price, like the insurers' data. If price information does become available, consumers will use it. I will discuss in chapters 9–12 how to make this happen.

Medical Travel

The concept of medical travel is also called medical tourism. But that seems oxymoronic—like friendly fire. Whatever you call it, it is one of the fastest growing segments in patient-paid health care. People are traveling from everywhere to virtually anywhere for everything from face-lifts to liver transplants.[6] The reasons are higher quality and lower cost. A living-donor liver transplant that would have cost $450,000 in one of South Florida's top hospitals costs only $58,000 in one of New Delhi's equally capable hospitals. Against such savings, the typical $1,500 roundtrip airfare is trivial. Here are some examples of comparative prices of other medical procedures:

Procedure	U.S. Retail Price	U.S. Insurer Cost	India Retail	Thailand Retail	Singapore Retail
Angioplasty	$57,262–82,711	$25,704–37,128	$11,000	$13,000	$13,000
Gastric Bypass	$47,988–69,316	$27,717–40,035	$11,000	$15,000	$15,000
Heart Bypass	$122,424–176,835	$54,741–79,071	$10,000	$12,000	$20,000
Heart Valve Replacement	$120,138–159,325	$71,401–103,256	$9,500	$10,500	$13,000
Hip Replacement	$43,780–63,238	$18,281–26,407	$9,000	$12,000	$12,000
Hysterectomy	$20,416–29,489	$9,591–13,854	$2,900	$4,500	–
Knee Replacement	$40,640–58,702	$17,627–25,462	$8,500	$10,000	$13,000
Mastectomy	$23,709–34,246	$9,774–12,118	$7,500	$9,000	$12,400
Spinal Fusion	$62,778–90,679	$25,302–36,547	$5,500	$7,000	$9,000

Prices include hospital costs, airfare, and hotel rooms.
SOURCE: U. Kher, "Outsourcing Your Heart," *Time*, May 21, 2006.

Pennsylvania's Amish have been traveling to Mexico for years to purchase cut-rate medical care.[7] Last year, India alone received 150,000 medical tourists from the United States, Europe, Africa, and Asia. There, patients can go under the knife of American-trained doctors in Joint Commission International accredited hospitals for a fraction of the cost of numerous surgical procedures back home. Evidencing the increased demand for Indian health care, American medical travel companies have begun to offer package deals that include airport pickup, translation services, and airline bookings.[8]

Many of these international hospitals are accredited by the Joint Commission International, using the same standards applied by its sister organization, JCAHO, in the United States. Some Indian hospitals have reported success rates as high as 99.6%. Wockhardt Hospital CEO Vishal Bali has told me that his facilities specialize in cardiac, orthopedic, neurological, and minimally invasive procedures, performing thousands of each service every year. Sixty percent of its 550 super-specialist doctors were trained in the United States, Great Britain, and Australia. Wockhardt is an associate of Partners Harvard Medical International and emphasizes maximum quality, proper credentialing, and leadership in its chosen fields.

McKinsey and Company, the global consultancy, studied the medical travel industry and found the patients it interviewed were uniformly very satisfied with their care, expressing no hesitation in going abroad again for treatment or in recommending their friends and relatives to do so.[9] American insurers have begun to take notice. Mainstream carriers such as Blue Cross/Blue Shield of South Carolina, Aetna, and Cigna are providing coverage for lower cost health care abroad. In early 2009 Wisconsin's Anthem Blue Cross and Blue Shield began a trial program covering treatments at India's Apollo Hospitals. A cardiac bypass procedure there can cost a tenth of the $100,000+ price in the United States. The patient gets care reputed to be world-class; zero deductibles and copayments; travel and concierge assistance; airplane tickets for himself and a companion; and follow-up care back in the States.[10]

Medical travel-oriented providers aren't only to be found abroad. Galichia Heart Hospital, a private Wichita provider, charges a flat $10,000 fee for a common open-heart procedure for which its neighboring hospitals charge as much as $35,000. As its founder, Dr. Joseph Galichia has trumpeted, "This isn't just a good rate. It's a world-class rate." Dr. Galichia isn't looking only for uninsured American patients but also Canadians and Brits who are tired of waiting in long queues under their own countries' free national health programs.[11]

Medical travel is a sign that patients faced with financial incentives to shop for care will go to great lengths—and distances—to find high-quality, low-cost care.

Retail Generic Drugs

Wal-Mart made national headlines in 2006 by announcing it would begin selling several hundred generic drugs for only $4 for a thirty-day supply. The list of drugs has subsequently grown, and Wal-Mart has added the option of ninety-day supplies for $10. The event was historic in that it marked the first time in modern American health care that prescription drugs were being sold by a major retailer on the basis of price. Even so, Costco's membership clubs have more quietly been selling prescription drugs for years with only minimal markups.

Prescription drug customers have descended in droves on Wal-Mart pharmacy counters. Competitive responses by other large pharmacy retailers have followed. CVS Caremark, Rite-Aid, King Soopers, and other national and regional chains now offer similar programs. Even Walgreens, the flagship for high-retail generic drug prices, is now offering its Prescription Savings Club with four hundred drugs priced at $12 for a ninety-day supply. Walgreens has said the program has been "extremely successful" in retaining and acquiring customers.[12]

Wal-Mart has brilliantly targeted uninsured and underinsured retail shoppers who have to buy their prescription drugs with their own money. Many were already Wal-Mart customers. It has equally brilliantly undercut a key profit driver for other retail pharmacy chains—generic drugs. In recent years pharmacies have learned that because generic drugs are so cheap to buy at wholesale—often $2 or $3 for a ninety-day supply—they can mark them up many, many times and still price them well below the brand name drugs they replace. They have been able to do this since consumers have become habituated to prescription drugs costing a lot of money and never being advertised by price. That's because the pharmacies' focus has, until now, been on the vast majority of consumers who have health insurance with fixed-dollar copayments and thus couldn't care less about how much drugs actually cost.

Wal-Mart's move has exposed the seamy underbelly of that strategy by publicly pricing many generics based on their cost rather than the old industry standard of pricing what an unknowing, unmotivated market would bear. Wal-Mart recognized that, between the number of people with high-deductible health insurance and those without any insurance at all, there is a market of more than sixty million people who care a lot about retail drug prices. They are more than willing to use their well-honed consumer shopping skills to purchase drugs the same way they buy tires, soap, and DVDs.

Another key aspect of the Wal-Mart drug-pricing revolution is what doctors are telling me about their patients' behavior. Patients are increasingly asking them about generic drugs, specifically to take advantage of Wal-Mart's prices. Because of the incessant barrage of drug company sales reps giving away free drug samples, doctors have long tended to prescribe the most expensive brand name drugs automatically, even when lower-cost generics can do just as well. (There are no generic sales reps to tell them this.) Nothing is more effective at changing such doctor behavior than a patient asking for help saving money.

Sweating in the background are the major pharmacy benefit managers (PBMs) that sell many billions of dollars of mail order and retail drugs to the 250 million Americans who have health insurance through their employers or other insurers. PBM profit models have become heavily dependent upon their ability to sell generics at inflated prices. Fortunately for the PBMs, their consumers—the patients—don't care about drug prices, only the copayments. And most of their actual customers—employer human resource managers and health insurer contracting agents—are far less sophisticated than American retail shoppers. They continue to be largely clueless that they are overpaying by often vast amounts. This has allowed the PBMs to charge generic prices to their clients that can exceed retail prices to the public by factors of ten or more for some drugs.

I know this challenges the idea of sophisticated supply chain managers squeezing every penny out of their corporate purchases.

But such processes are nowhere to be found in the behavior of employers in contracting with their PBMs. When asked why, managers' answers essentially boil down to "We've always done it this way." This entire PBM business model is long overdue for some of economist Joseph Schumpeter's creative destruction. (Full disclosure: My consulting company, Hyde Rx, is such a creative destroyer.)

I don't want to go overboard in praising Wal-Mart's consumer strategy. Even as Wal-Mart has made the prices of many generics highly transparent and very cheap, I have noticed it charging high margins on many other generics not on the $4 list. Many of them are commonly used drugs. Also, Wal-Mart's Sam's Club sibling has removed drug pricing information from its website, making it difficult for customers to get pricing information on other drugs without actually buying them. Consumers with multiple prescriptions may not be saving as much money as they think.

Nonetheless, the lesson here is that the average American consumer, empowered by the responsibility and authority to spend his own money, is smarter than the highest-IQ bureaucrat—corporate or government—when responding to clear price signals associated with what he needs to buy.

The OTC Drug Market

It may surprise you to know that most FDA-approved medications consumed by Americans are purchased over the counter (OTC) without a prescription. OTCs are a $17-billion-a-year market that accounts for 60% of the quantity of all drugs sold in the United States.

For many years consumers have used their own money to purchase powerful, effective, and safe OTC drugs from drugstores and supermarkets. These drugs are effective against more than four hundred different medical problems, and many are as effective as prescription drugs. They contain more than one thousand active ingredients and are used in more than 100,000 products.[13]

OTC drugs include more than seven hundred products that required doctors' prescriptions within the past twenty-five years. Some of the newer ones, like Prilosec OTC, Claritin, Zyrtec, and their generic cousins, are available in full prescription strength, having been approved by the FDA for meeting four criteria for OTC sales:

1. Low potential for abuse or misuse
2. Can be used for consumer self-diagnosed conditions
3. Can be appropriately labeled for consumers
4. Can be used safely and effectively without the need for a doctor

You might wonder why such drugs ever required prescriptions. The answer is that by going the prescription-required route drug companies were able to charge far higher prices for them. It is only when drugs' patents expire that some of them move to OTC status because drug companies hope to leverage successful brands that would otherwise lose relevance in the prescription market.

Consumers have found OTC drugs to be a low-cost alternative to prescription drugs for many of their medication needs. Not only are the drugs much less expensive than most Rx meds, but consumers also don't have to pay a doctor to prescribe them. Increasingly, patients are learning to ask their doctors about OTC alternatives to prescription drugs, something that doctors are often delighted to recommend. Consumers have a long history of effective self-diagnosis and treatment, not to mention consumer savviness that serves them well in meeting their medical needs.

Non-Traditional Medicine and Dietary Supplements

The assertion that consumers won't obtain preventive care if they have to pay for it is challenged by the market success of the complementary and alternative medicine (CAM) industry. According to a 2008 study by the National Center for Complementary and Alternative Medicine (NCCAM), approximately 38 percent of U.S. adults and nearly 12 percent of U.S. children use some form of CAM.[14] CAM includes, among many other things, naturopathy, acupuncture, massage, aromatherapy, chiropractic, dietary supplements, herbal medications, and traditional remedies. Most such services are not paid for by health insurance.

Estimating the amount of money spent on CAM is difficult. The most authoritative study is more than a decade old, and the estimates in it are far from precise. But even in 1997, spending on such therapies by the U.S. public was estimated at between $36 billion and $47 billion.[15] Of that, between $12 billion and $20 billion was paid by consumers as professional fees to CAM providers. These alone were equivalent to about half of what consumers also paid directly to physicians that year and more than the amount they paid for their hospitalizations.[16]

Much has been written about the effectiveness of CAM, both pro and con—much of it con. George D. Lundberg, former editor of the *Journal of the American Medical Association* (*JAMA*) put his own view succinctly: "There's no alternative medicine. There is only scientifically proven, evidence-based medicine supported by solid data."[17] With this simple statement, he condemns most CAM treatments to the nether reaches of quackery and faith healing. The unintended irony is that he does the same for at least 70% of what licensed medical doctors do, since, as I have discussed previously, so little of their own standards of care have ever been scrutinized in scientific studies to see whether they really work. The widespread belief by consumers that CAM works may well be little more than a mass placebo effect (although placebos work, too). But the point is that these consumers are spending huge after-tax sums from their own pockets on preventive care and believe it to be helpful. Maybe they would do the same for regular allopathic medical care if it were also available at reasonable, transparent prices and without the poor customer service and excessive bureaucracy they now face.

Consumer acceptance of CAM belies the myth that Americans won't seek preventive care unless insurance pays for it. What it also suggests is that the medical establishment has failed to make its own preventive services available in a sensible, accessible way to consumers.

Lasik Eye Surgery

Every year in the United States, about 800,000 patients have Lasik vision correction procedures performed at a cost of $2.5 billion.[18] Lasik is the most frequently performed surgery in the United States, but because it is considered a medically unnecessary or cosmetic procedure by most insurance companies, it exists almost exclusively in the patient-pay market.[19] Lasik, a procedure performed by medical doctors (ophthalmologists), is a highly competitive business. Prices range from less than $1,000 per eye to more than $2,500. Competition has resulted in a real price decrease by almost half over the past twelve years.[20]

According to an analysis by the American Society of Cataract and Refractive Surgery of nineteen worldwide patient studies, Lasik patients have a 95.4% satisfaction rate with their procedures. The FDA reports only 140 negative cases between 1998 and 2006. Normally, patient satisfaction rates for medical procedures are not a reliable indicator of quality. Patients are not in a position to determine whether their heart function, for example, has improved as much as it would have if their doctors had performed standard-of-care surgery. And for many other conditions, patients do well regardless of diagnosis and treatment. That is because of the body's ability to heal itself without—or in spite of—outside intervention. That is another reason so many doctor mistakes are never caught.

Lasik, however, is one of those procedures where the patient is essentially as capable as any professional evaluator of determining the quality of outcomes related to diagnosis and treatment. Normal vision impairment is not something that corrects itself, so any adverse quality outcome is normally detectable by patients. They either can see as well as they were told to expect—pain and complication-free—or they can't. I hasten to add that not even with Lasik can patients determine whether their treatment left them more prone to long-term complications, which a doctor might better be able to determine.

That said, it appears that Lasik customers have done a pretty good job of demanding and obtaining better care than is normally delivered by most insurance-dependent doctors. The RAND Corporation says that atrial fibrillation patients get appropriate care between 20% and 50% of the time. Breast cancer patients do better, with an 85% rate. So a 95.4% success rate for Lasik is exceptional by any standard. I had the procedure done in 1997 and am one of the satisfied patients, even though the doctor had to perform a do-over on my left eye because of initial under-correction. Still, I was happy because I was able to end thirty-five years of wearing contact lenses. And the do-over was included in my original price—not something you normally experience with insurance-covered surgery.

Despite the high approval rates (and the encouraging fact that patient satisfaction is tracked), it seems that the relatively few disgruntled Lasik patients make a lot more noise about their unhappiness than patients receiving other medical and surgical procedures. Discontented Lasik patients put up websites, complain to newspapers, and write their own critical first-person accounts.[21] Some complain of truly serious complications and others of not quite achieving the 20/20 vision they expected. They expect more because they've paid for it, and that gives them the standing to speak out. I suspect this phenomenon will cause more doctors to look at each Lasik patient as an opportunity to avoid being featured on *60 Minutes*.

Lasik providers often offer patient financing to let them pay by the month. Some doctors even provide money-back guarantees and lifetime warranties, which should make their colleagues in the insured world nervous. Some providers are engaging in what looks a lot like bait-and-switch. They prominently advertise Lasik for only $250 per eye, without disclosing that hardly anybody actually pays such a low price. Instead, patients are subjected to up-selling to higher cost options, such as wavefront analysis and bladeless eye flap incisions. These add-ons can increase the costs to $1,500 per eye or more (which is still less than the $1,975 per eye I paid for much less advanced technology in 1997).

Caveat emptor is important in buying health care, just like anything else. A lot of people who believe the system should be inherently benevolent won't like this notion. To date, that belief has given us a health care system that delivers too much low-quality, overpriced, third-party-paid health care.

Letting consumers take control means expecting them to take responsibility. That requires that they realign their highly practiced consumer skills to include something that has long been outside their scope—health care purchasing. But the Lasik example tells us something else: under a health care system in which consumers control the money, *price matters*. Once a prospective consumer is satisfied that the quality is there, price will be the determining factor in whether she buys from one provider or another. That is why you see ads for $250 Lasik. These may be misleading (although some people do indeed pay that rate), but the real point is that the providers have quickly adapted to what they know consumers care about. Time and the courts will end misleading business practices in medicine, just as they have in other businesses. But under a consumer market-based health care system, price will become a key factor in determining both the supply and the demand for health care services.

Lasik may be a microcosm of what we can expect from a more patient-centric health care system. Not all of it is rosy just yet. Yes, Lasik prices have dropped over the years, despite great improvements in the technology, while prices of insurance-funded services have soared. And yes, the high rate of patient satisfaction is encouraging. But it's still hard to know in advance who are the best Lasik surgeons with the best facilities and, most important, who are the ones with the best outcomes. There are now several accrediting bodies working to identify the best doctors. But the industry has a long way to go before it can report uniformly collated outcome statistics and make them publicly available. Still, Lasik is a dynamic, patient-pleasing industry that is already punishing abusive and corrupt providers and rewarding those who receive good word-of-mouth from their patients. I expect that quality assurance and reporting systems will advance quickly and, as technology continues to improve, prices will continue to fall even further.

Gastric Banding

Gastric banding is a surgical procedure in which a silicone band is used to constrict the stomach in obese people who want to lose weight. The use of bariatric surgery for weight loss has exploded from virtually nothing in the early 1990s to more than 200,000 procedures per year in 2007. To a great extent, the marketing and delivery of gastric banding services has paralleled that of Lasik, as is evidenced by aggressive TV, billboard, and print advertising and the spread of free-standing, investor-owned outpatient surgery centers performing the procedure. The surgery is offered for prices ranging from $15,000 to $40,000, with the most common price being around $17,000.[22]

Common problems resulting from obesity include cardiovascular disease, certain cancers, and the wide array of maladies that result from obesity-related diabetes. For many people who have been unable to diet and exercise their way to weight loss, gastric banding has been, literally, a lifesaver. A January 2008 article in *JAMA* reported that the procedure essentially cured Type II diabetes in 73% of the adults treated.[23] There is also substantial evidence that the procedure can pay for itself in terms of reduced medical expenses in as little as two years.[24] Nonetheless, there is also evidence that bariatric weight loss may be temporary for many people unless they also permanently modify their dietary and exercise regimens.

As with Lasik, few commercial insurers cover gastric banding. Still, some government programs, including Medicare and the military's TRICARE program, now pay for it. Otherwise, like Lasik, it is primarily a voluntary consumer purchase. Although some policy analysts might argue for expanded insurance coverage for the procedure, I would suggest another approach. Under our current system of health insurance, people who fail to take personal responsibility for their health by maintaining normal weight are required to have their medical costs subsidized by those who do. This perpetuates moral hazard. Requiring health insurance to cover gastric banding would be an unnecessary extension of that subsidy.

A better approach would be an insurance system in which healthy behavior is financially rewarded and unhealthy behavior penalized. Obesity is, with few exceptions, the result of personal behavior. So is preventing and eliminating it. As I will detail in chapter 11 on my proposed American Choice Health Plan, a better approach would be a system of insurance premium reductions for people who keep their weight in a healthy range. Every insured person who could periodically demonstrate healthy weight and body mass measurements would receive a premium discount or rebate equal to the actuarial estimate of reduced medical costs.

Thus, people who are obese would have two choices: They could remain obese and pay higher premiums over their lifetimes to cover the average increased medical costs that will predictably result, or they could lose the excess weight and receive a rebate check or premium discount from their insurers. They could even use the newly available funds to pay back the money borrowed for their gastric banding. Or they could forgo the $17,000 surgery and change their diet and exercise behavior to lose weight and achieve the same personal and financial results. Not only would this approach provide substantial financial incentives for the obese to lose weight, it would also remove the unfair subsidy burden from those who have been taking care of themselves all along.

The amount of the premium reduction or rebate would be established by each insurance company based on its own actuary's calculations. If the above two-year payback period turns out to be real, then the individuals investing in their own gastric banding would receive a 50% return on that investment every year they keep their weight within a healthy range.

Such an approach would both obviate the moral hazard of insuring bariatric surgery while encouraging its use for those who can most benefit from it.

Retail Store Medical Clinics

Since their beginnings in Minneapolis in 2000, small, limited-service retail medical clinics positioned in large retail chain stores have seen rapid growth. These clinics provide walk-in treatment by nurse practitioners for a limited range of basic medical conditions, such as immunizations, sore throats, ear infections, and flu.

Since the first QuickMedx (now MinuteClinic), just under a thousand such clinics have opened in twenty-five states across the country, most in suburban areas.[25] The early innovators were entrepreneurs backed by private capital. Now the action is focused on such big players as Wal-Mart (with outsourcing and co-branding with local hospitals and Revolution Health's RediClinic unit)[26], CVS Caremark (having acquired MinuteClinic), and Walgreens (having acquired Take Care Health Systems). These giants now control much of the business and are aggressively pushing expansion. Although physically and operationally separate from onsite pharmacies, there are increasing co-marketing approaches, such as offering pharmacy discounts for clinic patients.[27]

One element in the evolution of these clinics is particularly noteworthy from a health policy standpoint—how they get their revenue. Retail clinics were originally conceived as cash-only retail businesses that offered low, flat-rate customer pricing ($35 in the case of the original MinuteClinic in Minneapolis) with no insurance billing. It soon became clear, however, that this price, though significantly below the equivalent cost of a regular doctor visit, actually represented a price *increase* to most patients who had insurance. Their normal copayments for such visits were usually only $20 or so. Thus, though the retail clinics represented a significantly lower price overall, anyone with insurance saw it as the quite the opposite. This tended to attract only the uninsured and those eager to see a provider immediately rather than wait for doctor appointments.

The clinics have since responded by offering insurance billing, but with a significant increase in administrative effort, cost, and accounts receivable. This change further highlights how the widespread coverage of normal consumer purchases by insurance has created perverse incentives and economics that retard price-based innovation in the market for health services delivery. It is another unfortunate consequence of the muddling of the concept of catastrophic insurance with that of prepayment for normal consumer services. Even this is rapidly changing, however, with insurance deductibles now topping $1,000 for the average American. Price is becoming important.

According to media accounts, patients appreciate being able to walk into clinics during evening and weekend hours and be seen by a nurse practitioner after brief waiting times—a welcome change from the normal doctor visit experience.[28] Only about 20% of customers pay cash—although Wal-Mart says that 55% of its clinic customers lack health insurance.

Unsurprisingly, medical doctors have been less than enthusiastic about this retail clinic innovation. One of the more commonly voiced complaints is that the clinics further fragment an already poorly co-ordinated medical care system. This has been the stated position of, for example, the American Academy of Pediatrics, which opposes the clinics outright.[29] Others more pointedly claim that only doctors should provide such medical care. They point out that lesser trained practitioners may miss complications or fail to refer patients to more appropriate providers. Such claims are belied by decades of studies showing that nurse practitioners consistently provide quality at least equal to that of doctors. And they do it with lower cost and superior customer satisfaction.

Usually unstated are doctors' concerns that they are facing competing providers of high-quality care who provide better customer service for a lower price. Pediatricians tend to be among the lowest-paid doctors. They are often burdened with seeing thirty to forty patients per day. You might be tempted to be sympathetic to their plight, especially when their years of medical training are being so readily trumped by nurse practitioners with far fewer years of training. The solution is not to suppress true innovations like these clinics but to rationalize the entire medical delivery system so that each provider can either find his proper niche or depart for more productive endeavors.

Rationalizing the system will help resolve the growing primary care physician shortage. We will need pediatricians more than ever for patient conditions that only they are trained to treat. Harvard Business School professor Clayton Christenson says that such innovations as nurse practitioners will allow the normally lower-paid primary care doctors to move up the food chain. They will do this by sending fewer patients to specialists while charging higher fees for providing higher value-added services.[30]

This will all seem harsh to those who see medical practice as more a social calling than economic endeavor. But it is the reality we—and they—must face if we're ever going to see a truly effective, high-quality medical care delivery system that is available and affordable to all. Anything that requires highly trained personnel to deal with low-intensity problems is wasteful. Overall, retail clinics are a low-cost, consumer-friendly approach to treating minor medical problems. And consumers are using them in numbers sufficient to attract big players with deep pockets. According to Margaret Laws of the California Health Care Foundation, "The clinics are the latest big example of how you could think about consumers and what their needs are, rather than a health care system exclusively designed around the needs of providers."[31]

The Medically Savvy Amish

The Amish and Mennonite religious communities of Lancaster County, Pennsylvania, have already figured out what consumers will quickly learn under a consumer market-based health care system: Health care can cost a lot less if you're willing to pay cash upfront. A *Wall Street Journal* article by Joel Millman reported how church elders from these faiths were able to negotiate hospital rates as low as 28% of the national average for procedures such as hip replacements, appendectomies, and C-sections. These groups spend $5 million a year for health care in Lancaster County, all of it without the insurance coverage they have foresworn as part of their rejection of much of the secular world. In exchange for 50% up-front payments and a pledge not to sue for malpractice, one local hospital has agreed to all-inclusive package pricing for various procedures, regardless of the hospital's actual costs for an individual case. By being better, more reliable payers than most insurance companies, these Anabaptist communities were able to negotiate rates even lower than those paid by some insurers.[32]

These religious groups learned the art of medical cost negotiation after years of crossing the border into Mexico for cut-rate care. As a result, health care providers from Tijuana and other border cities make regular marketing trips to Lancaster County to present their prices, services, and patient testimonials to prospective patients. This information has put these careful consumers in a strong position to negotiate more effectively with the local hospital. In a telling comment, the CEO of the Heart of Lancaster Hospital, Lee Christenson, said, "If you're paying out of pocket, you'll hunt for bargains." He concluded, "The Amish won't pay for health care they don't need."

Hyde Rx Services Corporation

My own consulting practice is in an industry sector that is a microcosm of almost everything that is wrong with health care, the pharmacy benefit management (PBM) industry. Although I may be fully in the throes of cognitive dissonance, I'm anything but hypocritical. My proposed American Choice Health Plan would utterly destroy my business by making it unnecessary. Let me explain.

Let's say you're the CEO of a large national company and want your employees to have company-sponsored health benefits. You want to avoid the headaches of fifty different state insurance regulatory regimes, so you opt to self-insure under federal ERISA rules that preempt state oversight. By self-insuring, you are putting your company into the insurance business, which neither you nor any of your managers know much, if anything, about. So you hire benefits consultants and insurance brokers to come in and tell you how to do it. Most likely, they will tell you to do it almost exactly the way every other self-insured employer does it. That's because neither you nor your consultants have any incentive to be truly innovative or, God forbid, actually run your health insurance venture like the new line of business that it is. I will discuss the reasons for this in chapter 4.

The consultants will generally help you hire two different kinds of companies to administer your health plan. First, you'll need a third-party administrator (TPA) to manage your medical benefits. The TPA will contract with medical providers, enroll your employees, and process their claims for hospital and doctor services. Second, you will need a PBM to do the same things for your prescription drug benefits, but with pharmacies instead of doctors. Why two? There are several reasons, but none of them is very good. It's best to just accept it as yet another one of those historical accidents that are embedded in, and contribute to, our dysfunctional health care system.

Because you now have a separate administrative structure for your pharmacy benefits, you need to craft the employee drug benefit pretty much distinct from the medical benefits. That is easy enough, as long as you don't care about having common deductibles, out-of-pocket spending limits, coordinated benefits, or combined utilization and financial reports. That's not a problem, since you, the CEO, will turn over the management of all this to your director of HR, who has exactly zero background in running an insurance company. Thus, such considerations usually won't rise high enough to be on anyone's radar screen anyway.

Your consultants will tell your HR manager that the best way to pick a PBM is to send out an RFP (request for proposal) to the usual suspects. Each PBM will send back the answers to many detailed questions. These will cover AWP discounts, MAC rates, dispensing fee schedules, and other minutiae that allow PBMs to avoid the single question that RFPs never seem to ask: "How much will my company and my employees spend on drug benefits next year?" It's a lot like buying a car based on which dealer claims to offer the lowest markup, cheapest interest rate, and biggest discount on maintenance costs—but without ever telling you the actual price you will pay for the car. The big PBMs will tell you that they get great prices on drugs because they buy them for so many millions of their clients' employees. This is a true statement. They also tell you that they can pass the savings on to you, the client. That, too, is true. They can. But alas, they don't.

Virtually 100% of PBM profits come from the difference between what they actually pay for drugs and what they charge their clients and members for them. In disappointingly few cases do these PBMs make money by delivering their clients the drugs their members need at the lowest available prices. Instead, they make the most money when their members buy the most drugs with the highest markups—currently generic drugs. RFPs rarely ask about real markups. Instead, they ask about such irrelevancies as the percentage discounts they will give you from a drug's average wholesale price (AWP). Without going into the details, let me just say that the inside joke in the pharmacy industry is that AWP means "Ain't What's Paid." It's an artificial metric that has virtually nothing to do with what you would normally expect to pay for a drug—either at wholesale or retail—with or without a "discount."

PBM drug markups come in three varieties: (1) retail spreads; (2) mail service pharmacy profits; and (3) manufacturer rebates. Retail spread is the difference between what a PBM pays a retail pharmacy for a drug dispensed to a member and the higher amount the PBM turns around and charges its client—either an employer or insurance company. In general, the spread is relatively small for brand-name drugs but often huge for generics. Mail service profits result from PBM ownership of mail service pharmacies their clients' members use. Manufacturer rebates are direct payments by brand-name drug makers to reward PBMs that direct their clients' members to their drugs rather than those of competing manufacturers. Rebates also have included switching fees that drug makers pay to PBMs that successfully switch members from a drug that's about to go generic (and become a lot cheaper) to a replacement brand drug that will end up costing a lot more. (I described the clever eight-step process by which the brand-name drug manufacturers do this in my book, *Prescription Drugs for Half Price or Less*, pp. 96–101.)

The relative importance of each of these revenue sources has changed in recent years. After suffering lawsuits and extremely bad press that bared revelations of rebate chicanery, PBMs stumbled upon an even more lucrative profit model that simultaneously cast them in a far better public light—as long as the light isn't too bright. Now the lion's share of PBM profit comes from markups on generic drugs, whether sold by their captive mail service pharmacies or by independent retail pharmacies. The PBMs proclaim the value of lower cost, equally effective generics by encouraging their members to use them to replace their expensive brand-name drugs. That's fine as far as it goes. But it turns out that generic drug wholesale prices are usually so incredibly cheap that PBMs can mark them up anywhere between three and twenty times and still tell their clients they are saving money against the brand alternatives.

Although the high-margin generics are indeed cheaper than equivalent brands, the PBMs somehow fail to tell their clients that their employees can often find the same drugs at lower prices from existing retail and independent mail order pharmacies *while paying their full retail prices*. Employees just need to know where to shop. A prime example was reported by *The Wall Street Journal*. The General Motors Corporation was paying its PBM $181.22 for a three-month supply of generic Zantac dispensed to GM employees. At the same time, anyone with a prescription could buy the same drug from Wal-Mart for $78.62 or from Costco for only $22.00. (At the same time, the independent mail service pharmacy I recommend to my clients was charging only $13.71.)[33] Most employers don't have the financial resources of a General Motors. (No, wait, now I guess they do.)

Fortunately for the PBMs, their consumers have no incentive to shop around for better prices. Any drugs they buy from a non-

PBM pharmacy won't be covered under their employer's insurance plans. Also, most employees pay only fixed-dollar copayments for their drugs, regardless of their actual price. If an employee pays $10 for a generic drug prescription, she really doesn't care whether its real price is $13 (the approximate overall average cost of generic prescriptions before PBM markup) or $181.22. The employer client just pays the difference without ever realizing there was one.

PBMs also have insurance companies as clients, and the dynamics are similar, except that the PBMs will often share their largesse with these customers. That way it's easier for the insurers to go along with the PBM model than to take more innovative approaches.

With more blockbuster brand-name drugs losing their patents and going generic, the PBMs have ridden this generic profit model to new heights of success—all on the backs of their clients and members. It is probably the largest, most successful industry in America that fundamentally depends on the ignorance of its customers.

I started learning all this several years ago via my health industry consulting practice. I had been involved in starting and operating a small chain of retail pharmacies owned by my HMO company, Peak Health. But that was before PBMs came to full fruition in the late 1980s and after we had sold the company. As I learned about PBMs, it dawned on me there might be a better model. If successful, it could even destroy the current one. It would benefit everyone, with the obvious exception of all current PBMs, as well as the brand-name drug companies. But they could all use a healthy dose of market discipline.

In one of my periodic fits of entrepreneurial recidivism, I changed my consulting practice, Hyde Rx Services Corp. (HRx), to focus on helping my clients adopt a new model for employee prescription drug benefits. Unlike mainstream PBMs, HRx doesn't get any markup on drugs from any of the fifty-five thousand contracted retail and independent mail service pharmacies used by our clients' employees. Instead, we charge our clients who are on the program a fixed, per-member-per-month management fee. HRx's stated goal is to help clients and their employees get the drugs they need at the lowest possible cost. Not marking up drugs helps achieve that, but it's a relatively small part of the story. Mostly, we work to help employees change their behavior in how they buy their drugs. That requires two things—incentives and information.

Here's how we do it. First, we encourage each of our employer clients to replace their fixed-dollar copayments with equivalent co-insurance, which means their employees will pay a percentage of each prescription's actual price but with an annual cap on total out-of-pocket expenditures. That provides the incentive for employees to care about how much their drugs actually cost, but it doesn't tell them how to go about getting cheaper drugs. That requires the information component, which we like to deliver face-to-face with each client's employees.

We start by telling the employees that 80–90% of them will be able to spend less money on their drugs during the following year than they did during the previous one. Next, we tell them how to talk to their doctors. We suggest that they say something like, "Doctor, before you reach for your prescription pad, please take a look at this list of questions to see whether you can help me save money on my drugs, because I now have to pay a big percentage of my actual drug costs." Invariably, even doctors who stay up nights figuring out ways to screw insurance companies respond positively to this request. They are oriented by training and habit to serve their patients, and nothing is more effective in eliciting that service than a patient asking for help. Without that request, the doctor will usually assume the patient doesn't care about cost. When a doctor realizes a patient does care, it becomes much less easy for him to give the patient a handful of free drug samples along with a prescription for the same, invariably expensive stuff.

Here are the "Seven Questions," which we also print on the back of each member's HydeRx ID card:

Doctor, can I save money with:

1. Alternatives to drugs?

2. OTC drugs instead of Rx?

3. Generic drugs?

4. Lower-priced brand drugs?

5. Tablet-splitting doses?

6. Ninety-day mail order Rx's?

7. Extra free samples?

The questions are arranged in order of importance, from highest savings to lowest, ranging from how to avoid drugs altogether down to minimizing the cost of any regrettably necessary brand-name drugs. We then discuss each question with the employees, giving concrete examples. We also provide reassurance to everyone, from blue-collar factory workers to Harvard MBA CEOs, that it's okay to ask these questions. Their doctors will respond positively. We have yet to hear of any doctor doing otherwise.

One of our earliest clients for this service came on board more than five years ago. After taking the account from one of the huge, traditional PBMs and providing our training to the employees, we waited nervously for the initial results. When the first month's utilization reports came in, my heart sank when I saw that the number of prescriptions under Hyde Rx had actually risen a few percentage points, despite the alternatives suggested by the first two questions (alternatives to drugs and OTC meds). The real shock, however, came when I looked at Rx claims costs. Total expenditures had plunged by nearly 50% from the previous month—again, for *more* drugs. As the year progressed, the number of prescriptions continued to climb, and the total expenditures leveled out at about 62% of costs under the previous PBM—a 38% savings for both employer and employees. This pattern has repeated itself with each of our clients since then when they have changed to coinsurance and employee training.

What happened? The coinsurance incentive and the consumer information worked. The employees descended on their doctors like biblical locusts. Many got replacement prescriptions for lower-priced drugs, especially generics and some over-the-counter medications that were also covered by the employer at our behest. Then they bought the drugs from their pharmacies and discovered they were now paying average generic drug coinsurance of only $2.60 per prescription, which contrasted with the old $10 generic copayment or the $30 brand-name copayment. The $2.60 resulted from their now paying 20% coinsurance on an average generic prescription drug price of only $13. Again, we make money from our fixed management fee, not from marking up drugs.

The members discovered that they could now pay much less than they had previously to control their blood pressure, cholesterol, depression, asthma, diabetes, and allergies—especially if they had been previously prescribed brand-name medications. Various studies have shown that patients are price sensitive about prescription drugs, just as they are about everything else. So our patients' compliance with their doctors' treatment and prevention recommendations went up, and total drug costs went down.

In other words, we turned the drug purchasing responsibility over to the actual consumers. They—motivated by both personal health *and* price—started taking better care of themselves at lower total cost, both to themselves and their employers. On average, the 35–40% savings figure has held up across the board. We still see room for savings improvement to at least the 50% level, because not all our clients' employees have taken advantage of the "Seven Questions."

What would the PBM world look like under a universal consumer market-based health care system? It would disappear entirely, having been entirely rendered obsolete by consumers who no longer need them. With consumers controlling their own money, doctors wouldn't even need to be asked the "Seven Questions." Physicians would have heard them so often that it would become second nature to incorporate the answers to the questions into their practices.

Patients wouldn't need a PBM to tell them where to buy their drugs and how much they had to pay for them. Instead, they would seek pharmacies with the lowest prices.

Pharmacies would compete on price and customer service. Internet-savvy patients—virtually everyone within ten years—would easily be able to find the lowest-priced pharmacies in the entire country—or within walking distance. The smart PBM employees who realized they would soon lose their jobs would depart early for other opportunities. The really smart ones would retire on the profits from having shorted their employers' stocks. Personally, I hope to be living off the proceeds of a small bookshop specializing in hard-to-find first editions of this book. It could be a classic by then and, alas, extremely rare.

Consumer-Driven Health Plans

Consumer-driven health plans (CDHPs), including HSAs, MSAs, HRAs, and other high-deductible health insurance now account for 20% of all individuals under sixty-five with health insurance in the United States. It is also the fastest-growing segment of health insurance.

How well has this increased exposure to high deductibles and individual responsibility resulted in bringing consumers better, lower-cost health care? Consumers with HSAs versus people in non-CDHP plans are more likely to ask their doctors about the costs of recommended treatments (52% vs. 33%), to choose lower-cost options (36% vs. 23%), and to use lower-priced mail order for buying prescription drugs (43% vs. 30%). They are also more likely to track their health care expenses (72% vs. 40%), estimate future expenses (38% vs. 22%), and discuss expenses with their doctors (38% vs. 27%). They are about 50% more likely to participate in wellness programs and are slightly more likely to use preventive services and equally likely to receive necessary services and comply with prescribed treatment. Savings due to reduced utilization averaged $1,074 per member for CDHP groups when compared with groups having standard insurance benefits.[34] In other words, consumers with increased responsibility and incentives are more likely to extend their normal consumer skills to buying health care, much like they do with virtually everything else.

Another salutary aspect of CDHPs is that they promote consumer savings. According to an estimate published by the AMA, Health Savings Account balances totaled $9.4 billion by the end of 2007, only two years after the authorizing legislation.[35] This suggests that consumers will indeed put money aside against future medical expenses if afforded the same tax advantages as employer-based insurance and if given the option of paying their normal medical purchases themselves.

Not everyone, however, is happy with their CDHPs. In general, enrollees are less likely to recommend the coverage to others (38% to 45%). There are at least two reasons for this. First, despite the much lower insurance premiums charged for high-deductible health insurance, many consumers have been either unwilling or unable to put the savings into Health Savings Accounts or other reserve funds from which they can later pay their normal medical expenses. When they have such expenditures without the savings to pay for them, they have had to make them at the expense of other personal budget items, usually things that are much more pleasurable than health care. When, however, employers fund HSA accounts, as two-thirds do,[36] or workers set aside their premium savings in HSA accounts, consumers are better able to pay their recurring health care costs without having to reduce other expenditures.

A second, and greater, problem with the current CDHP concept is that it is almost impossible for consumers to do the one thing that makes a consumer market possible—to find out the price of health care products and services before they are purchased. This is an unfortunate artifact of the growth of managed care, Medicaid, and Medicare during the last three decades of the twentieth century, which made even minor medical expenses subject to insurance coverage. With consumers no longer asking about prices, providers stopped providing them.

What has replaced the once efficient price mechanism is the wasteful, opaque, and highly arbitrary billing and collection system now used by virtually all providers and insurers. In that system, there is literally no such thing as price. Instead, insurers use complex formulae containing thousands of variables and literally millions of rules that only computers can calculate. They determine how much a given insurer will reimburse a given provider for a given set of services. Doctors have increasingly suspected insurers of using these mechanisms to systematically underpay them. The American Medical Association has sued Aetna and Cigna over the use of a database it says was rigged to underpay doctors on out-of-network claims for more than a decade.[37]

Nowhere in this system is there an opportunity for consumers to know how much almost anything will cost. Largely as a result of past reimbursement methods, doctors now routinely charge more than twice as much as they actually collect. Their "prices" are like a hotel's rack rate off-season—irrelevant.

Estimates of the total cost to the health care system of this parasitic billing and collection system have run as high as 31 cents of every health care dollar spent.[38] If we could eliminate it and replace it with competitive, transparent pricing, we could eliminate literally hundreds of billions of dollars of annual waste. The cost of processing a medical bill would become trivial, comparable to that of a credit card transaction.

Even more powerful would be the effect of consumers shopping by price as well as quality. Providers would then actively seek ways to provide the highest quality health care more efficiently for the lowest prices. This would give rise to innovations in technology, practice standards, and management procedures. Unfortunately, nothing in our current health care system encourages such a change. A consumer market-based system would require it.

Federal Employee Health Benefits Program (FEHBP)

If you are a federal employee or retiree, my American Choice Health Plan may sound familiar. It should, because the wide choice of health plans available under American Choice is partially modeled on the Federal Employee Health Benefits Program (FEHBP) that covers most civilian employees and retirees of the U.S. government. Nationwide, FEHBP now offers a choice of 269 different health plans.[39] Although no employee has that many individual options (Iowans have twenty-four), each has a wide choice of plans available that includes high-option benefits, HMOs, PPOs, consumer-driven plans, and high-deductible health plans in which the government will even fund an employee's Health Savings Account.

The FEHBP began in 1960 by an act of Congress, but its multiple-choice consumer structure owes more to historical accident than to clever legislative design. Back when it came time for Congress to enact a global health benefit plan for all federal employees, few of the myriad agencies and labor unions involved were willing to give up their own established plans. So Congress grandfathered them all in. This created a supermarket of health plans that has proliferated ever since.

Every government employee eligible for FEHBP has an annual opportunity to select any offered plan. She must stay in that plan until the next annual open enrollment period. FEHBP is managed by the federal Office of Personnel Management, which selects plans, negotiates premiums, and provides an in-depth website (www.opm.gov/insure/health/index.asp) that allows each FEHBP member to compare available plans, member satisfaction rates, quality ratings, and prices before choosing the insurance option best suited to her personal needs and circumstances.

FEHBP's major innovation is that individual employees always get to choose the best combination of plan costs, features, and service from among many competing plans. If an employee's chosen plan subsequently fails to live up to its promises, the member is free to leave and buy another one during the next open enrollment period. There are no limitations or waiting periods for preexisting conditions.[40]

This ability of individual customers to vote with their feet has created a strong incentive for participating plans to focus on their customers' needs. As a result, federal employees complain far less about their health insurance, because they can simply change to more appropriate plans. The effectiveness of this market discipline may be the main reason why relatively few employees actually do change plans—less than 5% each year.

FEHBP has demonstrated that consumers are fully capable of making rational choices in purchasing health insurance within the structure of a robust, competitive market. Unfortunately, it has failed to do so in a way that achieves effective cost control. In 2009, for example, the only thing that kept average FEHBP premiums from increasing by double digits was the government's tapping into FEHBP's reserve funds—not something it can do every year.[41] Even so, the employee share of the premium for the most popular Blue Cross/Blue Shield standard plan (selected by 60% of FEHBP's eight million participants) rose by 12.9% for singles and 13.4% for families. According to Colleen Kelley, president of a federal employee union, "This is an enormous increase that erodes federal employees' standard of living."[42] There are at least three features of FEHBP that contribute to its inability to control costs (none are incorporated into American Choice):

1. *Employer Contribution Basis*: FEHBP is not a defined-contribution program. That is, the federal government does not contribute a fixed amount to each employee's health insurance purchases. Instead it pays *the lower* of 72% of the weighted average premium of all employees *or* 75% of each employee's actual premium, regardless of the actual plan chosen.[43]

   This creates a strong bias for employees to choose plans with high premiums instead of plans with high deductibles. The government pays the lion's share of any higher premium but keeps most of any savings from lower-premium selections. FEHBP does offer high-deductible plans that include contributions to member health savings accounts. Employees have avoided such plans because they get to keep so little of the resulting premium savings for their HSAs. With that kind of contribution structure, it is unsurprising that fewer than twelve thousand of the eight million federal employees chose high-deductible plans in 2008.[44] If FEHBP were a true defined-contribution program, it is likely that the high-deductible plans with health savings accounts would be far more popular. Members would be able to apply the full amount of premium savings to their personal HSAs against future health care purchases. That could provide a major push toward more individual responsibility for controlling health spending while continuing to deliver excellent insurance coverage.

2. *Community-Rated Employee Contributions:* Currently, FEHBP requires every employee choosing the same plan to pay the same premium contribution, regardless of the employee's age, gender, geographic location, or acceptance of personal responsibility for healthy living. This is an example of an employer charging employee premiums on the basis of pure community rating, a problem-plagued approach I discuss in more detail in chapter 4. Thus, the 2009 total Blue Cross annual premium contribution for a twenty-two-year-old non-smoking government worker in low-cost Iowa making $26,000 per year is the same ($5,387 per year) as for an obese sixty-four-year old government executive chain-smoker making $125,000 in high-cost Boston.[45]

Under a more equitable premium-setting mechanism based on member age, gender, location, and personally controllable health risk factors, the younger worker with the healthy lifestyle would pay only a small fraction of the amount paid by the older, highly paid, overweight executive with a two-pack-a-day habit. The older worker would be financially penalized for continuing his self-destructive behavior. Or he could avoid the penalty by stopping smoking and losing weight. FEHBP's pure community rate simply won't work for the kind of nationwide, universally accessible, prevention-oriented health insurance program we need.

3. *Excessive Coverage Requirements*: FEHBP requires richer than necessary insurance coverage for such normal, low-cost consumer purchases as primary care, preventive services, and most prescription drugs. This obviates virtually any need for beneficiaries to shop for medical care goods and services by price. Dropping such benefit requirements from health insurance would allow—and virtually require—a competitive, affordable consumer market in medical services and products to emerge to offer high-quality care.

Despite its fundamental shortcomings, FEHBP has demonstrated that consumers can intelligently navigate a robust and competitive health insurance market when empowered with the money, the information, and the choices that allow them to best determine how to meet their own health care needs.

The Medicare Drug Program

The government's Medicare program for the elderly and disabled is facing massive problems with lack of cost control and an impending crisis in its funding. Ironically, a signpost to the way out of its problems may be Medicare's own Part D prescription drug benefit program that debuted in 2006.

For its first forty years, Medicare had no prescription drug benefit. That coverage gap was finally addressed with the 2003 passage of the Medicare Prescription Drug Improvement and Modernization Act (MMA). The MMA decreed its Rx benefit program would begin in 2006 and would be offered and administered only by competing private health plans. There were howls of protest at the time, claiming that turning over Part D to the private sector would fail because the government would not be allowed to negotiate drug prices for its beneficiaries. Instead, the program has been a remarkable success.

It has enjoyed strong popularity, with beneficiary satisfaction rates remaining high throughout the program's first three years.

One of the marked features of Part D is the wide range of benefit choices available to beneficiaries. Basic Medicare Part D coverage is hardly comprehensive. It includes significant deductibles up front and the notorious "doughnut hole" in the middle that can leave beneficiaries paying thousands of dollars in drug costs. Had Congress passed Part D as a government-run program, this basic plan would have likely been the sole benefit option. That would have been as much as the government could afford to provide within its budget constraints.

Initially, there was concern that there would be wide swaths of the country in which no private insurer would be available. This prompted Congress to allow CMS, the Medicare agency, to offer coverage itself in such areas. There was an explosion of private health plan offerings, however, with residents of even sparsely populated Wyoming having an annual choice of at least fifty different private drug plans. These options range from the bare-bones basic plan up to coverages that eliminate the deductible and doughnut hole. Prices vary widely, with each beneficiary being able to choose the combination of benefits and premiums that best fit her own circumstances.

Most striking is that the privately insured Part D program costs have been lower—much lower—than the government originally projected.[46] In every program year thus far—2006 through 2009—average beneficiary premiums have been significantly below initial government estimates. In 2003, for example, the government estimated that the 2009 premium cost to beneficiaries would average $44.12 per month. The actual number, based on plan bids as of August 2008, was only $28. That's 37% below the original estimate. Also, fully 97% of the 2008 beneficiaries had choices of 2009 plans that offered either no premium change or a decrease in premiums.

Many opponents of the private-sector approach preferred the traditional administration by the CMS bureaucracy of a single benefit plan. That would have virtually guaranteed that government-set premiums would have been at least as high as the government's estimates. Private insurers have aggressively competed with widened choices. They have generated huge savings and achieved a high level of customer satisfaction. And any beneficiaries who are unhappy with their plans have the option to change to any other plan once a year.

Medicare's Part D success at offering consumer choice and reining in costs is in stark contrast to the rest of the Medicare program. It offers a striking example of many of the principles that would allow a regulated market-based solution for health insurance for all Americans.

These are some of the more significant examples of sizable segments of health care in which patients are daily utilizing their consumer skills to purchase high-quality health insurance and health care at affordable prices. There are many others, including huge or growing industries in prescription eyewear, dentistry, cosmetic surgery, and concierge medicine. They drive a thriving sub-economy of health care that behaves much like the efficient consumer market economy in which we buy almost everything else. These examples should put an end to the frequently heard mantra that health care is just too important, too complex, or too technical for mere consumers to navigate on their own. The only thing preventing the emergence of such a consumer market on a wholesale basis is the structure of our current system. It prevents consumers from getting answers to their two key questions: Who are the best providers, and which of them is cheapest? That, as I shall explain, is fixable.

Is Health Care a Right?

A central thesis of this book is the necessity for America's consumers to be granted the authority, the responsibility, and the accountability necessary to enable them to obtain the health care they need. A related issue that has been long debated in this country is whether Americans also have a right to health care.

Is health care a right? I wish it were. It would be so much simpler if all Americans could exercise their right to health care as they do with their freedoms of speech, assembly, and religion. As with constitutional protections, if health care were a right, my exercise of the right to medical care would not limit your ability to do the same thing. The supply would be free and limitless. Any question of infringement would be swiftly dealt with by the courts. Well, if not swiftly, then at least surely. This use of the word "right" is consistent with its common definition as the sovereign ability of humans to pursue their own ends free of government infringement as long as those pursuits do not infringe on the rights of others.

The salmonella in the peanut butter for medical care is that, unlike our constitutionally protected rights, it is hardly free and endless. When I sit in a doctor's examining room or lie in a hospital bed, no one else can do it at the same time. I have to move on and free up those specific resources before the next patient can use them. Medical care is a scarce resource, like housing, 1955 Chevys, and all-natural charcoal. Medical care requires significant investment. Doctors must pursue many years of advanced education while enduring large costs—both opportunity costs and current ones. Establishing modern medical practices and hospitals is an increasingly capital-intensive engagement. Operating costs can be staggering. So no, health care is not a *right* as we normally use the word.

A closely related question is whether health care, as a scarce resource, is a public good that should best be provided by the government. For any good to be a public one, it must satisfy two requirements: It must be non-excludable *and* its consumption must be non-rivalrous. My apologies, but that's the way the economists put it.

Non-excludability essentially means that a public good, once produced, can be consumed equally by free riders as well as paying customers. *Non-rivalrous consumption* means that one person's consumption of the good does not limit the ability of others to do the same thing. An example of a public good is national defense. It is non-excludable because it covers everyone in the country under its protective umbrella, without regard to whether they have individually paid for it. Also, its consumption is non-rivalrous, in that one person's benefit from the advantages of national defense in no way inhibits the similar benefit by anyone else.[47] In other words, it's not a public good if its use can be limited to paying customers *or* if nobody else gets to use it when you do whether you paid for it or not.

Medical care is, therefore, not a public good but an economic good—that is, an "object or service that has value to people and can be sold for a non-negative price in the marketplace."[48] That's more economic geek-speak for the fact that it's something real that somebody has to pay for. It has scarcity and a measurable value to each consumer. If we're going to solve the problems of health care's delivery, affordability, and availability, we must come to grips with this reality.

Forget for the moment the semantics of medical care's status as a basic human right, a public good, or an economic good. Shouldn't it still be something that everyone should be able to obtain in a society as wealthy as ours? In my opinion the answer is yes. I haven't seen anyone—right, left, or center—opine that we should let people die in the streets for lack of essential medical care. I think most of us believe that all Americans should be able to obtain it. It's necessary for the life, liberty, and pursuit of happiness that, as Jefferson put it, *are* our inalienable rights. But medical care's status as an economic good means that we must seek to achieve this goal while meeting our competing needs and desires for other necessary economic goods.

Therefore, the question is not whether health care should be available to all. Rather, it is how it should be provided in the most efficient and effective way while least infringing on our ability to meet our other priorities. History tells us that the best way—the only way—to do that is via the mechanism of properly regulated markets.

You may have noted that I rarely, if ever, use the term "free markets" in this book. I consider myself a practicing lower-case libertarian[49] and don't see anything wrong with the term "free markets" when intoned with the intellectual resonance of a Milton Friedman. The term too often, however, connotes an assumption that free markets operate in the absence of government regulation. That's not the way it works, because even the freest markets require the rule of law to function properly at anything more than the most simplistic, elementary level.

Without a basis in law—read regulation—truly free markets may still exist, but only in the primitive forms of informal and black markets or of illegal piracy and criminal enterprises in which property rights, contracts, protection from theft, and other essential elements are enforced, often arbitrarily, by violence, corruption, and, by definition, lawlessness. Legitimate markets of the complexity necessary to sustain major economies cannot exist without law and regulation to ensure property rights, enforceability of contracts, rights of (at least) commercial speech and assembly, a sound currency, public infrastructure, a stable banking system, orderly bankruptcy procedures, national defense, social and economic safety nets, domestic and international trade policies, efficient capital formation, prevention of corruption and criminality, protection from unacceptable negative externalities (e.g., environmental damage), and resolution of significant market failures. These and other government functions are the desiderata of "free markets." Economists Charles Kindleberger and Robert Aliber have suggested that such regulation originally arose as a means to *reduce* the costs of doing business, not to impede business.[50]

The trick, though, is for regulation to permit markets to function without unnecessarily interfering with the free exchange of information and value that makes markets more effective than any other known method for creating and distributing economic goods. The central problem in health care is that it presents a market failure, but instead of government having identified and corrected it to allow markets to function, it has dived in largely to replace that function. And in doing so, it has stepped outside of its appropriate role. One purpose of this book is to suggest how to set that aright so that, although you may not have an inalienable right to health care, you should be allowed freely to obtain it on an affordable basis without having to sacrifice your other essential needs.

CHAPTER 4

Health Insurance:
What's Wrong With It and
What Needs to Be Done About It?

A recent CNN/Opinion Research Corporation poll revealed that most Americans are happy with their health insurance coverage but unhappy about the cost. The poll did not query those without health insurance, but presumably most of them would have been unhappy on both counts. In reporting the poll's results, CNN's polling director Keating Holland said, "It suggests a prescription for health care reform that Americans can swallow—start by addressing health care costs while allowing Americans to keep their current coverage and their current health care providers."[1] For reasons I hope to make clear in this chapter, his statement is the equivalent of saying we can solve the obesity problem if we can address its harmful aspects while allowing Americans to remain fat.

Virtually all of the problems we are experiencing in our current health care system are a result of a deeply flawed health insurance structure. In this chapter, I will explore how health insurance works, what goals we should demand that health insurance deliver, why employer-based insurance is dominant, and what this all means for crafting a new system to meet those aggressive goals. The discussion will necessarily require us to delve into some rather technical aspects of insurance you may have been perfectly happy to have ignored. That includes looking more closely at the uninsured, the critical issue of adverse selection, the pros and cons of group versus individual insurance, the various methods by which insurance premiums are priced, and an analysis of mandated insurance purchases. Discussing these subjects is unavoidable, because the devil is indeed in the details if we want to emerge with a truly functional health care financing and delivery system. The good news is that there is no math beyond simple arithmetic. And there won't be a quiz.

Perhaps the most frequently cited symbol of our health care problems is the 45.7 million Americans who have no health insurance. That number comes from the Census Bureau's annual estimate for 2007.[2]

The implication that many critics would have us draw is that these are people who can't afford insurance or are simply too sick to work for employers that offer it. Although that number certainly includes a lot of these people, they are actually a small minority of the total uninsured. Let's take a look at what we know about the uninsured, who they are, why they lack coverage, and what all this suggests about how we might correct the system's problems.

The Uninsured Problem

Getting a handle on the breakouts of who has insurance and who doesn't is not easy. There are multiple estimates, assumptions, and figures produced by various government and private organizations. For example, the Centers for Medicare and Medicaid Services (CMS) estimated 2004 Medicaid enrollment at 56 million, compared to the Census Bureau's 37.5 million. Nonetheless, one of the most comprehensive analyses of the uninsured is contained in the 2005 Census Bureau's Current Population Survey by the U.S. Department of Health and Human Services (HHS), using 2004 figures.[3] The total estimated number of the uninsured in this analysis was 45.8 million, virtually identical to the 2007 figure of 45.7 million. It provides a breakdown of estimated insurance coverage in the United States, as well as the number of uninsured. I have included population coverage figures in the table below:[4]

Sources of Health Insurance	Population Covered, 2004	% of Total U.S. Pop.
Employer-based group coverage	174,000,000	53.6%
Individual private coverage	16,900,000	5.2%
Medicare	39,700,000	12.2%
Medicaid/SCHIP	37,500,000	11.6%
Military/Veterans coverage	10,700,000	3.3%
Uninsured	45,800,000	14.1%
Totals	324,600,000	100.0%

Note: Total Population Covered exceeds the estimated U.S. population of 293,191,511 "because individuals can have more than one type of insurance either simultaneously or sequentially during the year." On the basis of actual population, the number of uninsured was 15.3% of the total population.

The uninsured by income were as follows:

Income	% of the Uninsured	% of Total U.S. Pop. In Each Income Category
Below Poverty	25%	13%
100-199% FPL	28%	18%
200-299% FPL	19%	17%
300-399% FPL	11%	14%
400-499% FPL	6%	11%
Above 500% FPL	11%	26%

Note: The Federal Poverty Level (FPL) in 2004 was $9,310 for a single individual and $18,850 for a family of four.

It is interesting that 53% of the uninsured are below 200% of the poverty line. Many of those people are eligible for Medicaid or SCHIP although not everyone with poverty-level income is eligible for Medicaid. A 2001 study reported that 27% of those eligible for Medicaid had not availed themselves of it and were otherwise uninsured.[5] Assuming that still holds, then an estimated 13,870,000 of the 45.7 million uninsured are actually eligible for Medicaid coverage if they just sign up. One interpretation is that the uninsured Medicaid eligibles are mostly healthy and will wait until they become ill to go through the daunting bureaucratic challenges of obtaining Medicaid coverage. An additional possible explanation is that many of them avoid those bureaucratic hurdles by either seeking free care or going without needed care. Either way, the safety net is there for them—they just haven't climbed the bureaucrat's ladder to jump into it.

The Census Bureau study also reports that 6.9 million uninsured workers and dependents have declined to purchase available employer coverage. These people are presumably eligible to enroll during subsequent annual open enrollment periods. They are in a similar situation to the uninsured Medicaid eligibles. They can get insurance if they need the benefits but only at designated times during the year.

Also of interest are the healthy uninsured who are earning well *above* the poverty level. A *Wall Street Journal* article reported that three-quarters of all uninsured people describe their health as "excellent" or "very good."[6] If we assume that their good health makes them eligible for individual health insurance and that those with incomes above 300% of the poverty level can afford to pay for it, then another 21% of the uninsured, or 9,870,000 people, have affordable access to individual health insurance but have not elected to purchase it.

Unlike the uninsured Medicaid eligibles and those who haven't yet taken advantage of their employer's insurance, these people will find themselves unable to obtain individual insurance if they wait until they are sick to try to buy it—*unless* they live in states that offer guaranteed-issue individual insurance or heavily subsidized high-risk insurance pools to the otherwise uninsurable (I have not estimated their numbers).

Taking into account these uninsured people who can actually get insurance if they want it, the table below suggests that, of the 45,657,000 uninsured in 2007, two-thirds, or 30,640,000 are *voluntarily uninsured*. That is, they have access to coverage *and* are able to afford it. They just haven't chosen to obtain it, partly because of bureaucratic barriers, partly because of free riding, and partly because health insurance is too often overpriced and a poor value. I acknowledge that there is likely some double counting involved with the uninsured employed group. Also, my numbers assume that employed people with access to insurance will be able to afford it if they really need to buy it, which may not be true in all cases. Even so, the number of uninsured who could be insured if they chose to be is a substantial portion of the total. And these figures do not include any allowance for approximately half of all the uninsured who will be that way for less than a year before obtaining insurance through new jobs or other sources. One survey by the Congressional Budget Office, using 1990s data, estimated that only 16% of the uninsured remained so for more than two years, thus indicating a lot of fluidity among the actual individuals counted in the uninsured numbers.[7]

Category of Uninsured in 2007	Total in 2007	%
Total Uninsured	45,657,000	100.0%
Uninsured but Eligible for Medicaid	13,870,000	30.4%
Uninsured but Eligible of Individual Insurance	9,870,000	21.6%
Uninsured but Eligible for Employer Insurance	6,900,000	15.1%
Total Voluntarily Uninsured	**30,640,000**	**67.1%**
Total Involuntarily Uninsured	**15,017,000**	**32.9%**

That leaves a total of the *involuntarily uninsured* at about 15,017,000 people. These include those who can't afford insurance, those who aren't eligible for any employer or government program, and those who are uninsurable on any basis because of medical conditions that make individual insurance unattainable. This is still a substantial number, but at 5% of the population, not nearly as dire as the forty-six million so often bandied about by the pundits.

The State-Mandated Uninsured

We need one more adjustment to the number of the involuntarily uninsured to take into account those people forced out because of unnecessary state benefit mandates. There are altogether more than 1,900 such mandates among the fifty states, which have driven up insurance premiums by as little as 20% in some states and as much as 50% in others.[8] The insurance trade group AHIP estimates that 20–25% of the uninsured have had to forgo coverage because of the higher premiums for mandated services that many people consider optional or medically unnecessary. These include infertility treatments, chiropractic care, wigs for cancer patients, and drug rehabilitation services.[9]

Using the lower 20% figure in AHIP's estimate, about 9,131,000 of the 15,017,000 involuntarily uninsured could afford coverage if the states were to remove such mandates and allow insurers to cover only essential health care. That leaves just under 6 million people who could be classified as the hardcore uninsured, or less than 2% of the population. Removing the effects of double counting would increase this figure somewhat, but the point still holds that the number of truly hardcore uninsured is a small fraction of the total forty-six million Americans who don't have health insurance. I hasten to add that the forty-six million figure is very real and a big problem no matter how we slice it. By itself, however, that number greatly overstates the magnitude of the problem.

Category of Uninsured in 2007	Total in 2007
Total Involuntarily Uninsured	15,017,000
Less: Uninsured Due To Benefit Mandates	9,131,000
Total Hardcore Uninsured	**5,886,000**

If all our problems in health care could be reduced to the single issue of getting insurance for six or seven million hardcore uninsured—or even fifteen million involuntarily uninsured—that would seem to be eminently solvable without our having to engage in wholesale health care reform. Unfortunately, that is not the case. The problem of the hardcore and involuntarily uninsured is real and serious, but even more serious are our rapidly escalating and uncontrolled medical costs, the unreliable quality that is killing more than 300,000 Americans every year, and the people who refuse to live healthy lifestyles and then consume 75% of our health care dollars. All of these major dilemmas are symptoms of a much deeper problem in the very structure of our health insurance system. Any attempt to reform health care without addressing that will be like fixing a leaky faucet on the *Titanic.*

If our dysfunctional health insurance system is at the heart of our problems in health care, then what goals would we want an ideal health insurance system to accomplish? To what extent has the current system failed to meet these goals? And why is health insurance the way it is instead of the way we want it to be? These are among the key questions I'll try to answer in the remainder of this chapter.

Goals

The purpose of any kind of insurance is to spread the risk of individually unaffordable losses among many players who are, more or less, equally likely to suffer such losses. Insurance does this by combining their risks and their expected costs into common funding pools from which payments are subsequently made to the players who incur losses. Almost anything can be insured, as long as the frequency and amount of loss are reasonably predictable, actual major losses occur only to a minority of members, and there are enough insured members willing to buy into the system to provide statistical confidence and financial sustainability.

Most people, including politicians and pundits—with ideological extremists excluded—would probably agree, albeit with some quibbling, on the following eight wish-list items for an American health insurance system. I listed a summary of them in chapter 1 and will provide more discussion here.

1. *Universal Availability*: Everyone in America should have access to affordable health insurance, regardless of individual health status or history. This point recognizes health care's unique status among life's necessities: There is virtually no distinction

between necessary and luxury services based on price level. That is, high-cost medical services, rather than being luxuries, tend to be just as necessary as the low-cost ones. Therefore, most people require insurance to be able to afford consuming the full range of necessary services. Making insurance affordable to everyone requires the recognition of two unmet needs. First, we need system change to bring spiraling costs under control. Second, we must have comprehensive social safety nets to support the poor and the disabled.

Many people would prefer dropping the word *availability* and just going with *universal health insurance* by requiring everyone to buy it. Mandated universal coverage, however, is neither attainable, desirable, nor—fortunately—necessary, as I will address in the last section of this chapter.

2. *Sustainable Value and Affordability*: Whatever we do with health care reform, we must include mechanisms that will get spending under control while encouraging innovation that perpetuates quality and productivity improvements. Preferably, these mechanisms will emerge automatically from a reformed system. That will end the failed, futile efforts of policymakers, regulators, and bureaucrats to achieve cost control by rule making. We must permanently stabilize health care costs as a sustainable portion of GDP and especially as a sustainable portion of personal budgets. Otherwise, we will face an imminent future of rationed medical care and/or declining living standards. Then only the wealthy will enjoy the kind of health care access most of us take for granted today. Health insurance alone will not be able to achieve affordability. But it can be structured to enable mechanisms that will. And at the very least we can configure it so that it will stop contributing to the problem by hiding prices, misallocating resources, empowering unhealthy behavior, and paying more to doctors who harm patients than to those who cure them.

3. *Free Rider Prevention*: Any insurance plan that allows anyone and everyone to enroll must also prevent them from gaming or free riding the system by delaying their insurance purchases until they become ill and know they will receive more in benefits than they pay in premiums. Any insurance system that fails in this—absent external subsidies—will quickly sink into a terminal progression of adverse selection, greater payouts, higher premiums, more adverse selection, yet greater payouts, and so on until collapse. To prevent this vicious cycle while allowing universal, voluntary access, we must have enrollment and underwriting rules that place the costs of such gamesmanship squarely on the gamesmen.

4. *Voluntary Participation*: Many if not most advocates of universal insurance believe it is necessary to require everyone to purchase health care coverage in order to keep free riders from destroying universally accessible insurance. It isn't. Others believe we should require everyone to get insurance because it's good for them. That is paternalism, which fails to accept individual priorities and choice. There are well-proven mechanisms that can be utilized to prevent free riding without forcing people, for the first time in the history of our country, to purchase something from public or private third parties (and inefficient ones at that) as a condition of living in the land of the free.

5. *Financial Protection*: Health insurance, as any other type of insurance, should protect us against the unaffordable costs of involuntary, unpredictable events. Over the past four decades, managed care and Medicare have muddled this concept by introducing coverage for once-inexpensive items like doctor visits, laboratory tests, and prescription drugs. It is important to recognize the difference between prepayment for such normal, predictable consumer purchases and insurance coverage against extraordinary medical events. With the exception of a few fully integrated health care systems (e.g., Kaiser), the prepayment

approach has added layers of excessive cost while obscuring prices from consumers. In crafting health insurance reform, it is essential to make a distinction between necessary insurance that virtually everyone needs and prepayment, which should be optional.

6. *Choice of Insurance and Providers*: People want choice. They're used to it because it is functional. Choice recognizes that different people have different needs, different priorities, and different financial means to meet those needs and priorities. Health care is no exception. Some will argue that allowing for choice in health insurance plans will only confuse people. Yet federal employees currently navigate 269 different annual choices of health insurance plans. The residents of Wyoming are able to choose from fifty different Medicare drug plans. The citizens of tiny Switzerland have a choice of ninety different health plans. Making choices does require more consumer effort than accepting a one-size-fits-all standard. Fortunately, Americans are probably the most demanding, discriminating, and skilled consumers on the face of the planet. Those abilities can be just as useful in purchasing health insurance and medical care as in buying cars, computers, big screen TVs, and blue jeans. At bottom, choice is necessary to allow consumers to demand and to act on information about products—and their sellers—that will best meet their individual needs.

7. *Portability*: One of the major disadvantages of group insurance is the lack of portability that would allow each person to own his own health insurance policy, regardless of who he works for and whether he is unemployed, retired, eligible for government-sponsored coverage, or just taking a long sabbatical. The average American changes jobs eleven times during his career lifetime, often involving periods of unemployment and moves to employers that provide no health coverage.[10] Currently, some former employees have access to the partial portability of CO-

BRA coverage. But it offers no choice of benefits (only those their former employers chose). It causes adverse selection that drives up insurance costs for the remaining employees. With limited exceptions, it is very expensive (especially for younger people). And its availability is only temporary. Lack of portability is one of the biggest causes of millions of Americans lacking health insurance. It also promotes productivity-robbing job lock, in which employees become trapped in jobs they hate for fear of losing coverage—especially when they have dependents requiring expensive medical care. True portability of coverage will go a long way toward resolving all of these problems.

8. *Personal Responsibility for Prevention*: Health insurance should provide incentives for people to manage their own health risks, which include weight, smoking, alcohol consumption, blood pressure, cholesterol, blood sugar, and other individually controllable risk factors. Most readers might assume this means expanding insurance coverage for primary and preventive health care. It does not. Managed care's having done that over thirty-five years has failed to achieve a pandemic of healthy living. The awkward fact is that most preventive medical services cost more than they save. We need another approach.

Why and How Has Health Insurance Failed to Meet These Goals?

To answer that, it is necessary to delve into how we got where we are, explode a few myths in the process, and identify the key weaknesses we need to fix while recognizing any strengths of the current system that we wish to preserve.

Adverse selection is perhaps the single most important aspect of insurance for politicians and policy wonks to understand when pursuing health insurance reform. Adverse selection is the tendency of people with poor health to apply for or continue health coverage more frequently than people in better health.[11] It is at the heart of the free rider problem.

Health insurance—indeed all insurance—relies on the Pareto Principle. That principle avers that, at any given time, a small percentage of insured people will incur a large percentage of total medical claims. It is more commonly called the 80/20 rule. It means a large percentage of relatively healthy members must be present in an insurance pool to fund the costs of the relative few who need expensive care. Achieving a proper balance of healthy and unhealthy members is absolutely essential to the ongoing sustainability of any insurance pool. Any insurer that fails to anticipate and limit the natural tendency toward adverse selection will inevitably get a risk pool that contains too few healthy individuals to pay the bills, a condition that Milliman actuary Bruce Pyenson has dubbed the 70/20 rule. Unchecked, adverse selection leads to a financial death spiral of excessive costs, higher premiums, and a further exacerbation of adverse selection as healthier members increasingly exit the pool for more affordable alternatives. Pyenson describes this as "the insurance equivalent of a run on a bank."[12]

There are only two cures for an adversely selected insurance pool. First, the insurer can eliminate the risk imbalance by imposing underwriting controls before its capital is exhausted (i.e., before it goes broke). Second, it must alternatively fund those losses with subsidies from either external sources (e.g., government) or internal ones (e.g., other profitable lines of business).

Adverse selection risk permeates the issue of health insurance. That's why you'll see it cropping up repeatedly in the discussions that follow.

Group Insurance

Currently, there are two basic types of medical insurance: group insurance and individual insurance. For anyone seeking to achieve effective reform, it is necessary to understand both.

Group insurance is what most Americans are familiar with. Nearly two-thirds of Americans under the age of sixty-five are enrolled in group coverage through their employers.[13] Employer-based group insurance dates back to the post-Civil War era—if not earlier. But it only began to achieve prominence during the 1930s. That's when Blue Cross and Blue Shield plans and other insurers emerged to enroll members on a wholesale basis through their employers.

In 1943 the dominance of employer insurance was frozen into place by a wartime federal income tax ruling that excluded employer-provided health benefits from workers' federal and state income taxes, as well as FICA and (later) Medicare payroll taxes. Eventually codified into law, this provision did not extend similar treatment to individuals and self-employed persons purchasing their own health insurance. They have to pay with after-tax dollars. The advent of Medicare and Medicaid in the 1960s further expanded the concept of tax-free group coverage to the aged, disabled, and poor.

Many health policy commentators point to the tax benefit as the primary reason why group insurance is now the dominant model. That oft-repeated proposition is not correct, however. With or without the tax advantage, other phenomena are at work that naturally favor group coverage over the one-at-a-time individual variety. Even if tax treatment had always been the same for everyone with health insurance, group insurance would still be the dominant mode for insuring Americans. Although the tax benefit may have cemented group's natural preeminence, there are at least five reasons why group insurance would be dominant without it:

1. *Lower Administrative Costs*: The wholesale nature of group sales keeps selling and administrative costs relatively low as a percentage of premiums. Individual insurance, with its requirements for medical underwriting and individual sales efforts, has been the much more expensive variety to sell and maintain.

2. *Low Adverse Selection Risk*: Employer groups are assembled for purposes that are largely independent of an individual employee's desire for health insurance. This reduces the risk of adverse selection, since there are barriers to entry for those whose primary need is health insurance. This eliminates the need for detailed

medical histories of each worker and family member, which considerably reduces underwriting costs while allowing coverage to be offered without exception to all employees and dependents.

3. *Predictable Medical Costs*: The medical costs of large groups tend to be much more statistically predictable than those of individuals and are thus relatively easy to price.

4. *Healthy Risk Pool*: Employed people, having to be physically and mentally fit to work, tend to be healthier than unemployed people (especially the poor unemployed), which further lowers medical costs and premiums. This factor and the previous three all cut the costs of selling, underwriting, administering, and paying for health benefits under group insurance. As a result, a much higher percentage of the premium dollar goes directly to health benefits in group than individual insurance. This reflects the higher efficiency of the former—at least under the current system.

5. *Appearance of Employee Affordability*: Employers directly pay significant amounts of employee compensation in the form of health insurance premiums. In 2007 employers paid an average of 84% of the premium for single coverage and 72% for family coverage.[14] This makes such coverage appear to be more affordable to employees, even though the employer contributions come out of fixed employee compensation pools that include total wages, salaries, and fringe benefits. The high level of employer contribution tends to ensure participation by a large percentage of employees, regardless of health status or history, which further reduces any tendency toward adverse selection, because healthy workers are much more likely to enroll. In general, the higher an employer's contribution, the higher healthy employee participation in health insurance will be. This reduces the cost of health insurance for everyone.

For all these reasons, group insurance has natural advantages over individual insurance, which is why it has become institutionalized as the overwhelmingly favored model. The advantageous tax treatment may have reinforced that position, but it did not create it.

An employer can offer group insurance in one of two ways. First, the employer can purchase coverage from an insurance company, or second, it can bypass insurers and self-insure its own employees' health care risks. In general, smaller employers must settle for purchased insurance because they lack the numbers of employees necessary to predict their costs actuarially. Most large employers self-fund (self-insure). Self-insurance now covers 55% of America's workers.

Self-funding offers significant advantages for companies large enough to do it:

- *State Regulatory Exemption*: Self-insured employers are exempt from most state insurance regulations. They enjoy far more flexibility under federal ERISA rules in establishing benefits outside of state-mandated minimum benefit requirements, premium rate-setting rules, premium taxes, and other burdens. This state of affairs is particularly advantageous to multi-state employers that, under ERISA, are able to offer standard benefit plans and rates across all states without regard to local requirements.

- *Favorable Selection*: The opposite of adverse selection is favorable selection, in which relatively healthy individuals or groups can place themselves in the position of not supporting sicker people. With self-funding, employers with younger, healthier employees can sometimes favorably select themselves out of larger and less advantageous insurance company risk pools, thus reducing *their* costs of coverage while increasing them for the remaining members of the insurance company pools.

- *Return on Prevention Investments*: Self-funded employers directly benefit if there are any health care savings that result from their investments in smoking cessation programs, subsidized gym memberships, chronic disease management programs, and other health promotion activities. Such savings could otherwise be diluted by the larger number of members of insurance company pools.

- *Improved Cash Flow*: There are cash-flow benefits for employers that pay health expenses when due rather than upfront via health insurance premiums to an insurer.

Despite the advantages of self-funding over commercial group insurance, self-funding does nothing to control medical care inflation.

I will later discuss the lack of cost control as a problem with all group insurance, but another issue bears discussion here: the chronic under-management of self-funded programs by employers. An employer's decision to elect self-funding involves taking on all the responsibilities of operating a full-fledged health insurance company for its employees. These responsibilities include:

- Conducting actuarial modeling and review
- Designing benefit plans
- Setting premiums
- Performing ongoing competitive benefit and premium analyses
- Setting up health promotion programs
- Managing the underwriting function
- Buying reinsurance
- Managing eligibility
- Implementing utilization and disease management programs
- Preventing member fraud
- Negotiating and contracting with providers
- Coordinating benefits with other insurers
- Adjudicating and paying claims
- Detecting and preventing provider fraud
- Conducting claims audits

- Producing and analyzing financial and utilization reports
- Performing other functions necessary for any well-run insurance company.

In effect, self-insuring is the same as setting up an insurance company subsidiary, albeit with streamlined marketing, sales, and regulatory compliance functions.

Unfortunately, few if any of the companies doing this have the expertise or experience necessary to do it effectively. Instead, virtually all self-funded employers treat self-funding as a purchasing function to be run by their largely unrelated and unprepared human resources (HR) departments. Their managers rarely have operational health insurance experience.

The primary mission of HR has traditionally been to field a capable workforce by effectively managing these functions:[15]

- Hiring and firing
- Labor law compliance
- Employee orientation and development
- Labor relations
- Performance management
- Compensation
- Retirement benefits
- Health and welfare benefits.

Historically, obtaining health benefits has long been an insurance purchasing function, with the HR department making a periodic decision about which health insurer to use. HR managers, in turn, have traditionally relied on insurance brokers and employee benefits consultants to recommend insurers based on benefits, services, and prices.

It has usually been the broker or benefits consultant who introduces the opportunity to take advantage of self-funding. The HR manager then takes it to her boss, often the CFO, who vets it with the other C-level executives, including the COO and/or CEO. Often, the higher the review, the less involved the executive, particularly with an issue as insomnia-inducing as purchasing health benefits. In this review process, the advantages of self-funding are presented and sometimes quantified, with most large employers then adopting the approach. The decision to have HR continue to manage the new health benefits regime is usually automatic, especially since that's the way almost everybody else does it. Without really thinking about it, management makes the decision to start and operate an insurance subsidiary as though it were still a health benefits purchasing function. It's not.

C-level executives tend to pay little ongoing attention to the performance of these quasi-subsidiaries other than periodically to bemoan the ever-increasing medical costs at Business Roundtable meetings. Ironically, although companies manage their self-funding as a purchasing function, not even companies with exquisitely developed supply chain management processes actually utilize them in buying what is often their largest and certainly most out-of-control expense—medical care. HR managers are rarely held accountable for their contributions to bottom-line performance. Most are thought to do a good job if they just show annual health benefit cost increases (i.e., trends) even slightly below national averages.

There is often a conflict between the responsibility to provide for a motivated and satisfied workforce and running an effective in-house health insurance company. As a result, insurance decisions often end up being made according to whether they will result in complaining phone calls to HR from employees rather than on what is in the overall best interest of the employer and its employees.

HR managers almost always rely on employee benefit brokers and consultants to advise them on implementing and managing their insurance functions. Experienced health insurance and managed-care operators in these disciplines are almost as rare as in HR. Too often these advisers and the contractors they recommend have their own agendas, which aren't always focused on delivering the health benefits employees need at the lowest cost.

To manage the insurance function, employers invariably hire pharmacy benefit managers (PBMs) and third-party administrators (TPAs)—often divisions of major health insurers—thinking they will get the same performance and attention to key issues these vendors apply to their own insured lines of business. They don't. Engaging the average PBM to structure and manage your pharmacy benefit is like giving Offices 'R' Us the unlimited authority to decide what office supplies you will buy and in what quantities; you are going to be buying a *lot* of overpriced office supplies. All the while your supplier is telling you how you're saving by *his* being able to buy high volumes cheaply—and all without the client having to pay any administrative fees.

And even with fine print disclosures, employers rarely question benefits consultants and brokers who accept commissions, fees, rebates, cruises, and resort vacations from the PBMs, TPAs, and reinsurance companies they recommend to their HR clients. Self-funded employee health benefits are perhaps the most under-managed resource that employers buy.

Problems with Group Insurance

Despite its longstanding dominance, group health insurance, whether self-funded or provided by outside insurers, suffers from major flaws that are increasingly exposing its fundamental unsuitability as an even partial solution for effective health care reform. This is true for all employers, no matter the size.

1. *Lack of Portability*: One of the major failings of group insurance is its lack of portability. This shortcoming shackles an employee's coverage to an employer at a time when the concept of a lifetime career with a single employer has gone the way of Arthur Anderson, subprime mortgage-backed securities, and analog TV. Non-portable insurance has become an anachronism in an era when people change jobs as often as they change cars. The lack

of portability artificially locks people into jobs they hate. Those who lose them due to layoffs or illness often lose the means to obtain one of life's basic necessities, even if they can otherwise afford it. Lack of portability is a significant contributor to the problem of the uninsured in this country.

2. *Large Employer Bias*: Group insurance is enormously biased in favor of larger employers. In 2004, 71% of firms with fifty or more employees offered employee health insurance whereas only about 50% of small companies did so.[16]

Small business has long been the economic engine of our country, producing all of our net new jobs. Yet group insurance has increasingly served to foul that engine. Take the example of two people working two identical jobs with identical health insurance from their employers. A person working for a small company can easily pay twice as much for the same coverage enjoyed by his identical colleague working at a large company. That's because small groups' lack of risk pool size makes them susceptible to huge year-to-year pricing swings—mostly upward. With smaller groups, just a few sick employees or dependents can raise rates for the entire group to the point of unaffordability for all.

That size disadvantage also deprives small firms of the ability to self-insure. They are locked out of the freedom their large competitors enjoy to escape completely from the punitive health benefit mandates imposed by all states. This factor alone has been estimated to drive up insurance costs by 20% to 50%, depending on the state.

Many small employers have cut benefits, hiked employee premium contributions, and increased deductibles and copayments. Many others have reached the breaking point. With state and federal regulations providing no options to all-or-nothing defined-benefit insurance, many employers have been forced to go the "nothing" route. Even when employers could have continued contributing meaningful amounts to their employees' health insurance, they have had to completely drop all health insurance benefits.

As insurance premiums soar, many employers are changing insurers, restricting options, and cutting benefits in an increasingly desperate attempt to maintain coverage. Employees may be exceedingly price conscious in all other aspects of their economic lives, but their employers give them no say in matters of price, choice, or quality of insurers or providers.

Annual changes in insurers are not unusual. They frequently require employees to change doctors while paying more for the privilege. Many employees find their only choice is to continue being played as pawns or dropping out of employer coverage altogether. Many younger, lower-paid employees are doing the latter.

3. *Contingent-Workforce Ineligibility*: The past three decades have witnessed explosive growth of temporary and part-time employment as the U.S. economy has continued its shift from manufacturing to service-based industries.[17] The U.S. Bureau of Labor Statistics says these so-called contingent workers represent a substantial portion of the workforce, with nearly 80% of all employers hiring them.[18] The problem is that few contingent workers are covered by employer group insurance programs. These workers are entirely on their own if they want to find affordable health insurance.

4. *Lack of Employee Choice*: Less than half of all employer insurance programs give employees even minimal choice of insurers, benefits, medical networks, or how much they pay.[19] Instead, employers put all these key decisions into the hands of human resource executives who, however capable, aren't allowed to know the individual health needs of their employees because of HIPAA requirements. Even though an increasing number of large private employers are offering consumer-driven health plan

options, 83% of public employers fail to do so. Their HR managers have decided that their employees should not have such choices.[20]

5. *Moral Hazard*: Group insurance creates moral hazard by subsidizing unhealthy personal behaviors. Employers seldom charge higher premiums or out-of-pocket charges to employees who smoke, abuse alcohol, or are obese—even though these and other personally controllable health risk factors account for 75% of all health care costs. Group insurance also financially discriminates against young, lower-paid workers who are forced either to subsidize their older, higher-paid colleagues or to go without insurance altogether, which many do. Although many of these younger workers are making rational decisions by dropping such artificially overpriced coverage, a widespread urban myth says they do so because they're young, foolish, and think themselves invincible. The available evidence suggests otherwise.

6. *Poor Accountability*: As pointed out above, people with group insurance usually have no choice of insurers. As a result, their insurers have no real accountability to them. This allows some insurers to unilaterally delay and deny valid claims, drop providers, hide behind impenetrable bureaucracies, and otherwise behave in a high-handed fashion while dealing with their members. Their abused members have no choice of taking their business elsewhere. Group insurance has also hidden from its members the prices of insurance and medical services. This has removed any individual knowledge, concern, or ability to care about or control them.

7. *Misstated Total Compensation*: Employer insurance mischaracterizes employer contributions as an employer-paid benefit. Such costs are really just a diversion of a portion of the employees' total compensation, which creates the illusion that employer insurance is in addition to employee compensation, when it is, in fact, part and parcel of it. Like squeezing a water balloon, if you in-

crease health insurance costs, you decrease take-home pay. This phenomenon creates a Catch-22 for younger employees who decline or drop employer coverage. Although they may save on the unfairly high payroll deductions required of younger workers, they entirely lose the "employer's" share. They thus relinquish a significant portion of their own compensation to the employer's bottom line.

8. *Cost Control Failure*: The above problems are all bad enough, but perhaps the worst aspect of group insurance is that it has utterly failed to control health care spending. To the contrary, it has fanned the flames of medical inflation by promoting moral hazard, by insulating employees from any knowledge or concern about price or medical necessity, and by granting a virtual blank check to medical providers to provide excessive, low-quality care at ever-increasing prices. Attempts by some employers to promote wellness and restrain spending generally fail to recognize where the true locus of the interest in health lies—with the individual workers and consumers who should be making the critical choices about their own health and how their compensation is spent. Instead, employers have adopted an increasingly paternalistic model with human resource managers making the key decisions for their employees.

9. *Administratively Inefficient*: I discussed above that group insurance is relatively efficient when compared with current forms of individual insurance, but that's like arguing that Mussolini was a better leader than Hitler. The McKinsey Global Institute has estimated that all these separate employer health insurance arrangements require $75 billion in non-value-added underwriting, marketing, sales, billing, and administrative costs that are ultimately borne by the employees and that could be better diverted to increase employee pay.[21]

For these and other reasons, employer-based group insurance is inherently unsustainable. The only reason it hasn't completely collapsed already is that most employers have been able to increase employee take-home pay despite the much larger percentage increases in health insurance costs. Excessive health care inflation, however, won't allow this to last forever, and for many smaller employers it has already ended.

Andrew Stern, president of the Service Employees International Union, has assessed the situation succinctly:

> We have to recognize that employer-based health care is ending. It is dying in front of our very eyes. It was a good friend. It served America well in the twentieth century. We love it dearly. Employers, to their credit, lived with it for a long time, despite all of the distortions that it has created, but it is collapsing in front of our eyes. It may still be breathing, but anybody who can look into the future says this employer-based health care system is over in America. If we don't say that, we are just going to keep building on a very unstable foundation that is not really appropriate.[22]

The huge government group programs Medicare and Medicaid have, over their four-plus decades of existence, exacerbated virtually all of the problems of employer group insurance. And they have created major new ones of their own, which will be detailed in chapter 5.

The dominance of employer and government group coverage has locked out multitudes of self-employed individuals, part-time workers, the unemployed, the early retired, many small business employees, and others either too sick or too poor to purchase individual insurance on their own.

From a human standpoint, the worst result of group coverage has been the forced herding of fifteen million Americans into the ranks of what I call the involuntarily uninsured while making health insurance an unacceptably bad deal for another thirty-plus million. From an economic standpoint, the worst thing group insurance did was prevent the emergence of a viable consumer market for health insurance and medical services. By transferring the purchasing and payment responsibilities to third parties—employers, insurers, and governments—this system gave doctors and hospitals a virtual blank check for medical care without effective controls on utilization, quality, price, cost, or waste. This has happened despite massive top-down efforts of a plethora of government and corporate bureaucracies to rein it in, which I will discuss in chapter 5 and other chapters.

For a while during the last three decades of the twentieth century, the growth of employer-friendly HMOs and then managed care helped to reduce unnecessary hospital costs drastically. But the recent decline of managed care has brought a resurgence of waste and unnecessary, inappropriate care. It has left behind a new tradition of insurance coverage for services and products that had once been considered normal consumer purchases, such as doctor visits, lab tests, X-rays, and prescription drugs. The theory was that such coverage would prevent illness and result in major savings. Not only did that not happen, but such coverage removed the last remnants of consumer concern about health care prices. Managed care never did anything to deal with the underlying inflationary dynamics of health care's distorted economics. Once hospital waste was eliminated from the system, the true nature of unbridled health care inflation came roaring back.

The lack of a consumer market option also removed any need for hospitals and doctors to compete for patients on the basis of quality, price, or value, much less customer service. This has been a major driver of the inexorable rise of health care costs for the past four decades and is why you're only 50% likely to be getting the current standard of medical care from your doctor or hospital. There is simply too little accountability to consumers and patients by insurers, employers, doctors, and hospitals that are more responsible to each other than to their ultimate consumers.

Group insurance has turned into a terrible way to protect people from the unaffordable costs of necessary medical care. Of the eight goals listed earlier for health insurance reform, it meets only three: It is at least nominally voluntary; it prevents adverse selection; and it provides financial protection. It fails the tests of universality, cost control, choice, portability, and prevention. It's enough to make one wonder why so much policy verbiage is spent on trying to preserve it.

Individual Insurance

Individual insurance is by far the smaller category of health insurance in the United States, consisting of about eighteen million participants—just 6% of the U.S. population. Individual coverage requires an insurer to enroll people one at a time via an application process, requiring considerable sales and underwriting efforts that significantly drive up the cost of acquiring members, each of whom is required to pay his own premiums without the assistance of an employer or, by extension, the IRS.

Normally, an insurance broker will refer an individual applicant to an insurer in return for a 20–30% commission on the first year's premium and a declining amount thereafter. Each applicant is required to complete a lengthy application form that includes a comprehensive medical history. The application is reviewed by an insurance company underwriter, who determines whether the applicant represents a risk more or less equal to that of other pool members.

When concerns or questions about an applicant's health arise, the underwriter will often interview him directly and may even require a physical exam and a release of medical records for a more thorough review. Those who are essentially healthy but at greater than normal long-term risk, such as smokers, will usually be required to pay higher premiums. Some applicants for whom there are other concerns may be accepted but only subject to coverage limitations for preexisting medical conditions. Those who represent too high a risk of loss will be denied insurance altogether, including applicants with a history of cancer, heart disease, diabetes, or other potentially expensive medical problems.

The reason for all this scrutiny is the need to prevent adverse selection, to which individual insurance is particularly vulnerable.

Without careful underwriting procedures to control risks, insurers fear being deluged with unhealthy applicants who would skew pool risk to unsustainable levels by driving up claims experience, increasing premiums, driving out healthy risks, and ensuring the inevitable death spiral I described previously.

Individual insurance, as currently structured, operates at a significant disadvantage to group insurance:

1. *The Underwriting Barrier*: Because of the necessity of careful underwriting to ensure a sustainable risk pool, individual insurance is unavailable to anyone with a serious medical condition.

2. *Sales and Administrative Inefficiency*: Because of the high sales and administrative costs associated with the individual insurance business and because successful applicants initially represent a better-than-average risk pool, the medical loss ratios—MLRs, the percentage of premium revenue actually spent on health benefits—initially tend to be much lower for individual than for group insurance, on the order of 50–60% versus typical group insurance MLRs of 75–85%. Over time, however, the gap between individual and group MLRs usually narrows as the individually insured members age and gradually present a more standard overall risk profile.

3. *State Benefit Mandates*: Onerous state minimum benefit mandates require coverage for many services and products that most people might otherwise consider optional, unnecessary, or cheaper to buy on their own. These mandates, which are estimated to drive up insurance costs 20–50% depending on the state, result from the successful lobbying of state legislatures by special interest groups representing individuals and organizations that either suffer from these conditions or benefit from treating them. Their intent is to tap into insurance pool funds to obtain financial benefit for the limited number of people or providers represented by the special interests. Group insurance is also subject to state mandates, but larger employers can and do avoid them by self-

insuring and thus bypassing all such state requirements.

4. *The Tax Penalty*: Another factor that significantly drives up the real cost of individual insurance is that—unlike employer group insurance—it must be paid for with after-tax dollars. That's not just after federal and state income taxes, but also FICA and Medicare payroll taxes. Thus, it often takes $150 in before-tax compensation to pay the same premiums for individual insurance that a group plan can get for only $100.

5. *Rescission Practices*: One of the least salutary facets of individual insurance is the uncommon but sometimes nasty practice of rescission, which occurs when an insurer unilaterally and retroactively cancels a member's coverage. That can happen when a policyholder doesn't disclose preexisting medical conditions on his application and subsequently incurs claims tied to those conditions. Rescission can be entirely proper for dealing with outright applicant fraud resulting from lies on the application, but it can also result from an insurer's overzealous or unscrupulous reaction to unanticipated claims for members they thought to be healthy. It is particularly problematic for members who had dropped prior coverage in order to buy the lower-priced individual plan and then find themselves uninsured and, worse, uninsurable anywhere else.

Despite these shortcomings, individual insurance, even now, offers significant advantages over the group variety:

1. *Portability*: A major advantage of individual insurance is that it is portable, being owned by the individual, independent of employment status. No one has to give it up simply because she changes occupations, starts her own business, retires early, or becomes unemployed.

2. *Affordability*: Individual insurance is also surprisingly affordable for younger adults and children because it pools these people together and sets their premiums based on age. The younger you

are, the lower the premiums. Employers, on the other hand, use community-rated averages that discriminate against younger workers.

3. *Easy to Buy*: If you qualify, individual coverage can also be easy to buy. Online sites, such as eHealthInsurance.com and HealthInsurance.com, provide benefit comparisons and prices on multiple health insurance plans, along with the ability to apply online. For straightforward applications, some insurers offer almost immediate underwriting approval.[23]

4. *Consumer Choice*: People also have a much wider choice of available individual insurance companies—and medical providers—than is provided by most employers. That allows each individual to select a program that best meets his own particular needs. Many of these options are quite comprehensive and offer a wide variety of deductible, coinsurance, copayment, and tax-advantaged health savings account (HSA) options. Employer insurance rarely offers any individual customization of benefits and affordability.

5. *Cost Control*: One of the greatest advantages of individual insurance is its potential to encourage health care cost control. Although many currently insured members might not see it as an advantage, each person with individual insurance knows exactly how much her insurance costs. Employers tell their workers only the amount of the employee's share of the premium, thus making it appear to be much less expensive than it actually is.

How is this an advantage? It comes from providing the individual with much clearer pricing information upon which to decide the acceptable tradeoffs between paying more for insurance coverage and less for direct out-of-pocket expenses—or the other way around. It's an option almost never available on such a transparent and rational basis to employees with group insurance. By selecting higher or lower deductibles, individuals are allowed to make choices that can minimize their total health care expenditures based on their expected use of medical services. Such choices can provide strong financial incentives for people to seek the best providers for the lowest prices. Individual insurance gives each person the financial power to determine which health insurance *and* which medical services to buy separately in order to maximize benefits and minimize cost. The evidence is that consumers are responding to the wider range of deductible options by increasingly choosing high deductible health plans. According to a 2009 CDC survey, fully 44% of those with individual insurance have chosen such plans.[24]

This cost-benefit flexibility is greatly aided by the fact that buying normally consumed primary care medical services directly from doctors and other providers can be much less expensive than paying for it through health insurance. That's because buying it directly can bypass the additional burdens of insurance company overhead, profit, and the horrendously inefficient billing and reimbursement systems that unnecessarily afflict insured services. Thus, the more a person can buy normal medical care directly, the more she can save on total health insurance premiums and out-of-pocket expenses combined.

Despite the paucity of health care price transparency, there is also substantial and growing evidence that individuals with high-deductible health plans are applying their consumer skills to reduce their health care costs, particularly so for prescription drugs, medical imaging services, outpatient care, emergency services, and other frequently over-utilized services. It helps considerably that consumers can take advantage of insurer-negotiated provider discounts that allow them to pay as little as 40% of billed charges for their direct medical care purchases. Although the overall impact of HSA-induced cost control has not yet moved the needle very much on total health expenditures, the growing experience with high-deductible insurance offers promising evidence of the potential for consumer-motivated cost control in health care.

6. *Healthy Living Incentives*: The opportunity for savings can also be a powerful financial incentive for personal prevention and healthy living while improving one's ability to be prepared for an unpredicted, expensive medical event. That is because the savings from such rational consumerism can now be set aside in tax-exempt individual health savings accounts against a time when extraordinarily expensive medical events do occur. Furthermore, after an HSA has accumulated a sufficient balance to cover multiple years' worth of deductibles and other out-of-pocket costs, ongoing savings beyond that can be used by the person for...well, anything. My own son, for example, now has enough money in his HSA to cover more than two years' worth of his $5,000 insurance deductible. That gives him 100% coverage if he ever suffers from a skiing accident or some other unexpected, expensive medical event. He has a strong financial incentive to stay healthy—and to wear his ski helmet.

7. *Out-of-Pocket Tax Benefits*: The availability of HSAs in recent years has also alleviated some of the punitive tax burden of individual insurance. It has allowed individuals to use pre-tax dollars for their out-of-pocket health care expenses—but not for insurance premiums. This further rewards people for routing their health care dollars away from fully taxable insurance premiums and toward tax-exempt direct expenses. It is significant that even this modest change in tax rules in 2004 has helped make HSA-compatible health insurance one of the fastest-growing segments in the field, in spite of a widespread lack of public knowledge about the benefits and availability.

Even given individual insurance's portability, more rational pricing, and especially the potential to help control health care spending, the combination of high selling and administrative costs, the necessity to exclude high-risk applicants, the burdensome state-mandated benefits, and the punitive tax treatment have resulted in individual insurance being almost everyone's last choice for health insurance.

These deficiencies, however, are not inherent to individual coverage but have been imposed by the distorted rules of our current Babel of health insurance practice, law, and regulation.

Individual insurance is actually far more amenable to universal availability than group insurance. The only real issue for universal individual insurance is figuring out how to avoid adverse selection without making participation mandatory—a readily solvable problem using time-tested techniques.

All the problems the current system imposes on individual insurance would disappear under a reformed system of (1) universally available individual insurance without regard to preexisting medical conditions; (2) reasonable adverse-selection controls; (3) simplified, transparent medical provider pricing; (4) a level playing field on taxes; and (5) the elimination of unnecessary benefit requirements. Under such a rational system, individual insurance could shed all of its unnecessary burdens and emerge as the most efficient and effective mechanism to achieve the goals we seek.

Individual coverage could meet all of our eight goals. Here's the final scoreboard for group versus individual insurance:

Goals	Individual Insurance	Group Insurance
1. Universal availability	Yes	No
2. Sustainable value and affordability	Yes	No
3. Voluntary participation	Yes	Yes
4. Adverse selection prevention	Yes	Yes
5. Financial protection	Yes	Yes
6. Choice of insurance and providers	Yes	No
7. Portability	Yes	No
8. Personal Responsibility for Prevention	Yes	No

Quibblers can argue that it's not quite that clear-cut. A small number of large employers do indeed offer a wide choice of plans and providers (e.g., the federal government), but virtually no small employers do. And to the extent that employers promote high deductible plans, they do provide some incentives for cost control. These are, however, limited exceptions.

Nonetheless, Can't Group Insurance Be Preserved?

Assume, for the moment, that there is a way to offer private, voluntary, universal health insurance without creating an adverse selection death spiral. The question arises as to whether such a system can coexist with our current group-based insurance system. During a transition period, it probably could. Long term, it cannot. The primary reason is that employers with disproportionately older or sicker members would be able to save money by shutting down their group plans and dumping their members into the individual system, creating—you guessed it—adverse selection. At the same time, employers with younger or healthier employees would figure out that retaining their group plans would be less expensive than supporting their members' participation in the new individual plan. They would stay with the group plan—at least until their risks rose to a level where it made sense to convert to the individual plan—thus creating yet more adverse selection.

If you seriously think it's necessary to preserve employer group insurance, you might argue that we could simply augment it with government-subsidized, guaranteed-issue individual insurance. Then everyone could have insurance. There would still be serious adverse selection, but at least we would have the taxpayers' deep pockets behind the bad risks. This is one of the options that has been considered by the current Obama administration.

There are at least three very good reasons why this is a very bad idea. First, it isn't necessary to burden taxpayers with the excess costs of such adversely selected individual insurance. There are much better, more efficient, and less costly ways to do it, as I have outlined in chapter 1 and will discuss in chapters 9–12 in more detail. Second, it does nothing to get group medical costs under control. It would merely put a failing system on life support without curing its fundamental disease. Third, what such an approach will create, in effect, is a creeping single-payer program. People who get sick will tend to gravitate from private to public insurance. Eliminated is the concept of a Pareto-ruled insurance program, replaced instead by a taxpayer-funded entitlement with an ever-increasing drain on the public fisc.

But, you ask, why stick it to the taxpayers at all? Why not do as the state of Michigan does and just require a nonprofit Blue Cross plan to offer the high-risk individual insurance and pay for it from the profits it earns from its group insurance business? Or follow the Colorado model, which recoups the losses of its guaranteed-issue individual insurance plan, Cover Colorado, with annual assessments on all the other health insurers operating in the state? True, this does spread the risk of the otherwise uninsurable across the entire insurance pool, but it still does nothing to restrain health care costs. Somehow, if health insurance is to survive without forcing us into reduced standards of living, we will have to address the cost problem, and none of these programs can do that. Neither will the vain hope that increased coverage for preventive services or the use of electronic medical records will save any money any time soon. I discussed the former in chapter 2 and will cover the latter in chapter 8 with my discussion of single-payer insurance.

Ah, you might say, all the government would have to do is enact a play-or-pay rule in which employers would either have to provide employee health benefits or pay a tax or penalty into the government's program. That won't change the game at all since employers will now have an even more straightforward metric against which to measure the benefits of keeping versus eliminating their group insurance. If it's cheaper to pay the penalty and be done with the insurance hassle, employers will do so with a clean conscience, knowing that their employees now have the alternative of signing up with the government program. You will still have healthy employee groups staying with employer coverage and unhealthy ones going with the government's. It's a one-way street, driving sick people into the government program and leaving the healthy with their employers or private insurers. The government program would quickly become a black hole for external subsidies. And, once again, neither the employer insurance sector nor the government entitlement sector would have done anything to deal with out-of-control medical inflation. Any way you slice it, group health insurance would still be an economic and social dead end—as would the government-subsidized program.

A lot of institutional and social inertia is wrapped up in employer coverage, not to mention Medicare and Medicaid, which suggests the need for a transition period wherein everyone is given a choice of staying with the current program he's become used to or changing to an individual plan under a new, rationalized regime. Such a transition program would be rife with risk, problems, and unintended consequences, but if it's politically necessary, it should be as brief as possible.

Some policy wonks argue that employers will want to retain their group coverage. Indeed, group insurance brokers, pharmacy benefit managers, third-party administrators, employee benefits consultants, and group insurance companies that depend on group insurance for their livelihoods may well want to do so. However, it is unlikely that employers themselves will want to follow suit. Given an opportunity to get out of running their own declining health benefit plans that give them no competitive advantage, they would be irrational to resist moving to a more sensible system that improves quality and finally gets costs under control. They should readily opt out of group coverage in favor of a universal individual plan that meets all eight of our stated goals. True, we haven't seen any such enthusiasm to date, but that's because no one has yet presented a superior alternative. That's what I'm trying to do here.

A Troubling Conclusion—Market Failure

All this analysis suggests something interesting, if not profound. Even without tax benefits, group insurance, despite its fatal flaws, would still be a free market's dominant solution to the need for health insurance. That's because group insurance is the most efficient, self-emerging market method for forming large insurance pools. Individual insurance is also a market response, but its inherent deficiencies when compared to group insurance have thus far relegated it to a bit-player role. Yet, in principle, as I have shown above, individual insurance represents a far superior approach, assuming we can resolve the universality problem. If you're an advocate of free markets, this leads to an unhappy conclusion about health insurance: There is no naturally occurring way that markets will ever spontaneously emerge to offer insurance to everyone in an economically self-sustaining manner. *Laissez-faire* just doesn't work to produce universally available health insurance. The system will always fragment itself into separate, stratified risk pools—one consisting of those who can obtain market-offered insurance and the other of those who cannot. The latter will always either go without insurance or require artificial programs with external subsidies in an economically self-defeating cycle of adverse selection and failure.

In a purely libertarian society, such a *laissez-faire* approach might be acceptable. In ours, there is a widespread acceptance of a broader social, moral, and even economic responsibility to ensure all Americans have the ability to consume necessary medical services without facing financial ruin or worse. The highest and best way to fulfill this responsibility is to change the rules to allow individual insurance to function in a regulated market setting that can offer universality, affordability, portability, and all the other goals described above. The most efficient way to accomplish that would be to reform the regulation of health insurance in a manner consistent with what I will detail in chapters 9–12 as the American Choice Health Plan.

Health care is an intensely personal and undeniably emotional life-and-death subject. But in a lawful, free, market-oriented society like ours, that should argue for more individual choice and control, not less. Medical products and services are subject to the same dynamics of supply and demand as every other economic good. If health care providers are allowed to compete in selling their services to consumers, then the resulting market can function to meet their needs more effectively, more efficiently, and more humanely than can ever occur under a government command-and-control system.

Throughout much of the last century, many prominent economists believed that both capitalistic market-based nations and centrally controlled economies could flourish equally. We now know this was never true. Only market capitalism, operating under the rule of law, is sustainable on a long-term basis. Well-regulated markets, however imperfect, have been repeatedly shown to be the most effective means to meet most of the needs of most of the people most of the time, which only adds to the argument that regulated market capitalism should be looked to as a big part of the solution to health care—not something to be further eroded.

Thus far the *ad hoc* combination of group and individual insurance and the masses of people with neither have not achieved any sort of stability or sustainability. We need to—and can—craft a new insurance system that will.

Premium Rate Setting

I have held off getting into how insurers and employers price their insurance premiums because it can be mind-numbing. Long ago, I was a managed-care actuary, but even I find the subject less than scintillating. Nonetheless, understanding this aspect of health care is necessary for anyone hoping to undertake health insurance reform.

Numerous premium rate-setting methods are used by health insurers, whether private, governmental, individual, or self-funded. These generally boil down to five types: community rating, adjusted community rating, experience rating, self-funded costing, and individual underwriting. Here's a brief discussion of each:

- *Community Rating*: When an insurer charges the same premiums to everyone it insures, that is called community rating. The term derives from the fact that the insurer is basing premium rates on the average cost of treating all the members in its "community" of insureds. It is not, as some believe, based on the costs for the entire geographic community but only those members of the community the insurer actually expects to enroll.

Essentially, an insurer or HMO divides the expected total cost of insuring its entire enrollee population by the number of enrollees. That yields a per capita expense for the time period to be insured. To this, the insurer adds expected administration costs and desired profit margin. The total becomes something called the premium capitation rate. This capitation rate is then converted into actual premiums for different enrollee types, such as singles, couples, single-parents-plus-children, and families.

Under community rating, every family pays the same family premium. Every couple pays the same couple's rate. And so on. Different people enroll during different months of the year and then normally pay the same premium for a full year. Insurers usually establish a slightly higher premium for February enrollees than January enrollees to take into account the slightly higher inflation rate for the later members.

Community rating for the full premium is rarely used these days. It has an inherent tendency to be less competitive than the more commonly used experience rating. That, in turn, creates adverse selection in enrollment. Community-rated insurance is a relative bargain for older, inherently higher utilizing people whereas younger, healthier people tend to find it too expensive for their needs. As a result, many of the younger candidates will often decline to participate. Community rating was commonly used by Blue Cross plans between the 1930s and 1950s. Competition from experience-rated private insurers has led insurers largely to abandon the practice, especially for large employer groups.[25]

Community rating was required for federally qualified HMOs during the 1970s and early 1980s. Now, it is used only in highly regulated state markets and for some individual insurance plans, special high-risk individual insurance pools, and small group insurance.

Perhaps surprisingly, a form of community rating is still used by almost all employers in setting the employees' portion of premiums—but not the entire premium itself. Combined with an aging workforce, this has contributed to the increase in the number of Americans without health insurance. Here's how it works:

We know that about 22% of the forty-six million uninsured individuals have access to employer-sponsored and subsidized insurance, but they decline to take it. We also know that the increase in the uninsured over the past two decades has been "almost exclusively" from those who refuse to participate in employer-sponsored insurance rather than from reduced offerings of insurance.[26]

Add to this mix the fact that many of these voluntarily uninsured are younger employees who tend both to use fewer health services and to make less money than older ones.[27] With community-rated employee contributions, younger employees are being asked to pay more than their fair share to subsidize older workers who earn more. Many of the younger workers just don't see this as a good value, so they opt out of coverage.

Now, the demographic pig-in-a-python that is the baby boomer generation is nearing retirement. Average workforce aging combined with community-rated employee health premium contributions are making health insurance increasingly unaffordable for the young. This fact may actually account for most of the increases in the uninsured.

Community rating first arose as an egalitarian idea, but it ironically achieved decidedly unequal benefits. It is not a good way to pay for health insurance.

• *Adjusted Community Rating (ACR)*: The calculation of adjusted community rating starts out similarly to community rating. All premiums are based on the expected costs of the insurer's entire population, without looking at the specific health experience or status of any group or individual. In essence, the insurer calculates the same overall average per capita cost as with community rating. Similarly, the insurer adds a component for administration and profit to determine the premium capitation rate, as described above.

Before establishing the actual premiums to be charged, though, the insurer will make a series of adjustments to this capitation rate. These adjustments are based on characteristics of community subpopulations that affect health costs. For example, adjustments will usually take into account differences in costs by geographic region and by enrollee age, gender, and occupation. These adjustments recognize, for example, that health care costs in Boston are higher than in Denver; that older men cost more than younger men; that women cost more than men; and that farmers cost more than office workers. These adjustments are quantified by actuaries for each such factor and applied to the basic premium capitation rate before the actual premiums to be charged to each group or individual enrolling with the insurer are calculated.

Thus, an insurer would charge a group of one hundred employees in Boston consisting of female construction workers in their fifties more than a group of one hundred young male securities brokers in Denver, even though both groups might be based on the same base community premium capitation rate. It is important to note, however, that these adjustments are all broadly applicable statistical factors. Adjusted community rating does not take into account the specific health status or history of any group or individual in establishing premiums.

ACR allows insurers to offer insurance to a wide range of groups without pure community rating's high degree of adverse selection risk and its discriminatory treatment against the young, males, those living in lower medical cost areas, and those in less risky occupations. It is in widespread use by group insurance companies, HMOs, individual insurers, the Massachusetts Connector program, guaranteed-issue programs, and others.

- *Experience Rating*: Currently, most privately insured employer groups are charged premiums that vary from group to group based on each group's actual health expenditures and health status. This is called experience rating. When experience rating a new group, an insurer will either review an employer's cost data from the previous year or insurer, or, if that data is lacking, require detailed medical history questionnaires from each employee and dependent. Either way, the insurer will then base the premiums for that group on the actual experience and health risks of the members. Thus, for example, one group with a relatively high proportion of HIV and cancer patients will pay more than an otherwise identical group with no such morbidity experience. Experience-rated premiums can vary wildly from year to year, especially for smaller employers.

- *Self-Funded Costing*: Increasingly, as I have discussed above, larger employers have opted out of purchasing health insurance from commercial insurers in favor of self-insuring (or "self-funding"), in which they pay their employees' medical claims. According to the Kaiser Family Foundation's 2007 Annual Survey of Employer Health Benefits, 55% of insured workers were in partially or fully self-insured health plans in 2007. The percentages ranged from a low of 12% for employers with three to 199 employees and a high of 86% for those with five thousand or more employees.[28]

    There are several reasons for the growing popularity of self-funded plans, which I also discussed above. The big one is that self-funding is regulated by federal ERISA rules that allow an employer to provide a single nationwide health plan without being subject to every state's insurance regulations on minimum benefits, rating practices, and premium tax requirements.

    Each year, a self-funded employer's consulting actuary estimates total medical claims for the coming year. The employer then regularly deposits a portion of that total into a separate trust fund from which actual claims are paid. Deposits to the trust funds consist of both direct employer payments and employee contributions that have been withheld from employees' paychecks.

Because self-funding is based on the experience of single employer groups, albeit with backup reinsurance, it is arguably a form of experience rating. Since the enrollment pool consists only of the employees of a single group, however, self-funding could also be viewed as community rating. Furthermore, to the extent that an employer's contributions to the trust fund are calculated on the basis of the age and gender of each employee, it is also a form of adjusted community rating.

Before we go too far down a semantic rabbit hole, let's take a look at the key distinguishing feature of all self-funded employer plans. Although their respective total claims experience—and thus premiums—are actuarially predicted on the basis of previous costs and employee age and gender, the employer is always on the hook for whatever the actual claims are during the ensuing year. The only significant exception to this rule is when an employer purchases so-called stop-loss reinsurance against the risk of unpredictable, extraordinarily high claims during the period. Since reinsurance premiums are often calculated with an MLR (medical loss ratio) of only 50%, self-funded employers are incentivized to strike a balance between paying for catastrophic protection on the one hand and minimizing total plan costs on the other.

Common to virtually all group insurance plans, whether insured or self-funded, the employees' required premium contributions to be withheld from their paychecks are almost always assessed as a fixed amount per employee without regard to age or gender—that is, their contributions are assessed on the basis of pure community rating. In fact, federal laws prohibit employers from charging higher premiums to women than to men for the same benefits, even though women as a group are more expensive.[29]

Thus, in employer insurance programs—not just the self-funded ones—women tend to be subsidized by men and older employees by younger ones. On the gender subsidy question, there are public policy arguments on both sides. The most apparent one favoring the subsidy is that the inherently higher health care costs of women—generally related to reproduction—should be shared by both genders as a cost of continuing the species. Moreover, women carry much of the child-rearing burdens in addition to, or in lieu of, career responsibilities. And they tend to earn less than men, for reasons at least partially related to reproduction as well.

The less obvious flipside of the argument is that this approach can actually discriminate against women. Because women are paying less than their full cost, insurers and employers have a financial incentive to attract and underwrite men selectively and even to exclude or de-emphasize services aimed specifically at women, particularly during their childbearing years.

As for the issue of lower-paid young workers supporting their older and wealthier colleagues, I know of no serious economic or social argument that supports it. An economist acquaintance suggested that it's part of some sort of unstated intergenerational compact. Under her hypothesis, young workers make sacrifices now in favor of their older colleagues, knowing that they will be similarly sacrificed to by subsequent generations. This is the same argument underlying Social Security and one that is breaking down as the ratio of older to younger workers increases significantly as the boomers age. This problem is further exacerbated by younger workers who simply opt out of employer insurance altogether because the subsidy component makes it overpriced. I discussed this trend with a benefits attorney, who told me that there is no law or regulation requiring all employees to contribute the same amount. It appears that it's done that way because it has always been done that way.

- *Individual Underwriting Method*: Eighteen million people currently purchase individual health insurance. Except for states in which this market is heavily regulated to require guaranteed-issue policies to all applicants, the market is underwritten, meaning that applicants are screened by an insurance company underwriter for health conditions that may make them unacceptable for coverage. Such underwriting is often binary, in that the underwriter rules an applicant to be either acceptable or not. There are sometimes gradations of risk, short of outright rejection, that can exclude coverage for certain preexisting conditions and/or increase premiums. There is typically, though, little if any fine-grained risk adjustment for varying degrees of individual applicant health status. That's because even the best models for predicting individual medical costs are only about 20% accurate.

However differently each insurer may structure the benefit/premium product mix, all essentially work on the principle of allowing policies to be issued only to those with risk profiles within a preferred range. The premiums members pay usually vary by age, gender, and location of the policyholders—that is, they are based on adjusted community rating. They can also vary by health risk behaviors, particularly smoking. Because individually underwritten policies generally involve relatively high selling and underwriting costs, a higher proportion of premiums is required to pay for them than with group coverage.

Minimed Insurance

Any discussion of health insurance should include at least passing mention of minimed insurance, a relatively new type of individual health insurance that superficially appears attractive but which does little to provide protection against high-cost medical problems. Minimeds, also called limited-benefit health plans, are relatively cheap, highly profitable insurance plans that cover some primary care (e.g., a maximum of three to five doctor visits per year), minimal acute care (e.g., no more than $25,000 of in-hospital services at a maximum daily benefit of $300), and very low total benefit limits (e.g., $50,000).

Some of these plans claim to be available to anyone regardless of medical condition although the fine print—probably among the most unread text ever—will quickly disabuse anyone of the notion of a free lunch. To the extent such plans actually cover primary care, they offer nothing more than very expensive prepayment for normally consumed services. Most people would be much better off forgoing the minimed and finding one of the many doctors who will discount their rack rates by 50% or more for cash payment on the date of service. As for minimed hospital benefits, if a member experiences anything serious, he can easily end up with large hospital and doctor bills that are either excluded or beyond the maximum coverage of the policy. If someone is reasonably healthy, he would be much better off buying an individual high-deductible HSA-qualified insurance policy.

Why Not Mandate Health Insurance?

In my discussion of adverse selection, I mentioned the problem of sick people being more likely to buy or renew health insurance than healthy people. This tendency presents the central problem in reforming the health insurance system to allow everyone to buy coverage. A surprisingly large number of reform advocates prefer to address the adverse selection problem via the simplistic expedient of requiring everyone in the United States to purchase health insurance. Such mandates, though, won't work, may be unconstitutional, and—fortunately—aren't necessary to ensure universal access to affordable health insurance.

The state of Massachusetts is currently in the midst of an experiment that requires every resident to purchase state-approved health insurance. Enforcement is in the hands of the Massachusetts version of the IRS. The only exceptions are for people who successfully petition the state for the right to abstain on the basis that they can't afford it and no one else will pay for it. There are pages and pages of rules governing who can be allowed not to participate. For years, we've heard critics claim that health care should be a right. Mandates go them one better—health care as an obligation.

One might think of forced health insurance enrollment as a mandatory license to breathe. Indeed, once you see the price, sharp inhalations may be unavoidable. The glib but irrelevant argument-by-analogy is "you must have health insurance, just as car owners must have auto insurance."[30] But driving has long been viewed as a privilege subject to numerous regulations to protect the public safety. The requirement also includes the right to abstain from driving, and indeed there are almost 100 million non-driving Americans.[31] Everyone breathes. Also, the purpose of mandatory car accident liability insurance is to protect the victims of the insured drivers' mistakes, not the drivers themselves. Car insurance is not relevant to health insurance.

In any event, if health insurance mandates are no more effective than the automotive variety, why bother? Forty-seven states currently require drivers to have accident liability insurance, yet 14.6% of the driving public still doesn't purchase it. That's remarkably similar to the number (15.3%) who currently lack health insurance (see the discussion of the uninsured at the beginning of chapter 4).

A slightly deeper explanation offered by *New York Times* columnist Paul Krugman is that mandates to buy health insurance are "intended to deal with the problem of individuals who could afford insurance but choose to take their chances instead, then end up in emergency rooms, where taxpayers often end up paying the tab, if something goes wrong."[32] Although he does highlight the adverse selection issue, uncompensated ER care accounts for only 1.4% of hospital costs,[33] and even that limited problem is repairable by other, non-mandatory means, which I will discuss presently. The cost of uncompensated hospital care is not a sufficiently large problem to warrant something as intrusive as mandates to fix. Instead, mandates might be more appropriately viewed as the ultimate special interest perk for a health care industry that has been unable to overcome its own inefficiency and lack of consistent quality.

Overall, the advocacy of mandates has been surprisingly widespread and non-controversial. It is hardly news that the self-proclaimed liberal Krugman supports them. Or that the health insurance industry does.[34] What is remarkable is that prominent proponents of market-based solutions and limited government regulation have so readily raised the white flag on the issue.

My brilliant Harvard Business School classmate and now professor Michael Porter has said, "In health care, where an individual can impose costs on society, the need for mandatory insurance is common sense" and then adds the obligatory, "Everyone who wants to drive an automobile, for example, is required to have insurance so that they will not inflict costs on other citizens if they have an accident."[35] Prof. Porter has admitted, however, that he, "can't think of a way to do it without mandates."[36]

One of Prof. Porter's HBS colleagues and ideological competitors is Regina Herzlinger. Equally brilliant, she is an articulate, longtime proponent of consumer-driven health care. She has concluded (reluctantly, she has assured me) that we need a system in which "to protect against bankruptcy because of medical needs, individuals are required to purchase health insurance that covers all expenses exceeding some percentage of their income and liquid assets." She does realistically acknowledge that health coverage mandates may not be any more effective than car insurance mandates and points out that more drivers lack auto insurance in the mandatory states than lack health insurance.[37] Even my friend, noted author and self-professed libertarian Charles Murray, has proposed a system in which "everyone, starting at age twenty-one, must...buy health insurance."[38] He has justified it as necessary to prevent adverse selection. He, too, tells me he has arrived reluctantly at this recommendation.

If there is any doubt about the groundswell of support for insurance mandates, no less a figure than Newt Gingrich, the *enfant terrible* of the political right, has stated with authoritarian certainty, "Everyone should be required to have coverage."[39]

It can get pretty lonely on the voluntary side of the health insurance aisle. But there are a few stalwarts. Cato Institute scholars Michael Cannon and Michael Tanner point to the inherent unenforceability of mandates. They cite the fact that neither the IRS nor the Census Bureau even knows who and where all our residents are. These agencies are in no position to determine whether everyone has health insurance or anything else. Twenty-seven million American residents don't file income tax returns, many legally, many otherwise. They also call attention to the problem of subsidy-seeking special interests who, with coverage mandates, can much more easily lobby for increased benefit levels for their own advantage, which would continue the process of further raising premiums above market-clearing levels and making them less affordable.[40] Indeed, one of the major criticisms of Massachusetts' mandated coverage is its requirement for extensive benefits beyond those that are both necessary and unaffordable to most people.

Another vocal mandate opponent, health care finance expert and writer Greg Scandlen, adds, "I disagree that any legislature would ever be content with limiting the mandate to catastrophic coverage. It would open the door to everything under the sun—as it has in Massachusetts."[41]

Stripped of its camouflage, the mandate argument boils down to this:

1. People without insurance are a burden on those who have it.

2. The uninsured are also foolish not to buy insurance because it's good for them.

3. We can't think of any way to make health insurance attractive enough for these people to buy it voluntarily.

4. We also can't think of any way to keep free riders from being a burden on the participants.

5. Therefore, we must force them all to buy insurance.

It's a very weak argument to support something as intrusive and precedent setting as health insurance purchase mandates. If you're having difficulty holding your own on this subject in cocktail chit-chat, try breaking the ice with the list of arguments against mandates offered below. Not only will you overwhelm your friends with your logic, you will likely never be burdened with such cocktail party conversations again.

1. *Historical Precedent*: Until now, according to the Congressional Budget Office, "The government has never required people to buy any good or service as a condition of lawful residence in the United States."[42] In a country based on individual initiative and a broad range of constitutional rights, a lot of people may not agree, now or ever, that we should support private insurers and health care providers with a public mandate.

2. *Ultimately Unaffordable*: Mandates do nothing to control medical cost inflation that regularly outstrips the Consumer Price Index (CPI) by a wide margin. If health insurance premiums continue to rise faster than income, then no matter how inexpensive government-mandated insurance may be initially, it will eventually become unaffordable. Over time, increasing numbers of people would find they are unable to pay, mandates or no.

3. *Taxation without Representation*: Insurance mandates in effect convert the voluntary purchase of a service into the coerced payment of a quasi-tax to a private third party. I'll admit it would certainly be much more efficient than levying a real tax, thus bypassing the whole hassle of congressional debates, presidential vetoes, electoral risks, special interest lobbying, and borrowing from the Chinese. But it would also be the first time that the United States has required a universal tax or similar payment that allows private third parties to specify the amount of the tax (i.e., the premium)—especially one that increases over time by uncontrolled and uncontrollable amounts. Although insurers' administrative costs and profits could be limited by regulation,

actual health care costs could not—unless we added outright rationing of care, as they have in Canada and the U.K.

4. *The Privacy Argument*: Many would see the mandate as an unjust intrusion into their private lives. They value their privacy and don't believe that either their employers or the government should know about their health purchases, status, history, or habits. Also, without a truly comprehensive government safety net for the poor and disabled, many people would still not be able to afford it. Thus, mandatory purchases would require exemptions, much as Massachusetts now requires intrusive disclosure of income, evictions, disaster losses, family problems, and utility shutoffs to justify *not* buying insurance.

5. *Poor Value and Choice*: Many people may find the available insurance choices to be of poor value and inappropriate for their needs. They would prefer to decide for themselves what they will buy and how much they are willing to pay to get it. Even for people who could afford it, many would look at a mandated plan and see a bad deal not worth its price. This would especially be the case if current employer insurance pricing mechanisms are maintained.[43]

6. *Subsidizing Inefficiency*: Many people will object to being forced to support an unresponsive, indifferent, inefficient health care delivery system that too often delivers poor quality care, kills many people, and will become even less accountable to consumers under a mandatory purchase system.

7. *Other Priorities*: Many people will find that alternate uses of their money are rationally preferable to having health insurance—such as food, housing, heat, a job, a business, reliable transportation, and college educations for their children.

8. *Religious Objectors*: Some people have religious beliefs that lead them to shun modern medicine (Christian Scientists) or health insurance (the Amish).

9. *Unneeded*: Some people have sufficient personal resources not to need insurance, particularly if they are savvy enough to negotiate prices and even shop overseas for higher-quality, lower-cost health services.

10. *Too Pro-Allopathic Medicine*: Some believe that alternative medicine, lifestyles, and therapies are preferable to our current system of so-called allopathic medicine. They may be willing to pay for the former while forgoing any claim to the latter.

11. *Threatens Civil Liberties*: We are a country founded on constitutional liberty, and most of us believe that we, rather than the government, are the best judges of what is good for us—and we are willing to accept the consequences of our own decisions.

12. *Doubtful Constitutionality*: Mandates raise issues of taxation without representation, a violation of the takings clause of the Fifth Amendment, and lack of due process.[44]

13. *A Special Interest Bonanza*: If you think we have too many state and federally mandated insurance benefits now, what do you suppose will happen when everyone is forced to purchase government-approved health insurance? Baldness treatments, perhaps? At least now there are some states, such as Idaho, with relatively few unnecessary benefit requirements. Under a universal mandate, any such opportunities for enlightened legislative restraint would vanish, as special-interest lobbyists would disgorge themselves and their campaign contributions onto a pliant Congress.

This is what we have seen in Massachusetts, where Governor Mitt Romney's original proposal for an affordable, bare-bones insurance plan was replaced by a rich range of minimum required benefits. According to a Massachusetts state agency report, unnecessary benefit mandates have added $1.3 billion a year in costs, equal to 12% of insurance premiums.[45] This has contributed to insurance still being unaffordable for some 200,000 to 400,000 uninsured Massachusetts residents.[46]

14. *Unenforceability*: There is no known way to enforce a universal health insurance mandate effectively. We couldn't do it through the IRS because many residents don't file tax returns, both legally and otherwise. The Census Bureau, constitutionally charged with counting every American resident every decade, consistently fails to locate and tally tens of millions of people. Even the Canadians have a 4–5% nonparticipation rate in the two provinces that require nominal premium payments.[47] I suppose we could try police roadblocks with medical ID checks.

15. *Better Alternatives*: Harvard economics professor and Obama adviser David Cutler has estimated that reasonably priced health insurance could result in a purchase rate of 98–99% without mandates.[48] This is even more likely if universal access is accompanied by proper adverse selection controls to minimize free riders. It is likely that a voluntary system, offering real consumer value without the opportunity for gamesmanship, would yield a higher number of insurance participants than would any mandate. Insurance should be something purchasers believe will make them better off than if they had not purchased it. Forcing people to buy insurance will never accomplish this.

Any mandate requiring everyone to buy health insurance would be unfair and unworkable. Fortunately, it is also unnecessary, as I will discuss presently. What we really need is universal access to health insurance that virtually everyone will actually want to buy—without the adverse selection problem. We can do that.

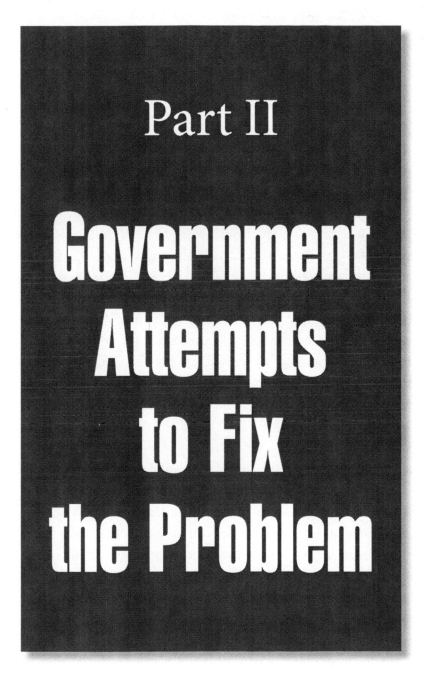

Part II

Government Attempts to Fix the Problem

PART II—GOVERNMENT ATTEMPTS
TO FIX THE PROBLEM

I described in the previous chapter the substantial issues and problems arising from the structure and practice of employer and individual health insurance. In the following three chapters I will discuss some of the most significant actions both federal and state governments have taken, often in direct response to these problems.

Some government programs, such as Medicare, Medicaid, and SCHIP, have provided much-needed services to millions of people excluded from private insurance, but they have also helped to greatly distort the organization and operation of health insurance and medical care in America. Another three programs promoting HMOs, self-funded employer insurance, and consumer-driven health care have provided incentives and empowerment for employers and private insurers to attempt to remedy the problems of excessive costs, burdensome state regulations, and tax inequities, but with inadequacies and unintended consequences of their own. A plethora of other government interventions, such as specialty hospital restrictions, certificate of need legislation, and any-willing-provider laws, have been enacted largely at the behest of specific provider groups to erect protective barriers against competition for their members. Other interventions have focused on increasing either the supply of or access to medical facilities and services. I call these laws the "quieter complications" because they have functioned largely outside the public eye while collectively having a major—largely negative—impact on the overall functioning of our health care financing and delivery system.

Whatever benefits these laws and programs may have delivered, their piecemeal nature has greatly exacerbated the problems originally caused by the market's failure to offer affordable health insurance to everyone. Many of the problems we now face are the unintended consequences of these piecemeal government fixes.

CHAPTER 5

Medicare, Medicaid, and SCHIP

The three main health-insurance-like benefit plans operated or sponsored by the federal government (other than for its own employees) are Medicare, Medicaid, and SCHIP. Together, these programs have done much to provide needed health care coverage to millions of people who would otherwise find it difficult or impossible to obtain affordable care. At the same time, they have had significantly unfavorable effects on the health care financing and delivery system as a whole.

Medicare

Prior to Medicare, one of the most serious effects of employer-based group insurance was that retirement often brought with it a loss of medical insurance. This contributed to the impoverishment of large numbers of the elderly who could not afford to pay for the burgeoning and increasingly expensive technology that was sweeping medicine during the 1950s and 1960s. A solution arrived in 1965 with the creation of Medicare. Medicare is now the largest public health coverage program in the United States. Elderly beneficiaries over age sixty-five make up 84% of those covered by Medicare. It also covers younger beneficiaries who are disabled or have end-stage renal (i.e., kidney) disease. Its expenditures in 2006 totaled $408 billion, about 3.1% of GDP. Current expectations are that Medicare will expand to absorb 6.5% of GDP in 2030 and 11.3% in 2081.[1] I expect to be around in 2030, so the future willingness of our proportionally smaller working generations to support that level of expenditure concerns me greatly.

Medicare has enjoyed widespread popularity for having brought much-needed medical coverage to millions of previously uninsured Americans. At the same time, Medicare has had perhaps *the* most destructive, distorting influence on the U.S. health care system of any single program. To understand that better, let's take a brief look at its history and operations.

To gain acceptance from a hostile medical community that had opposed it, Medicare was initially set up to be extraordinarily friendly to hospitals and doctors. Hospitals were reimbursed for their "reasonable costs." Doctors were paid their "customary charges." It was a virtual license to print money. The resulting explosion in health care costs unleashed a Pandora's box of corrosive effects that have done much to give us the health care system we have today. Medicare is now facing imminent bankruptcy while it effectively prevents the establishment of a genuine consumer market in health care. An increasing cadre of doctors is unwilling to accept it.

The problems started early. According to Robert Kulesher's account in an article in *Health Care Manager*:

> In the one year between enactment of the Medicare law in 1965 and initial implementation in 1966, the rate of increase in physician fees more than doubled, from 3.8% in 1965 to 7.8% in 1966. In the first year of Medicare's operation, the average daily service charge in America's hospitals increased by 21.9%. Between 1967 and 1971, the daily charges of American hospitals rose by an average of 13% per year.... Medicare's definition of reasonable charges also paved the way for steep increases in physicians' fees. In the first 5 years of operation, total expenditures rose...from $4.6 billion in 1967 to $7.9 billion in 1971. Over the same period, the number insured by Medicare rose only 6%, from 19.5 to 20.7 million people.[2]

Thus Medicare's costs ran out of control from the very beginning. Despite significant changes in hospital reimbursement methodology in 1983 and in physician payment methods in 1992, Medicare has continued to cause major financial headaches for doctors, hospitals, private insurers, Congress, federal budget officials, and taxpayers.[3]

Medicare's effect in promoting out-of-control health care costs is hard to exaggerate. By 2005 Medicare covered more than forty-two million beneficiaries and spent $327 billion in benefits.[4] Two years later it spent $427 billion. By 2017 it is expected to spend $844 billion.[5] The bigger the problem has become, the more the Medicare program has redoubled its centrally-controlled efforts to try to rein in costs. Medicare has been like a compulsive gambler who knows the dice are loaded against him but still hopes to recoup his losses on the next toss. It won't work.

Medicare's financial situation is dire. Its Hospital Insurance Trust Fund, supported by the accumulated payroll contributions of American workers, has repeatedly approached insolvency. Each time, it has been temporarily bailed out by higher taxes, lower provider reimbursements, or an unusually robust economy. Under current projections by its own trustees, it will run completely out of money in 2017.[6] Far worse, Medicare's total unfunded liabilities now exceed $70 trillion—a hundred times the mind-boggling $700 billion price tag of the 2008 TARP financial bailout bill.[7] The trustees have concluded with admirable understatement: "The financial difficulties facing …Medicare pose enormous challenges."

And that just accounts for the hospital trust fund. When all Medicare liabilities are tallied, the total present value of unfunded liabilities equals more than $70 trillion.[8] These obligations consist of Medicare's future requirements to provide care to its beneficiaries for which there has been no provision for the necessary funds to pay for it. Neither current taxes nor future government budget projections provide for sufficient revenues to cover the predicted costs. Former Federal Reserve Chairman Alan Greenspan has described the Medicare funding crisis as "several multiples more difficult than is Social Security."[9]

In fruitless attempts to rein in spending, CMS has resorted to ever more complex regulations. In total, they now stack three times higher than all IRS regulations. Just one recent rule change will expand the number of coronary angioplasty procedure codes that hospitals must use in billing Medicare from the current one to 1,170—for a single medical procedure.[10]

An increasingly targeted victim of Medicare's structural dysfunction has been America's health care providers. The storied days of 1960s largess are long gone. Even with its budget-busting economics, Medicare now fails to pay a sustainable price for the services it purchases from America's doctors and hospitals. It has become notorious for paying less than providers' costs. This mandatory discount has shifted costs dramatically from Medicare to private insurers. They, in turn, must pass on what amounts to an unlegislated tax onto employers and consumers.

A 2006 article in *Managed Care* pointed out some of the effects of this practice. In California, Blue Shield calculated that insurance premiums could be reduced by about 10% if hospitals could collect the same reimbursement rates from both Blue Shield and Medicare. Others have estimated that Medicare's cost-shifting has increased California's private insurance rates by 9.5%. In Washington State, hospitals collected about a quarter less from Medicare than from private insurers in 2004. They charged private payers $738 million extra to make up the difference.[11]

Likewise, doctors charged their private payers $620 billion more in order to make up for Medicare's niggardly payments. That's a total of $1.358 billion dollars just in Washington alone. It added an estimated $902 to the annual cost of a privately insured family insurance policy, equal to 13% of all private hospital and doctor payments. Most affected are those who have been forced by excess private insurance premiums to join the ranks of the uninsured. Nationwide, Medicare and Medicaid provider payment increases are lagging behind their actual cost increases, thus accelerating the rate of cost-shifting to private payers.

Congress has found it easier to extract needed program funding from America's often-maligned insurers than to enact the politically distasteful tax and Medicare premium increases required to make the system both solvent and equitable. (Note to Medicare-for-All advocates: Even with the shell-game legerdemain available to government accountants, not even Medicare will be able to shift costs from itself to itself under a single-payer approach that would replace all other insurance with a universal Medicare program. Unless you want to risk bankrupting providers on a wholesale basis, your proposal may well cost a lot more than you think.)

Medicare's Price Controls

One of Medicare's more far-reaching actions was the creation of the Resource Based Relative Value Scale (RBRVS) that dictates not just Medicare's payments to doctors but almost all doctor reimbursements by all payers nationwide. It is government price control and regulation on a grand scale that maintains an illusion of independent provider pricing.

Before 1992 and the creation of RBRVS, CMS reimbursed doctors on the basis of their "current, prevailing, and reasonable" charges (CPR). The intent was to reflect doctors' current market prices for their services. In reality, if the majority of doctors decided that a 20% jump in their fees was a "reasonable" thing to do, Medicare would pay them on the basis of CPR. Unsurprisingly, doctors regularly decided that it was eminently reasonable to increase their fees in amounts far greater than the prevailing Consumer Price Index. They prospered. Medicare didn't. CMS repeatedly tinkered with the CPR approach (in effect, applying CPR to CPR) to gain control of physician costs, but nothing worked. Between 1975 and 1987, Medicare reimbursement for physician services grew at a 15% compound annual rate.[12]

Government policymakers were desperate for a fix. As it turned out, the American medical establishment, in the form of the AMA, had itself unwittingly handed CMS one of the essential tools needed to rein in their doctors' inflationary practices. Since 1966, the AMA had begun publishing and periodically updating lists of thousands of standard Current Procedural Terminology (CPT) codes for every individual service that any doctor was known to do. By 1983 CMS had adopted CPT codes as its standard for all physician Medicare billing and in 1986 for all Medicaid billing. The AMA's largest source of revenue—significantly greater than member dues—is now the sale of CPT coding books and data files to physicians, who must purchase them every year or risk being accused of coding fraud by CMS.[13]

Then, in 1985, CMS contracted with the Harvard School of Public Health to determine the relative value of each CPT-coded procedure for each medical specialty. This followed the California Medical Association's termination of its own pioneering California Relative Value Scale because of antitrust concerns. The federal government had no such concerns.

In 1989 Congress mandated that CMS adopt a relative value approach to physician reimbursement. The relative values were to be based on the cost of providing the service rather than either the market value or the prevailing charges for those services. (Astute readers may have already questioned the use of the word *value* in anything based exclusively on cost.)

The entire system had to be budget-neutral—that is, CMS had to administer the system in accordance with a global budget established annually by Congress. With a single action, Congress removed all market determinations of both price and total demand, leaving only the supply of medical resources to seek its own level. This was to have serious consequences for Medicare's beneficiaries, America's doctors, and all medical consumers to this day, as we shall see.

Under RBRVS, each CPT code was assigned a relative value unit (RVU) consisting of separate variables for (1) the average amount of physician work required; (2) estimated practice costs including equipment and technology; (3) malpractice insurance costs; and (4) geographic cost variations.[14] The RVUs also factor in modifiers for the different medical specialties that say, as Dr. Benjamin Brewer puts it, "An hour of brain surgery is valued more highly than an hour of general medical care." [15] Finally, it applies a dollar conversion factor to each resulting value to calculate how much it will actually pay for each service that year. CMS changes the various RBRVS values periodically according to whatever factors it considers relevant or necessary. The American Medical Association chimes in once a year with recommendations and every five years with a major review of the system.

Initially, the RVU values resulting from these variable inputs could be checked against actual market prices to verify comparability. However, as the RBRVS system eventually displaced market pricing altogether, the determination of each variable became increasingly arbitrary over time since there was no longer any independent measure of its accuracy or appropriateness. Its increasing arbitrariness has rendered it irrelevant as any sort of measure of the true value of the services being paid for. One result has been increasing dislocations in medical supply—particularly in the decreasing number of primary care doctors. As a price regulatory mechanism, the original RBRVS was incredibly complex. Since then, it has become only more so. CMS continues to tinker, adjust, and modify RBRVS to take into account ever more fine-grained issues as it attempts to reduce the unintended consequences that have resulted from its previous versions.

Being congressionally mandated, the whole process is all highly political. It is thus susceptible to special interest favor seeking—but not market forces. CMS, aided by the AMA, does attempt to be objective in setting the relative values for all those services. It is, nonetheless, an arbitrary system that more closely resembles the old Soviet central planning and pricing regime than the more market-based system that has since replaced Gosplan, even in Russia. As the noted market economist and Russian Premier Vladimir Putin has said, "One doesn't have to be a particularly bright highbrow to see the obvious, that the market economy has major advantages over an administrative system." [16]

I'll spare you a description of the parallel ICD and DRG coding systems that CMS requires hospitals to use. Let it suffice to say that the ICD coding standard is currently undergoing an upgrade. It increases the number of its diagnosis codes from thirteen thousand to sixty-eight thousand and the number of procedure codes from three thousand to eighty-seven thousand.[17]

Let me summarize RBRVS to this point. Because the CPR exceeded the CPI, CMS adopted AMA's CPT, paid HSPH for RVUs, and created the RBRVS while simultaneously adopting ICD-9 to enable DRGs. OK?

Oddly enough, the essential problem with the RBRVS system is not that it is too complex. Quite the contrary. The issue is that it can never be complex enough to match the dynamic price optimization tendencies and mechanisms of a properly functioning market. There, the value to the consumer—the patient—is the critical determinant, not the arbitrarily calculated average cost of a service.

RBRVS's effects now extend well beyond Medicare and Medicaid. RBRVS has become the standard payment methodology for virtually all private insurers as well. Not even the largest private insurers have the clout to require doctors to bill them on a different basis than what the providers must use for Medicare. Thus, RBRVS's artificial rigidity and distorting effects have spread to all consumers. RBRVS continues to cause serious misallocation of resources throughout the health care system.

Medicare to Family Practitioners: Drop Dead

One casualty of Medicare's artificial payment scheme has been America's family practitioners. Since 2001 the CMS specialty modifier that determines the relative "value" of family practice doctors has fallen while that of, for example, anesthesiologists has risen.[18] Is that because family doctors have become less valuable, less useful, or less necessary than anesthesiologists and should therefore be paid even less? In effect, CMS says yes. The patients in need of primary care may think otherwise, but they have absolutely no say in the matter.

To make matters worse, primary care reimbursements have been repeatedly scheduled for steep reductions although last minute congressional actions have thus far staved off most of them. Nonetheless, "financially, family physician practices are bleeding to death," says Jim King, MD, president of the American Academy of Family Physicians.[19] As a result, while anesthesiologists earned an average of $185,000 per year in 2003, family practitioners made $140,000.[20] Neither is exactly a starvation wage, but family practice requires longer and more irregular hours, only one year less for training beyond medical school (four years as opposed to five), similar debt to finance, and considerably greater practice overhead that must be borne by payments from insurance, Medicare, and other payers.

Word has spread in the medical community and into the medical schools that Medicare's price control has turned family practice into an economic dead end. That is why, on the eve of massive baby boomer retirements and their growing demands for primary care, the number of medical school residents in family practice has been dropping for ten years. It peaked in 1997. The number of medical graduates going into family practice has dropped more than 50%. Doctors are rationally opting for specialties offering higher pay and better hours.[21] The American Academy of Family Practitioners has predicted a severe shortage of family doctors by 2020 if Medicare does not increase payments. Of course, if Medicare addresses the problem with higher payments to family physicians, the money will necessarily come out of the pockets of other doctors. Any way they work it, RBRVS requires CMS to decide which specialties are more important than others.

If a viable market were setting rates instead of government civil servants, it is highly unlikely that the growing demand for family medicine would result in fewer primary care doctors. This may be something to consider before advocating that Medicare be given the power to "negotiate" drug prices with the pharmaceutical manufacturers.

Among practicing family doctors, some are opting out of Medicare entirely. They are refusing to take Medicare patients on any basis—with some even refusing any insurance payments either. They simply bill their patients directly, requiring them to seek their own insurance reimbursements. In 2007, 17% of Medicare-age consumers reported having "a big problem" finding a new primary care physician, as opposed to 13% only two years earlier. A 2008 study by the Texas Medical Association found that only 38% of Texas primary care physicians and 58% of all the state's doctors were taking new Medicare patients, versus 78% for all doctors in 2000. Nationwide, the study reported that only 600,000 of the country's 1.5 million doctors are now willing to treat Medicare patients.[22]

Other doctors have figured out that if Medicare won't pay them reasonably for their normally billable services, they'll just do more of them. Many now require an office visit for almost everything. That includes many small matters, such as prescription refills that would normally be handled over the phone. Unlike lawyers, doctor can't charge for time spent with patients on the telephone or otherwise outside the presence of the patient. Their message: "Okay, Medicare, remember all the stuff we used to do for free because you paid us okay for the other stuff. Well, if you're going to stop paying us for the other stuff, we're no longer going to do the free stuff. One way or another, you're going to pay us, at least as long as we decide to play your game at all." Such gamesmanship is costly, wasteful, and unnecessary.

America's aging baby boomers will nearly double our elderly population by 2030. Yet Medicare's skewed reimbursement formulas have severely restricted the income of doctors specializing in geriatrics. These are doctors who are almost completely dependent on Medicare for their income. The average income for specialty-trained geriatricians was $163,000 in 2005. Compare that with the $170,000 they could have made as general internists, without having to go through all the extra training.[23] Medicare's emphasis on acute short-term, rather than chronic long-term, treatments further handicaps these doctors.

Because of Medicare's preference for certain specialties, others are in danger of going out of existence entirely. About 140 of the remaining four hundred neuro-ophthalmologists—an increasingly critical specialty for patients with otherwise undiagnosable eye diseases—will be reaching retirement age over the next decade. With their Medicare reimbursement rates having been cut by some 20% since the 1980s, these doctors are unlikely to be replaced. New doctors are simply choosing higher paying surgical or other specialties. Additional specialties facing acute shortages include endocrinology, rheumatology, and pulmonology.[24]

Unless Medicare is dramatically reformed to become more responsive to actual patient demand, its heavy-handed price and demand regulation promises to yield critical shortages of primary care and specialty providers for an increasingly elderly—and ill—population. As the late Nobel laureate economist Milton Friedman has often been quoted as saying, "If you put the federal government in charge of the Sahara Desert, in five years there would be a shortage of sand."

The impact on doctors is one of the visible problems resulting from government price setting. Not so readily apparent are the thousands of American health care entrepreneurs who are failing for lack of any CMS reimbursement recognition at all. No matter how brilliantly innovative your health care service model may be for improving care and lowering costs, if you don't have an approved CMS billing code, you're DOA.

The United States has long been an entrepreneurial hotbed that has given us higher living standards and lower prices. Why isn't this happening in health care? Part of the reason is that CMS's price control policies won't let it. We can't pin all the blame on CMS. But without intending to, it is engaging in a silent form of health care rationing. It affects not only its own beneficiaries but everyone. It's not the kind of rationing in which people are told they can't have some ingenious thing that would improve and extend their lives. It's much more subversive in that they never know what they are missing if it was never allowed to exist.

In the name of reducing costs, Medicare has engaged in a corrosive form of price control. In doing so, it has severely damaged the entire health care financing and delivery system while preventing the emergence of any kind of market-based solution.

The Harvard economist Benjamin M. Friedman, in his insightful book *The Moral Consequences of Economic Growth*, has suggested a solution: "The key to changing these perverse incentives is to broaden Medicare to allow elderly Americans to choose among different medical insurance plans, presumably with differing extent of coverage and probably with differing prices."[25] I will address this point presently.

Medicare has provided much-needed medical care to America's elderly and disabled but with huge unintended negative consequences to both the health care delivery and insurance systems. Virtually concurrent with the creation of Medicare in the mid-60s came another massive government program, this one for America's poor—Medicaid—which has had its own unintended effects. This was followed in the late 1990s with the State Children's Health Insurance Program (SCHIP) in an attempt to extend medical benefits to children of near-poor and working-poor families not eligible for Medicaid.

Medicaid and SCHIP

Medicaid is a joint federal- and state-funded health care entitlement program for low-income people. Administered by each state, it was created in 1965 and now provides health coverage and long-term care support services to fifty-eight million individuals. Seven and a half million of them are also covered by Medicare.

Medicaid spent $304 billion in FY 2006. That was almost double the $159 billion spent in 1997. Medicaid accounts for about one-sixth of all U.S. health care spending and nearly half of all nursing home care. Overall, the federal government pays about 59% of Medicaid costs, with states paying the remainder. More than half of all Medicaid beneficiaries belong to HMOs or managed-care organizations.[26]

Eligibility for Medicaid is based on income and population category. Not all low-income individuals are eligible. The population categories that generally qualify are children, parents of dependent children, pregnant women, the disabled, and the elderly (usually in concert with Medicare). Maximum qualifying income levels differ from state to state and from group to group. In general, coverage for children and pregnant women is available at higher income levels than allowed for the disabled and elderly. They, in turn, are allowed higher incomes than parents of dependent children. Younger, able adults without children rarely qualify for Medicaid, even at the very lowest income levels.[27]

The federal government sets minimum Medicaid enrollment and benefit standards. It allows a state to use those or its own, more generous, standards. Funding is on a matching basis, depending on the state's relative wealth and the amount of money it contributes. Federal matching funds are paid directly to each state. The state then augments the funds from its own budget and administers the programs through its own or county agencies. Each state sets its own benefit levels and eligibility requirements and then administers the process, which includes marketing (usually called outreach), enrollment, eligibility maintenance, claims processing, and payment.

State benefit levels and eligibility standards have tended to expand and contract over time. They have usually followed the waxing and waning of economies and tax revenues. Some states, such as Tennessee and Missouri, have encountered significant problems trying to maintain their programs. Of late, California has had a particularly difficult time. It defied federal law in 2007 to enact an across-the-board 10% reimbursement cut for providers, putting at risk access to providers by the state's Medicaid beneficiaries. By early 2009 budget deficits in twenty-five states had forced cutbacks or proposed cutbacks in their Medicaid programs. Twelve states had also looked at cutting back their SCHIP programs for children. Already enacted cuts in both programs have eliminated 250,000 children from the coverage rolls. Proposed reductions would have affected millions more except for a major program expansion signed into law in February 2009 by President Obama.

Both federal and state governments have long tried to balance their constrained Medicaid/SCHIP budgets on the backs of doctors and hospitals. They have paid significantly less than even Medicare pays for physician and hospital services, which has further contributed to significant cost-shifting to the private sector. A 2003 study of the South Carolina Medicaid program revealed that primary care doctors were paid only 78% of Medicare rates, equal to 61% of private insurer rates. Specialty providers were even worse off, receiving 66% of Medicare rates and 52% of private insurance reimbursement levels. Moreover, some rates had not been changed in more than ten years.[28]

A study by Daniel P. Kessler, a professor at Stanford University's business school, calculated that California's hospitals could have charged their privately insured patients 10.8% less in 2005 if Medicare and Medi-Cal (i.e., Medicaid) had paid enough just to cover hospitals' costs.[29] Surprisingly for many, Dr. Kessler discovered that the government's low level of payments contributed far more to cost-shifting than did the hospitals' uninsured patients, who added only 1.4% to costs.

Medicaid further adds late-payment insult to low-payment injury for providers. An Athena Health study revealed that, while the top private insurers took 27–33 days on average to pay doctor claims, the New York State Medicaid program took 137 days. The private insurers resolved 96% of all doctor claims on the first attempt. New York's Medicaid program resolved only 57%. The insurers denied about 6% of claims. Medicaid denied 39%.[30]

In one of the more bizarre twists on cost-shifting, the General Accounting Office (GAO) has reported that at least twenty-nine states engaged in fraudulent schemes to pay providers "amounts that greatly exceeded established Medicaid rates" and then required the excess to be rebated back to the state governments. The purpose was to artificially inflate federal Medicaid contributions so that the offending states could then launder the extra funds to be used for other state purposes.[31] If the perpetrators had been in the private sector, they would likely have been jailed.

There has been another, even less salutary effect of Medicaid's niggardly reimbursement policies. The program has been transformed over the years from one intended to bring care and dignity to the poor into one in which low reimbursement rates have increasingly resulted in sick beneficiaries not being able to find doctors willing to treat them. Despite the lower fees and late payments, doctors, to their credit, have not tended to abandon Medicaid completely in large numbers. There is, however, substantial evidence of doctors limiting the number of Medicaid patients in their practices. And some do refuse to participate at all. Many states have resorted to cutting provider payments in lieu of reducing eligibility or benefits, despite evidence that such policies restrict beneficiary access to regular care. This has increased costly emergency room utilization.

Increasingly, toward the end of the twentieth century, Medicaid's coverage for the strictly poor exposed the problem of children in working-poor families above Medicaid's income cutoff levels who were without health insurance. In 1997 the federally legislated State Children's Health Insurance Program (SCHIP) was created as a new, non-entitlement, state-administered program. Its purpose was to subsidize medical care primarily for low-income children who are ineligible for Medicaid or any other form of "creditable coverage," such as private insurance. SCHIP gives states extensive discretion with respect to benefit design, eligibility standards, payment levels, and administrative procedures. States may use SCHIP funds to expand children's Medicaid eligibility or may operate SCHIP programs separate from Medicaid. They may also combine the two.

By mid-2006 SCHIP had enrolled 4.1 million beneficiaries and was spending $7.9 billion per year.[32] The program was greatly expanded in early 2009 and is expected to cover as many as eleven million children in working-poor families that don't qualify for Medicaid. Like Medicaid, SCHIP funding is on a joint federal and state matching basis.

Children who meet the various state income and asset standards are entitled to receive full benefits under both Medicaid and SCHIP. In some states certain people earning more than the required limits are allowed to pay premiums to buy in to Medicaid and SCHIP programs.

Medicaid and SCHIP are defined-benefit plans. Any recipients who earn even one dollar more than allowed by the eligibility standards are pushed off the coverage cliff and lose all their benefits. This "cliff effect" constitutes a high marginal "tax" rate (far in excess of 100%) for anyone losing coverage because of increased earnings. Because of the high cost of private health insurance, this provides an incentive for current or prospective beneficiaries to limit their incomes and savings and to hide or divert assets to stay within the eligibility guidelines.

Medicaid and SCHIP health care benefits are essentially free, involving neither premium contributions nor copayments for services, although small copayments are sometimes charged for some services or prescription drugs. It has been estimated that putting a price of zero on health care for these consumers has led to $50 billion in excessively utilized health services being consumed without regard to benefit.[33] Putting copayments even as small as $.50 to $3 on physician office visits or prescription drugs has yielded dramatic reductions in health services utilization. Medicaid beneficiaries, though, are as likely to eliminate necessary as unnecessary care. Medicaid patients react much more strongly to cost sharing than middle-class individuals in cutting their utilization, with potential adverse health consequences for those with health problems.[34]

There is evidence that Medicaid's expanded coverage since 1997 to cover low-income employed people has had a substantial crowd-out effect on private health insurance. In 1999 the percentage of children covered by private insurance was 65%. By 2004 it had fallen to 59%. During the same period the percentage of children on Medicaid rose from 22% to 29%.[35]

The widespread lack of effective Medicaid financial and claims controls has resulted in frequent fraud. In New York State alone fraudulent and unnecessary spending is suspected in 40% of all claims, totaling $18 billion a year.[36] A 2006 investigative article in *City Journal Magazine* covered the issue extensively and reported many of the findings that follow.[37] Nationwide Medicaid fraud is estimated to total $30 billion per year. There have been numerous cases of lax oversight, which has resulted in such abuses as doctors billing in excess of twenty-four hours per day, fake vendors being paid for phony invoices, pharmacists collecting for dispensing drugs to dead patients (who didn't get better but still reportedly voted in Chicago), home health providers being paid for hospitalized patients, $300 million of New York Medicaid payments going to medical transportation companies for unnecessary and undelivered services, Nigerian immigrants running a several-hundred-million-dollar ring of fraudulent medical equipment stores, a dentist billing for 991 procedures during a single day, and widespread physician bill padding.

Practically all of the reported state efforts to deal with fraud are aimed at catching the malefactors after they have perpetrated their scams. The more aggressive states, such as Texas and Kansas, have increased legal scrutiny to nail the bad guys. The thinking is that these measures will deter others from engaging in similar acts. Even when other states catch fraud, the punishment is often lackluster. Ohio accepted $409 to settle a half-million-dollar ambulance service overpayment and wanted only $155,000 to settle $3.4 million in over-billing by speech centers. Florida was unable to tell auditors whether it had even collected $133,000 in fines against one defendant. The state settled another $40 million fraud case for $100,000. It is not clear whether the initial fraud claims were overstated or the states just failed to pursue adequate payment.

The federal government and most states spend little on fraud detection and much less on improved administrative and claims adjudication systems that private insurers normally use to prevent fraud in the first place. The federal government's Medicaid fraud unit was reported in the *City Journal Article* to be vanishingly small, with a mere eight people and a non-salary budget of only $26,000. Medicaid fraudsters also prey on Medicare. Despite the fact that California has saved nearly $60 million by matching Medicaid and Medicare databases, only six other states have implemented similar procedures.

State attempts to rein in Medicaid costs have been met with heavily lobbied political opposition by unions, hospital administrators, and other special interests seeking to expand payments. This had been particularly a problem for such fraud-ridden services as home health care and nursing homes. Steven Malanga, the author of the above noted *City Journal* article, concluded, "In short, Medicaid, designed to provide health care to the poor, has become a benefactor of the health-care industry, a jobs program, and a gigantic arena of political manipulation."

One proposed solution for Medicaid fraud is for states to contract with private insurance companies to manage enrollment and claims adjudication. For years, large private employers have hired them to manage their self-funded employee health benefits. Florida's Medicaid program is undertaking just such an approach in an attempt to utilize private insurance companies' sophisticated fraud-fighting capabilities. Unless the states require these insurers to use the same fraud prevention and authentication procedures they use for their commercial clients, however, such programs will have questionable effectiveness.

Back during its first year of operation in the mid-1960s, Medicaid expenditures totaled $1 billion. Five years later, they were $6.3 billion. In 1977 they were $18 billion, and people were beginning to worry seriously. By 2007 they were $333 billion.[38] This 33,300% increase in Medicaid's costs over four decades occurred while the number of people living in poverty remained essentially flat as the poverty rate declined from 14.7% in 1966 to 12.3% in 2006. [39]

Medicaid's growth in expenditures is out of control. It is now the largest item in the California state budget. It consumes 25% of Florida's and more than 30% of Rhode Island's. Even with these problems, most states have been looking to enact program restorations, improvements, and expansions for acute and long-term care beyond current levels—or at least they were until the economic meltdown of 2008–09.[40]

Like Medicare, Medicaid was started with the best of intentions to assist a group in dire need of help, but forty years of uncontrolled health care cost increases, along with congressional and state expansion of eligibility and benefits, have created an unsustainable financial miasma.

CHAPTER 6

HMOs, ERISA, and CDHC

The United States government has enabled three major innovations in private health insurance design over the past forty years:
HMOs, self-insured employer plans (ERISA plans), and consumer-
driven health care plans (MSAs, HRAs, and HSAs). The first two
have had major impacts on private health insurance over the past
three decades. The third is coming on as strong this century as the
first two did during their early years.

The HMO Act

Less than a decade after the inauguration of Medicare and Medicaid and more or less concurrent with state and federal certificate of
need activities to control hospital supply (discussed below in chapter
7), the federal government launched a major effort to limit hospital demand to get health costs under control. The instrument was
the health maintenance organization, or HMO. In 1970 the federal
government began funding nationwide technical assistance for new
HMO development, which turned into full-blown financial support and regulation with the HMO Act of 1973. Key features of that
law included a preemption of the laws in many states that inhibited
HMOs, financial support for HMO development and operation, and
a mandate for employers to offer available federally qualified HMO
options to their employees.

Most people now take for granted that health insurance covers
everything from doctor visits to prescription drugs to hospital stays,

all for a relatively modest out-of-pocket copayment on the part of the patient, albeit with increasing deductibles of late. They forget, or never knew, that as recently as the 1980s health insurance was usually referred to as hospitalization insurance because that was all it covered. Hospitalized patients usually had to pay upfront deductibles plus 20 percent of any costs above that. Almost nothing outside of a hospital was covered. Routine doctor visits, diagnostic tests, X-rays, and prescription drugs were all considered normal consumer purchases, much like minor car repairs. They were also inexpensive. There were no outpatient centers providing surgery or exotic imaging services. They hadn't been invented yet, and insurance wouldn't have covered them anyway.

Ever entrepreneurial, America's doctors figured out a way around the lack of insurance coverage for most of what they did outside of hospitals. They just started doing it *inside* hospitals. They started hospitalizing their patients for virtually anything and everything. Did a patient want a physical exam not covered by insurance? No problem. Just write a "suspected diagnosis" in the patient's chart and admit her to the hospital for a complete workup. Got a bad cold and need bed rest? Where better to get it for a "suspected flu" than in a hospital where you can be waited on day and night? Minor surgery? How about ten days with a semi-private room? Blue Cross would pay the hospital. The doctors would be paid by Blue Shield—and at higher rates than they would have received from their patients for equivalent office visits.

Doctors made (and still make) virtually all decisions about where patients received treatment. As a result, health care consumers were put in hospitals far more frequently and kept there far longer than medically indicated. Sometimes that was even dangerous. Hospitals back then came nowhere near today's improved, but still miserable, ability to avoid medical mistakes and hospital-acquired infections. Nonetheless, excessive hospitalization was the "standard of practice" everywhere, so not many people questioned it. As for the hospitals, you can imagine they were "shocked...shocked that there was unnecessary utilization going on here." ("Your extra revenues, sir.")

Primary care was really cheap then, and most patients could afford it. But their doctors had figured out how to game the system to get more from the insurers. You may be thinking that the insurers must have hated this. *Au contraire!* All they had to do was tote up their costs and add another 20–25 percent for administration and profits and then watch as their bottom lines grew every year along with their costs. All the insurers were doing it, so everybody was a winner.

The employers writing the checks for the insurance premiums were not so happy, however. But they had an out, too. They just took the extra money out of their employees' total compensation pool, effectively diverting it from what would have been pay increases. The employees didn't notice because the combination of productivity improvements and inflation still gave them more take-home pay every year. They never even knew they were paying for their own health insurance since the same thing was happening to all employees everywhere. It all seemed normal.

And even if the consumers had realized it, there wasn't much they could have done about it. The problem was something economists like to call a negative externality. That's what you get when you're in a large party of restaurant diners who decide, before ordering, that each of you will simply pay an equal share of the final check. Splitting a common bill makes the Chateaubriand and first-growth Bordeaux much more inviting to each of you than if there were separate checks. Human nature almost guarantees that each diner, and thus the table, will spend more than would have been the case with each footing his own bill. This is especially so when they all see the first glutton ordering the lobster appetizer, 20 oz. rare steak, Chateau Mouton Rothschild, baked Alaska, and the Port.

The same thing happens with health insurance. When there is no personal financial brake on medical care demand or on indulgence in smoking, eating, alcohol consumption, or their consequent health care costs, people demand medical services that more appropriate personal and financial constraints would have rendered unnecessary. The big difference between the restaurant example and health insurance is that the diners feel the financial pain at the end of the meal, thus making them more likely to demand separate checks from then on. Patients with health insurance rarely see their full share of the bills so don't get the direct responsibility or the feedback that leads to different behavior.

It is important to recognize that American patients forty years ago weren't over-hospitalized by mere percentage points. No, it was by *factors* of three or four or more. What had started as a good faith attempt by insurers to provide financial protection against the unavoidable and unaffordable personal costs of serious illness came to be exploited by medical providers and turned into a major problem of runaway medical costs.

Helping fan this glowing ember into an economic conflagration, the federal government in the mid-1960s started pumping huge sums of Medicare and Medicaid payments into the system without any checks on unnecessary spending. And this was on top of the massive federal Hill-Burton Program support to help pay for the new hospital construction thought to be needed to keep up with the increased demand. In 1974 a congressional report concluded that "the massive infusion of Federal funds into the existing health care system" had severely distorted the health care market by "contribut[ing] to inflationary increases in the cost of health care."[1]

Entrepreneurs and capital markets came to realize by the 1960s that running hospitals could be a very profitable business, which gave rise to the rapid growth of for-profit chains. They, too, enjoyed an almost unlimited ability to fill new beds with paying customers—whether they needed the care or not.

By 1970 all of these developments led to a nationwide crisis in medical costs, with expenditures reaching a panic-inducing 7.2 percent of GDP, up from 5.2 percent a decade earlier. (Note: We panicked easily in those days. Health care consumed 16 percent of GDP in 2008.)

The HMO Act of 1973 was meant to put a brake on all this excess hospital utilization. The term "health maintenance organization" was coined by Dr. Paul Elwood, who had been promoting a health maintenance strategy since the 1960s. The basic idea of HMOs had been around since at least 1866. That's when the Tredegar Iron Works in Richmond, Virginia, hired a doctor to attend to the daily needs of workers and dependents who voluntarily paid 1 percent of their monthly wages into a medical fund.[2] The idea then, as now, was to allow workers to avoid the financial pain of unexpected health care expenses in favor of small, regular payments into a fund via regular payroll deductions and employer contributions.

The first organization now recognized as a true HMO, albeit forty years before the term was invented, was the Ross-Loos Medical Group in Southern California in 1929. It was followed in 1945 by the Kaiser Foundation Health Plan developed by industrialist Henry J. Kaiser and Dr. Sidney Garfield. Ross-Loos is no longer in existence, but Kaiser has grown to cover 8.7 million members from 125,000 employer groups in nine states and Washington, D.C. As a nonprofit organization, Kaiser provides doctor services through exclusive contracts with independent, for-profit Permanente Medical Groups. Hospital services are provided by wholly owned nonprofit Kaiser Hospitals and through contractual arrangements with independent hospitals.

The original HMO concept, though superficially similar to health insurance, was substantially different in important ways. Health insurance is a financial risk-sharing function in which premium payments are pooled from a large number of people. They then reimburse those relatively few individuals who incur health care expenses, often above a certain deductible level. Whereas an insurer might contract with doctors and hospitals to obtain discounted rates, insurers took no responsibility for making sure that insured person actually received care—or that care was provided in an organized, coordinated, and appropriate manner.

The HMO concept was to create single health care entities that merged the previously separate functions of medical insurance and medical service delivery. HMOs introduced the concept of prepayment for normally non-insured primary care (doctor office visits, outpatient prescription drugs, lab tests, and X-rays). Thus structured, an HMO would contract with members to provide, not just pay for, virtually all of their medical care needs directly for a single monthly payment.

HMOs collected these payments through their members' employers, which contributed the lion's share of the payments. Unlike traditional indemnity insurance that usually covered care provided only in hospitals, HMO member service contracts (rather than insurance policies) specified a comprehensive array of health care benefits. These included everything from primary physician office care (including ancillary services) to prescription drugs to emergency care to full, unlimited acute hospital care. All services were provided with little or no member out-of-pocket payments. When there were any, they were almost always in the form of nominal fixed-dollar copayments for doctor office visits and sometimes for emergency room visits. Whereas insurers sold insurance to insureds, HMOs sold prepaid health services to members.

The combination of direct service, prepayment, catastrophic financial protection (in effect, insurance), and comprehensiveness was considered necessary to support the two stated economic tenets of the HMO concept:

1. *Savings from prevention and health maintenance*: By providing a full array of non-hospital primary and outpatient care with little or no out-of-pocket expense, members would seek preventive care and early illness detection and treatment. This would prevent later, and far more expensive, treatments for full-blown diseases—thus, it was believed, saving a lot of money.

2. *Elimination of medically unnecessary hospitalization*: Doctors and patients would no longer have any financial incentives for

unnecessary hospital use, thus substantially reducing hospital utilization and cost. To reinforce this point, HMOs incorporated formal controls and financial incentives to make sure that participating doctors hospitalized people only when medically necessary.

The theory was that savings from prevention and reduced hospital costs would provide the funds for the HMOs to provide the expanded outpatient services while offering premium rates that were competitive with the then-dominant indemnity insurance companies. Taking into account the much lower out-of-pocket costs for HMO members, HMOs would save their members a lot of money on patient care while providing equal or better quality.

HMO Limitations

Despite their apparent promise to reduce health care costs dramatically while making their members healthier, HMOs came with significant limitations that reduced their attractiveness to many potential members. One of the most significant was that HMO members could use only their HMO's doctors. Each member would have her own primary care doctor—typically in family practice, internal medicine, OB-GYN, or pediatric medicine—who would be responsible for providing, directing, coordinating, and managing her care. Primary care doctors would decide when and which specialists a patient needed to see, whether for office or hospital treatment.

The patient and her medical records always returned to the primary care physician, who was responsible for overall coordination of care throughout the system. In an era of increased medical specialization and fragmentation, this coordination role was (and is) very helpful to guide and direct patients through the often confusing maze of medical providers. This approach was also effective in reducing unnecessary utilization of expensive specialists but often resulted in service duplication when a patient who really needed to see a specialist was first required to see her primary care physician to make the actual referral.

For all their advantages, HMOs clearly weren't for everyone, especially those who had longstanding medical relationships with doctors who were not in an HMO. HMOs frequently offered far fewer doctors in a more limited geographic area than the insurance companies, which paid for virtually any covered doctor service anywhere. As a result, most people joining an HMO had to change doctors. This initially limited their attractiveness and held down their growth.

HMOs and Dual Choice

The HMO Act of 1973 required employers to offer an available HMO only as an alternative employee choice to a more traditional insurance offering. Most HMO advocates considered this dual-choice feature to be essential to the success of HMOs. That way, no one was forced to join one. As we shall see, it was the elimination of dual choice in favor of HMO-only employee benefits that contributed significantly to the decline of HMOs and the downfall of their illegitimate offspring, managed care, in the early twentieth-first century.

When employers offered HMO and insurance options, each employee had to choose between the two during each subsequent annual open enrollment period. The choice locked him into his chosen plan until the next open enrollment period a year later. The HMOs' more comprehensive benefits, coordinated service model, and significantly lower overall costs were most attractive to employees who had no regular doctors and to those willing to change doctors and accept the limitations of the plan.

In the early years (late 1970s through much of the 1980s), a majority of employees had no desire to leave their established doctors or to subject themselves to an HMO's limitations in seeking all non-emergency care through a single primary care doctor. Many people felt they should be able to make their own judgments on how to manage their own health. That included the ability to choose their primary and specialty doctors and hospitals. Since the traditional insurers imposed no such limits, there was no reason for most people to switch. It was not unusual for an HMO to enroll only 10% to 20%—and often less—of a group's employees during the initial open enrollment period. Nonetheless, a well-run HMO could usually count on increasing those percentages year by year as it established its reputation and as the gap between insured program costs and HMO costs continued to widen.

Although HMO costs were significantly lower than insured costs, employers rarely shared in the savings. That was because the HMO Act required employers to pay the same amount toward an employee's HMO premiums as they contributed to the competing insurance premiums. Thus, when an HMO had lower premiums than a competing insurer, it was the employee who benefited, both from lower payroll deductions for his share of the premium and from lower out-of-pocket costs. Employers pretty much paid the same amount either way. Had the HMO Act included this equal contribution feature but without requiring employers to offer HMOs, it seems unlikely that HMOs would have achieved the foothold they did in the '70s and '80s. HMOs offered no financial benefit for employers and also increased their administrative burdens.

Initially, HMOs came in three flavors:

1. *Group Practice HMOs* provided physician services under contracts with either preexisting or newly formed medical groups. The medical groups could be either single specialty or multi-specialty group practices. They could be either exclusively HMO providers or offer services to both HMO and regular fee-for-service patients.

2. *Staff Model HMOs* hired their own salaried primary care doctors and, often, specialty physicians as employees of the HMO.

3. *IPA HMOs*, or Independent Practice Association HMOs, offered the widest choice of doctors, contracting with hundreds or thousands of individual and group practice physicians in private practice throughout a market area. IPA HMOs usually contracted with a single intermediary IPA organization, which

then took care of the actual doctor contracting and reimbursement arrangements.

Group practices and IPAs were usually paid a per-member-per-month capitation fee by the HMO. Capitation covered all physician services to HMO members. Medical groups would in turn pay their doctors according to whatever internal compensation system they had in place, whether salary or production-based. IPAs usually paid their doctors on a fee-for-service basis. IPAs normally held back 15–20% of billed charges until an end-of-year reconciliation to make sure there was enough money to go around. The remaining holdback balances, if any, could then be paid out to the doctors.

The most cost-effective early HMO models were the staff and more numerous group practice models. HMO primary care and hospital utilization controls were more successful than with the more dispersed, and often fiercely independent, IPA doctors.

Although some of the HMOs that predated the HMO Act of 1973 owned their own hospitals (e.g., Kaiser, Group Health Cooperative of Puget Sound, and later, Ross-Loos), almost all new start-ups relied on contractual arrangements with existing community and regional hospitals. Payments were most frequently on a discounted charge basis. Over time, rapid HMO growth began to give them the clout to negotiate fixed per diem, capitation, and all-inclusive diagnostic-related hospital payments.

Regardless of model, HMOs were responsible for ensuring their members received promised care in the most appropriate setting. Because patients' only financial responsibility was to pay the fixed-dollar copayments, they no longer received provider bills or submitted insurance claims. Thus, there were no denied claims with HMOs. As a result, members no longer cared about the prices of doctor office visits and ancillary services.

The lack of HMO claims denial was important. Prior to HMOs, bills from providers would often go directly to patients rather than insurers. Patients would then have to fill out insurance claim forms and submit them to their insurers with their bills or paid receipts. Insurers' claims examiners would determine whether the patient was eligible, whether the service was covered, and then calculate how much of the bill the insurer would pay. Claims were frequently denied for a variety of reasons, often because patients or doctors failed to check the proper box or to provide a particular piece of information. Growing dissatisfaction with insurance company claims procedures became a major marketing advantage for HMOs during the 1970s and '80s.

If a participating doctor rendered a service to an HMO member, it was automatically covered. It was the HMO's responsibility to make sure doctors were treating patients appropriately and in the correct venues. If HMOs paid their doctors on a capitation basis, providers were responsible for enforcing their own utilization.

Patients loved it. Member satisfaction rates were frequently in the high 90% range. HMO benefits were more comprehensive than they had ever before experienced. There were no longer any deductibles, coinsurance payments, claim forms, or denied claims. Patients just had to show up and get their services.

In that era, when most health insurance covered only hospital-related expenses, HMOs represented both a revolutionary and controversial approach that many doctors found threatening. The combination of organized medical group practice—an organizational form long-suppressed by organized medicine—and government promotion of not-for-profit HMOs, meant just one thing to many doctors—socialized medicine. Okay, maybe two things—socialized medicine and serious competition—not necessarily in that order of importance. This led many solo doctors to reluctantly and defensively join IPA HMOs. Their fierce independence and lack of cooperation was often a problem. One federally funded HMO in Albuquerque, New Mexico, Mastercare, actually shut down after its doctor-controlled IPA decided not to provide any discounts from its doctors' normal fees. Ironically, this occurred not long before HMOs began to convert to for-profit status and to greatly enrich their owners through public stock offerings. But at least in Albuquerque "socialized medicine" was stopped in its tracks.

Few of the traditional insurers comprehended the essential nature of HMOs. They often failed to understand that HMOs succeeded or failed by how well they rigorously eliminated unnecessary hospital use, coordinated patient care, managed provider resources, and tracked liabilities—often on a daily basis. Since their members almost always had an annual choice of another payer, HMOs had to focus on something else previously unheard of: member satisfaction.

The insurers' approach to claims tracking, risk management, and premium setting focused primarily on measuring their health care costs as a percentage of premiums—the medical loss ratio, or MLR. An insurer with a target MLR of 80% would therefore want to have 20% of premiums left over to cover administrative costs and profits. They would adjust premiums from time to time to maintain a target MLR. If costs went up, they might look more closely for claims they could deny. If that proved insufficient or unwise, they would simply raise their premiums.

As purely financial intermediaries, insurers had no way to control or influence the doctor and hospital services being provided to their members. There's a saying in business that if you don't measure it, you can't manage it. Insurers couldn't manage it, so they didn't bother to measure much of anything past the MLR. They also lacked the prepayment mechanism that let HMOs lock in doctor costs in advance. Insurers just paid bills as they came in.

Insurers didn't (and many still don't) track hospital use on a concurrent basis, waiting instead for the bills to arrive. Because the bills often arrived weeks or months after the services were provided, the insurers' accountants never really knew how much they owed. They had to estimate their actual expenses using historical information. They would book those estimates in a catchall liability account called IBNR, for claims incurred but not reported (i.e., not received). Good insurer accountants and actuaries put a lot of effort and resources into estimating IBNR because mistakes can be disastrous. An insurer that significantly underestimates IBNR wouldn't know that it needed to increase its premiums to cover its costs. That can quickly lead to financial impairment and, in extreme cases, failure and takeover of the insurer by the state insurance commissioner.

In effect, insurers assume that medical costs are natural phenomena they can reliably predict and price. HMOs, on the other hand, work on the basis that their members' medical needs are amenable to rational measurement and management to direct patients to proper care in the lowest cost setting.

Unlike the insurers' focus on MLR, HMO financial and operational managers delved much deeper into their costs. They would carefully track metrics for hospital utilization rates, the number of doctor visits per member, hospital admission rates and lengths of stay, hospital prices, and pharmacy utilization rates and costs. HMO inpatient care coordinators were in daily contact with hospitalized patients and their doctors. They regularly reported back to HMO medical directors with current hospital censuses, individual patients' status, estimated remaining patient days, and any issues requiring medical director follow-up with admitting or treating physicians.

At virtually any point in time, any capable HMO CFO could tell you almost exactly how much the organization owed for health care services used by its members up to that very day. It wasn't that hard because they had already paid their doctors via monthly capitation prepayments, and they carefully tracked exactly which members had been in hospitals every day and how much longer they were expected to be there.

Probably the single biggest difference between HMO and insurance company business models was that HMOs actually measured and managed these metrics against actuarially budgeted standards. If hospital utilization rates were getting out of line, the medical director would look for inappropriate admissions, excessive lengths of stay, or alternatives to inpatient care that might indicate a need for chats with the responsible doctors. If he found the higher medical utilization to be appropriate, that was a signal for the actuary to determine whether it was a temporary usage spike or a longer-term trend. This would alert the CFO to analyze the need for a premium hike. HMOs continuously measured, managed what they measured, and sought to improve ways of providing better patient service in the most appropriate setting at the lowest cost.

In effect, HMOs operated as though they actually were the providers. They worked hard to ensure appropriate allocation of re-sources to provide high-quality care. The reason HMOs were able to do this so successfully was that there was so much opportunity. The old system of indemnity insurance had allowed providers to become incredibly sloppy in over-utilizing expensive medical services on a grand scale. Economic self-interest had very effectively trumped doctor and hospital benevolence and social responsibility. It was the negative externality problem writ large.

Again, the economic argument for HMOs was based on lower costs through preventive medical care and lower hospital utiliza-tion. Unfortunately, savings from medical prevention didn't pan out. There were two reasons. First, individual health risk assessments by doctors or anyone else have a terrible track record of predicting a person's need for health services. Thus (Kaiser co-founder) Dr. Sid-ney Garfield's original concept of using multi-phasic health testing to direct patients to the most efficient care didn't work. Second, the cost of detecting and preventing nascent diseases almost always ex-ceeds the cost of treating the relatively few such diseases that would have emerged without such action. Thus, the term *health mainte-nance organization* turned out to be a misnomer.

The hospital utilization controls, though, were extremely ef-fective in saving money. It turned out that only about 25–30% of previous hospital use had actually been medically necessary. By the late 1970s new HMOs were springing up all over the country. They immediately began cutting hospital utilization for their members by 50–75%. By the late 1980s the lower premiums that resulted al-lowed HMOs to take major chunks of market share away from the indemnity insurers. Hospital administrators began feeling the pain of a new phenomenon—empty beds and even shuttered hospitals.

From 1990 to 2000 managed care consolidated its hold on American health care. As a direct result, the number of acute hospital beds in America fell from 3.7 per thousand population to 2.9—a 21.6% drop. Similarly, the average length of a hospital stay dropped from 9.1 days to 6.8, a fall of 25.3%.[3]

The most telling impact of HMOs was on the number of hospital closures. Nationwide, more than one thousand hospitals were shut down. The number of short-term, non-federal hospitals peaked in 1975 at 5,979—early in the government's push for HMO development. By 2000 the number had declined sharply, to 4,934. It has continued to slide since then.[4] The top-down hospital demand assessments mandated by Hill-Burton had been massively overestimated (see Hill-Burton discussion in chapter 7).

The savings generated by HMOs were immense and paid for the coverage of member outpatient benefits. They also generated healthy profits for many HMOs. Although the certificate of need programs had utterly failed to reduce hospital overcapacity (again, see chapter 7), HMOs were ruthlessly effective with their Schumpeter-style creative destruction.

In the early 1970s HMOs had been seen as the salvation of the health care system. The events of the next three decades seemed to justify that optimism. Employers began to embrace them enthusiastically—not that they really had a choice. Few people today remember the almost universally positive press that HMOs received during that era. For HMO managers of the day—like me—those were the good old days.

It wasn't until February of 1983 that the HMO movement became an industry. That was when Len Abramson's U.S. Healthcare floated its immensely successful initial public stock offering. By the end of 1983 five HMOs had gone public, including my own, Peak Health Care. Private investors began pouring money into HMO ventures. The initial 1970s rush for not-for-profit HMOs promoted by federal financial support was replaced in the mid-'80s by major inflows of private capital to develop for-profit HMOs. Investors also bought and converted most of the not-for-profit HMOs into for-profits.

Enter Managed Care

By the late 1980s the HMO concept had broadened—some would say diluted—into what we now call managed care. Managed care included traditional HMOs but became dominated by hybridized IPA/indemnity models. With names like *network HMOs*, *preferred provider organizations*, and *point of service plans*, these health plans offered much larger networks of doctors and hospitals. Some plans even allowed members to get services outside of the networks for a higher copayment.

This change began the effective re-indemnification of American health insurance, which rapidly accelerated as more traditional indemnity carriers—at least the ones that hadn't left the building—began offering HMO-like products. They continued, though, to use a primarily indemnity insurance management model, which largely replaced physician capitation and brought back the practice of providers having to bill insurance companies directly and wait for uncertain payments at indeterminate times.

Members of these new plans still got HMO-like benefits, for which they paid small copayments during doctor or hospital visits. Members rarely received any bills, and the critical distinction between real HMOs and the newer hybrids was completely lost on them. As long as the managed-care companies had the upper hand in negotiating ever more favorable rates with doctors and hospitals, they felt little need to put pressure on claims payments. Thus, their members rarely saw claims denials.

The 1990s saw a counterattack against managed care by providers who wanted to gain more negotiating leverage with the payers. Doctors formed large, single-specialty, near-monopoly medical groups in specialties such as orthopedics, oncology (cancer), and OB-GYN. Managed-care companies had little negotiating clout with them.

Hospitals went on a merger binge, reducing the number of players in many markets and gaining pricing clout in the process. Hospitals also indulged in the short-lived fad of acquiring primary care doctor practices. They wanted to have better control of their hospital admissions. They also wanted to provide a more united front in negotiations with managed-care companies.

Overall, these actions were successful in swinging the pendulum back in favor of the providers. They pushed through large rate increases for their services. Moreover, as managed care's market share peaked around 2000, it ran out of room to cut hospital utilization rates any further. Unfortunately for the managed-care companies, however, the employer market had become addicted to low health care inflation. It had become resistant to managed-care rate increases. At the same time, managed-care investors had become used to annual double-digit increases in company profits and wanted them to continue. It was a tough time for managed care executives.

Managed care had turned out to be a one-trick pony for medical cost control. Once managed-care companies had pulled the hospital utilization rabbit out of their hats, they had no encore. That left only one avenue for cutting costs and maintaining profits—the one involving increased claims scrutiny, fine-print coverage exclusions, and tighter prior-authorization requirements for expensive medical care. These developments completed the return to the bad old days of indemnity care. There were horror stories in the media and movies of cancer patients and others being denied necessary care. Claims were retrospectively denied because of technicalities, coverage limitations, or after-the-fact determinations that the care was unnecessary, experimental, or provided by the wrong doctor. Initially, the claims hit the providers. But once a claim was finally denied, providers increasingly turned to patients for collection. These new and unexpected liabilities understandably angered patients and their employers.

As public backlash emerged against these practices, "HMOs" were widely blamed, despite the fact that many of the real problems were with traditional indemnity companies disguised as HMOs or former HMO companies that no longer hewed to the HMO model.

These developments marked the beginning of the escalating war between providers and insurers over claims billing and collection. Before the rise of HMOs, the fees posted by doctors and hospitals represented the prices they actually expected to collect from patients and insurers. Even the early Medicare program paid doctors their fees if they were similar to other doctors' prices.

With the return of claims billing, insurers installed powerful computer systems programmed with complex rules to spot billing mistakes, gamesmanship, and misbehavior by health care providers and to kick out nonconforming claims. Doctors and hospitals responded by buying or contracting for their own computer systems to enable them to beat the insurers' systems and maximize their collections. That tit-for-tat battle has continued to escalate ever since.

One of the rules that insurers required was that no matter what reimbursement amount the insurers' computers might calculate for a provider claim, they would never pay more than a provider's actual billed charges. Also, in the early days of the battle, many insurers paid providers on a percentage-of-billed-charges basis. Providers responded to both of these rules with the simple expedient of raising all their posted prices above anything any insurer would ever pay. What little meaning health care pricing still had after the advent of managed care was utterly destroyed by this action. That is why doctors and hospitals today charge more than twice as much as they know they will collect from insurers, thus obliterating any meaningful connection between posted prices and actual collections.

You can see it every time you receive an explanation of benefits (EOB) from an insurer after you obtain a medical service. The first column of figures will show the provider's charges, the second the insurer's discount adjustment to those charges, and the third the allowable amount to be paid—often only 40–45% of the amount shown in the first column. It is now virtually impossible to determine the price of any medical service either before or after you receive it until the claim has been subjected to literally millions of provider and in-surer computer decision rules that will ultimately spit out how much is actually paid.

It is noteworthy that virtually no providers are now paid on a percentage-of-charges basis. CMS has replaced such practices with the various relative "value" and fixed-price requirements now used by virtually all payers. Yet the practice of setting sky-high doctor and hospital rack rates remains. I have repeatedly asked health care pro-viders why they do this. Their answers have all added up to, "That's the way everybody does it." It's a corrosive, vestigial practice that no longer has any reason for existence. It has remained because there has been no reason to change it to a more rational pricing model.

A New Dual Choice: Take It or Leave It

A primary reason for the emergence of hybrid managed-care models had to do with the dual-choice nature of HMO marketing. HMOs' limited physician availability had made it necessary for em-ployers to give their employees an alternative choice of indemnity insurers with no such restrictions. The problem was that HMOs were rapidly displacing these indemnity plans. As their share of an em-ployer's population shrank, indemnity plans were losing the ability to offer benefits at a price anyone could afford. This forced more and more people into the HMOs. Inevitably, employers started offering only HMOs, with no indemnity option at all. This forced employees into plans that made them change doctors and accept limitations on their ability to choose how, where, when, and from whom to receive care.

Quite understandably, many of the employees forced into HMOs didn't like it. They tended to aim their displeasure at the HMOs themselves. This, in turn, drove demand for more flexibility by the HMOs in allowing wider physician choice, which was one of the key reasons for the creation of various hybrid HMO/indemnity models I described above. It allowed members to go outside HMO pro-vider networks in return for higher copayments. Many such plans reintroduced deductibles and coinsurance (i.e., percentage patient payments), making them even more like the old indemnity companies. This change resulted in less control of provider utilization and costs by the managed-care companies.

By the end of the 1980s the former classification of HMOs into staff, group, and IPA models was in tatters. It was used only by federal regulators to enforce the dual-choice mandate. Managed-care plan types had morphed into combinations of the three, as well as preferred provider organizations (PPOs), point of service plans (POS), and hybridized versions of all of them. Managed-care membership exploded from nine million HMO members in 1980 to more than fifty-four million in MCOs by 1990. "HMO" had become a generic term with a diminishing relevance to its original concept as an alternative to traditional insurance.

Despite the emerging problems, MCOs by the mid-1990s seemed to have finally tamed medical inflation. Medical costs actually fell by 0.8% in 1996. That was well below both the CPI increase (2.9%) and the growth in worker wages (3.3%). It was the only time that has happened in at least the past forty years.[5]

HMOs and MCOs were very effective at eliminating unnecessary and expensive hospital utilization, but the underlying causes of excess health care inflation had never really abated. They had been merely camouflaged by the rapid reductions in hospital costs from the growth of managed-care market share. Simply stated, hospital utilization rates during that period were dropping faster than provider prices were rising.

The more that managed-care organizations loosened member access to doctors, the less control the MCOs could exercise over doctor behavior with respect to providing only covered and approved services. This, tied with an increasing pressure on MCO care managers to control costs through claims denials, made patients financially responsible for the inappropriate behavior of their doctors. That was the beginning of the end for managed care's dominance.

The managed-care movement had shot its hospital savings bolt by around the year 2000. Then the previously buried medical inflation monster rose from its grave, pulled the MCO stake from its heart, and once again rampaged across the economic countryside.

By 2009 a majority of employers had abandoned formal managed-care plans in favor of PPO-based plans. PPOs and their POS derivatives—"point of service" plans—were increasingly looking and behaving like the indemnity plans of yore. There was a big difference, however. Unlike the indemnity insurers of a generation past, the new insurers are now covering primary and preventive care, physician office visits, lab tests, outpatient radiological procedures, prescription drugs, and a raft of similar, often state-mandated, benefits. These are the HMO-like benefits that people used to consider normal consumer purchases in pre-HMO times—not something to be insured against.

Whereas thirty years of managed care delivered a temporary reduction in medical cost inflation, it almost completely destroyed what had been a strong consumer market for affordable consumer medical services. We had completely muddled the concept of insurance as protection against unpredictable, unaffordable events. We had replaced such insurance with a combination of consumer service prepayment and insurance against unaffordable risks.

Also, the once-vaunted health maintenance that was supposed to prevent diseases and lead to an outbreak of healthy living didn't work. One of the few successes—reduced cardiac death—resulted almost completely from the widespread use of only two new drug classes—statins and beta blockers. Otherwise, it had little to do with increased access to preventive medical services and healthier lifestyles.

Managed care may be effectively dead, but HMOs are not. Nor should they be. Just ask Kaiser and its 8.7 million members. Our mistake in the 1970s was believing that HMOs represented *the* answer to all our problems in medical cost, quality, and coordination. They may have been a one-trick pony from the standpoint of cost, but the HMOs that have stayed true to form and are offered to people who have other choices continue to provide a highly effective way to organize, deliver, and pay for medical care. They're just not the only way.

ERISA

Only a year after the passage of the HMO Act, Congress enacted the Employee Retirement Income Security Act (ERISA) of 1974, a federal law that regulates employee health and pension benefit plans in the private sector, which has been significantly amended over the years, most notably by COBRA and HIPPA. Its biggest impact on health care has been the freedom it has given large employers (especially those with multi-state operations) to bypass all the state-mandated health benefits. ERISA does this by allowing employers to avoid state-regulated health insurance in favor of self-insurance, or self-funding as it is more commonly called. This option has also freed these employers from state laws that require premium taxes, govern premiums, mandate underwriting requirements, and impose other burdens.

Only six million Americans were insured through self-funded plans when ERISA was enacted. Today, that figure stands at fifty-five million, representing 40% of all group coverage in the U.S. The remaining 60% are in fully-insured plans.[6]

ERISA has been a godsend to large employers from the standpoint of standardizing and simplifying regulation of their health benefit programs. Unfortunately, though ERISA does not specifically exclude small employers, it might as well have done so. That's because they lack the actuarial heft to predict health risks accurately and to fund them. The law of large numbers favors employers with thousands of employees over those with fewer than several hundred or so by providing the statistical basis for accurate cost forecasts necessary for self-insurance. Although large employers can self-fund with confidence, smaller ones will do so at considerable risk.

It bears repeating that smaller firms have long been the engine of job creation in the United States. In 2004, eighty-one million workers were employed by firms with fewer than five hundred employees. These workers constituted 60% of all private employment. Fully 98% of *all* firms started with fewer than five hundred employees.[7] Thus, virtually all of the thirty-eight thousand firms that now have more than five hundred employees (constituting the other 40% of firm employees) came at one time or another from the ranks of much smaller startups. Why then do we saddle these smaller employee factories with regulations and costs that often make it impossible for them to offer the health insurance they need to attract the best and brightest workers who will power their growth?

By exempting large employers from any concern about runaway state insurance laws, we have excused them from applying their substantial clout to oppose such measures when they first arise. Instead, the favor-seeking special interests have a clear path to the trough. They are too often unopposed in legislative hearings by those they harm—the small employers who were at work that day. For more on ERISA's impact on private health insurance and on the entire health care system, I refer you to my discussion of self-funding in chapter 4.

MSAs, HRAs, and HSAs

Patrick Rooney and John Goodman are hardly household names, but both have rightful claims to the title Father of the HSA. Goodman and Rooney may not have invented the concept of health savings accounts, any more than Paul Elwood invented HMOs—both concepts had multiple grandparents stretching back into the dim mists of history. Goodman is the president of the National Center for Policy Analysis (NCPA), a think tank headquartered in Dallas. The late Rooney was the Chairman and CEO of Golden Rule Insurance Company. Throughout the 1990s and beyond, Goodman and Rooney supported the idea of "medical IRAs" to provide a long-term solution to the looming funding crisis for Medicare.[8]

Rooney first met Goodman in 1990 and became a strong convert to the medical IRA idea. He subsequently poured more than $1 million of his and his company's money into a concerted congressional lobbying campaign. In 1992—the year I met John Goodman at a Cato Institute conference where we presented our respective ideas on health care reform—he and Gerald Musgrave published their book, *Patient Power*. It provided the intellectual backbone for the concept of high-deductible health insurance backed by tax-advantaged individual savings accounts to pay out-of-pocket medical costs.

The essential idea was to return to the concept of true health insurance in which consumers pay for normal medical expenses from their own funds, relying on their health insurance to pay for any big-ticket items. Because of the relatively high deductibles, the premiums on such insurance would be much lower. This, in turn, would allow consumers to bank the premium savings in their tax-advantaged medical savings accounts. It would then be used to pay for normal consumer purchases of doctor visits, diagnostics, and prescription drugs. By returning price to the health care purchasing equation, it would incentivize consumers to purchase only necessary care and to seek it from providers offering the best combination of quality and price—i.e., the best value. In a way, the underlying personal-responsibility philosophy of the medical IRA was the polar opposite of the HMOs' concept of the health plan's responsibility for covering everything a patient needed.

The most immediate effect of *Patient Power*, augmented by Rooney's relentless lobbying, was the inspiration of a slew of congressional bills—from both sides of the aisle. At first they didn't get anywhere, but Goodman's ideas helped crystallize a powerful force that effectively killed Hillary Clinton's health reform plan in 1993. It helped that HMOs were simultaneously delivering medical inflation rates at or below the CPI.

It wasn't until 1996 that Goodman's and Rooney's efforts paid off in a more proactive fashion with the passage of congressional legislation allowing a limited demonstration of medical savings accounts, or MSAs. This was to be a four-year experiment in which small employers and self-employed individuals could participate. The legislation capped the number of permitted MSAs at 750,000.

Unfortunately, the program was hamstrung by so many restrictions that only about 100,000 MSAs were set up during the program's first two years.[9]

Then, in 2002, the IRS issued a surprise ruling that allowed employers, including large ones, to establish MSA-like health reimbursement arrangements (HRAs) that removed many of the MSA's restrictions. The IRS did, though, impose restrictions of its own that have limited their adoption. HRAs can be funded only by employers—not employees—and neither the health insurance nor the employees' notional savings accounts are normally portable for employees who leave their jobs.

HRAs were a response to the limitations of MSAs and of FSA plans (also called "cafeteria plans" or Section 125 plans). FSAs permit employees to choose to have their employers withhold some of their pretax compensation in flexible spending accounts. These accounts can then be used for out-of-pocket health care and other qualified expenses. The problem with FSAs is their use-it-or-lose-it feature. Any balance remaining in an FSA account at the end of the year must revert to the employer. Thus, the employee loses it, even though it was funded with his own money. HRAs offer a way around that limitation, allowing employees to build up employer-paid funds from year to year, as long as they remain employed with the same company.

Encouraged by these limited advances, Rooney, Goodman, and Goodman's fellow NCPA scholars soldiered on with lobbying efforts, publications, and presentations pushing for even more flexible saving-based consumer health care programs. Those efforts resulted in the landmark HSA legislation of 2004. It removed many—but not enough—of the restrictions that had hampered MSAs and HRAs. The law allows anyone who purchases a qualifying high deductible health plan (HDHP) also to open and fund a health savings account (HSA) with a financial institution, usually a bank.

HDHP deductibles (2009) must be at least $1,150 for an individual and $2,300 for a family. Consumer out-of-pocket spending can be no higher than $5,800 (individual) or $11,600 (family). HDHP members who set up HSAs can contribute up to $3,000 per year for an individual and $5,950 for a family, without paying state or federal income, FICA, or Medicare payroll taxes on the deposits. For people fifty-five or older, an additional annual contribution of $1,000 is permitted.

Any payments from an HSA for qualified health care expenditures also incur no tax. Both people with individual insurance and employees with employer-sponsored HDHP insurance are allowed to set up and contribute to HSAs.

The HDHP/HSA program was kicked off in January 2004. By January 2008, 6.1 million Americans, or 2% of the population, were covered by it. To put that number into perspective, this is a greater number in four years than were newly enrolled by HMOs during the first eight years after the landmark HMO Act of 1973.[10] Today, HRAs and HSAs are constituents of a growing trend toward consumer-driven health plans (CDHP), in which consumers take a greater financial responsibility for spending their health care dollars wisely. HRAs and HSAs also constitute one of the more positive approaches by the government to inject a greater degree of market discipline into the health care financing and delivery system. Despite their early success, however, HRAs and HSAs suffer from significant disadvantages that seriously undermine their effectiveness.

Permitted levels of consumer-responsible deductibles and other out-of-pocket expenditures have been initially set at relatively high levels before the insurance must pay for everything else. These limits, however, are allowed to increase annually only at the general inflation rate—not the much higher rate of medical inflation we have seen for most of the past forty years. Unless medical inflation abates to something approaching general inflation, then it won't be very many years before the term high deductible health plan will be an oxymoron. Deductibles will become not so high when compared with other forms of insurance. Even HDHPs will gradually erode the concept of consumer responsibility for normal consumer health care purchases. That will turn it back into just another prepayment plan with real insurance behind it.

An even more insidious effect of this gap between medical and general inflation rates is that annual HDHP premiums must necessarily increase at even higher rates than medical inflation. The explanation is a little tricky, so let me provide an example.

Let's say that the Atlas Insurance Company offers an HSA-qualifying high deductible health plan with a $2,000 annual deductible and that the average person buying that plan is expected to incur $3,000 in health care claims costs during the year. Atlas will base its premium for the policy on its expected cost of $1,000 for the year (the $3,000 total claims, less the consumer's responsibility for the $2,000 deductible = $1,000). To simplify the example, let's assume that Atlas doesn't add a margin for overhead and profit. It therefore sets a premium at exactly $1,000 per year. Let's now assume that annual medical inflation (or medical trend as the actuaries call it) is 15%. Thus, the health services in the second year are expected to cost $3,450 (115% of $3,000 = $3,450). We will assume that the deductible remains at $2,000—a reasonable assumption, given current practices. That means Atlas will now have to base its second-year premium on a new expected cost of $1,450 (total second-year claims of $3,450, less the insured's $2,000 deductible = $1,450). Assuming no markup for overhead and profit, we see that the year-two premium for the same high deductible health plan is now $1,450—a 45% increase from year one, with no increase in benefits or health services utilization.

How could it be that a 15% increase in health care costs leads to a 45% increase in premium? Is the insurer gouging the poor member? No, it is merely recovering its actual claims liability with no profit or overhead. The problem lies in the fact that the insurer is adding the insured's entire second-year claims increase to the relatively small premium base from the first year. The base was small because the $2,000 deductible absorbed the majority of the first year's claims costs.

The math is simple, but the effect is traumatic. This is not a hypothetical example. Consumers today with HSA-eligible health plans are now seeing such unexpected increases in their premiums—every year. These increases are making originally low-cost HDHPs increasingly expensive and less affordable.

The easiest way to fix this problem is to permit insurers to increase the deductible each year by the medical inflation rate. That allows both the insured and the insurer to share in cost increases proportionally. That way, annual premiums can increase only by the medical inflation rate—rather than a much higher factor. It would be a simple matter for insurers to build such annual deductible increases into their insurance policy contracts, except for one currently insurmountable barrier—the law won't let them.

That's because, as I said above, the government allows maximum consumer out-of-pocket costs for HSA-qualified insurance to rise only at the general inflation rate—not the much higher medical rate. Unless the law is changed to permit greater out-of-pocket increases—or until medical inflation rates fall significantly—HSAs are seriously threatened. (Note to congressional opponents of HSAs: If you want to kill the program, you really don't have to do anything but wait.)

Despite the promise of HSAs and HDHPs to increase consumer awareness of and responsibility for health care costs, even the most aggressive attempt at individual state health care reform has largely ignored them. Massachusetts has set minimum benefit requirements for 2009 health plans that require primary care benefits for doctor office visits and low deductible limits for prescription drugs. Massachusetts also deems federally qualified HSA-eligible plans to be acceptable.[11] My search of the Massachusetts Commonwealth Connector website (www.mahealthconnector.org) in January 2009, however, failed to find any health plan labeled as HSA-compatible. Only after further searching on individual health insurer websites did I find a single Connector-authorized, HSA-compatible plan offered by an insurer in parts of western Massachusetts. That is hardly a ringing endorsement for consumer power.

Even the same federal government that had previously allowed and promoted HSAs has cut back its support where it counts most— for its own employees. For 2008 the federal Office of Personnel Management decided to limit its contribution to employee HSAs to no more than 50% of the deductible or 25% of the plan premium. This forced a 33% reduction in contributions for at least one employee group.[12] Said a government spokesman, "We're not schizophrenic. And neither are we." Okay, nobody really said that, but someone might as well have.

Perhaps the greatest threat to consumer-driven health care is the Center for Medicare and Medicaid Services (CMS). Its iron grip on national medical reimbursement rules effectively controls pricing throughout the health care system—for both government and private payers. This has given rise to our Rube Goldberg system of billing and reimbursement, which grievously afflicts us all and provides zero usable pricing information for consumers.

It is difficult to overstate the pricing problem. Without real pricing information, HSA owners have little ability to navigate the health care economy the way they were intended to. Essentially, every doctor's and hospital's "price" is a phony number. It may be entered on a claim form by a provider's computer somewhere, but it has nothing—absolutely nothing—to do with the amount that the receiving insurer or government program will actually pay. That is calculated after the claim has been scrutinized, screened, eviscerated, and recast by literally millions of decision rules in the payer's computer. Long gone are the days when a doctor's or a hospital's billed price was what they actually expected to be paid. Even worse, because Medicare promises serious penalties for anyone who charges private payers less than the government, providers artificially inflate their charges to everyone to make sure they don't inadvertently run afoul of Medicare's edict. Any consumer trying to shop price hasn't got a chance, unless he can find a doctor or hospital willing to negotiate price upfront.

Insurers are increasingly trying to provide rudimentary pricing information to consumers with online postings of actual reimbursement rates for many doctor and hospital procedures. These, however, are average rates that are a long way from actual provider prices a consumer can rely on in making a purchasing decision. Hospitals refuse to post the prices they're actually willing to accept from individuals because (I'm not making this up) they consider them proprietary. It's like Wal-Mart telling you its prices are a secret until you sign your credit card slip.

Without a complete, radical elimination of government price controls, consumer-driven health plans will never get us to a true market-based system that will force providers to offer prices that are not just transparent but also competitive, reasonable, and reflective of underlying value. Without that, consumer efforts will continue to be drowned like a tow sack full of unwanted kittens in a swamp of price disinformation—something no market can survive.

CHAPTER 7

The Quieter Complications

O ver the past century, many thousands of federal and state laws, regulations, and rulings have influenced or changed how health care is financed and delivered in this country. In this chapter I attempt to corral some of the most significant of these actions, most of which the general public has never heard about. Each item discussed has had a unique impact on the health care system, too often distorting it beyond anything a rational person might consider necessary, reasonable, or proper. Although not exactly a dirty dozen of abusive legislation, the list does provide an object lesson in unintended consequences that have cost us dearly.

Tax Policy

I described earlier how most health policy analysts now recognize that our current employer-dominated group health system was locked in as a result of a 1943 IRS ruling—later codified into law. It allowed wartime employers to get around wage controls in recruiting scarce labor. They were able to provide health benefits without including their cost in workers' taxable income. Individuals without an employer or government-sponsored plan have had no such advantage. They are required to pay their medical costs from after-tax income. When you spread this effect over the millions of workers whose employers don't provide health insurance—or are self-employed—you begin to realize why so many are unable or unwilling to accept such a heavy burden to insure themselves against financial catastrophe. The financial deck is simply stacked against them.

State Medical Practice Laws

Dating from the early twentieth century, state laws have given allopathic medical doctors a virtual corner on the market for the practice of medicine in the United States. We tend to take for granted that this physician monopoly is in the natural order of things. It is not. Originally designed to separate quackery from more scientifically-based medical care, these laws have standardized medical education, emphasized scientific research, licensed practitioners, and used the power of the state to shut down or marginalize competing approaches to medical treatment. To a great extent, these changes were once positive, putting an end to many practices that had no basis in demonstrated effectiveness. Many of the old practices had been positively harmful—witness the welcome departure of purging, bleeding, and blistering.

The watershed event of this revolutionary shift was the publication in 1910 of the Flexner Report, which set the course of medical practice, regulation, and education pretty much to this day. The report's author, Abraham Flexner, concluded that there was too much variation in medical schools and in the students they admitted. He recommended the standardization of curricula and of student admission requirements. Those recommendations have resulted in the university-based medical school and hospital model we see today. Interestingly—and perhaps tellingly—Flexner was not a doctor. He was an educational theorist who believed doctors to be a social instrument rather than an economic resource. He held that "the medical profession is an organ differentiated by society for its highest purposes, not a business to be exploited."[1] The growing economic impact of health care has substantially eroded this belief over the years. But Flexner's social argument still supports much of the philosophical and cultural underpinnings for today's proponents of medical care as a basic human right to be provided by government.

Please note that the comments that follow relate to the organization of the medical profession. They should not be interpreted to criticize the hundreds of thousands of doctors who serve professionally with dedication, skill, and utter devotion to their patients. Most of us personally know more than a few doctors who have made our lives more functional, less painful, and even possible. I am certainly among the beneficiaries of their care. One of my goals is to help enable them to perform at a higher level within a system that meets their own needs far better than the current one does.

The state medical practice laws that resulted from the Flexner Report (and subsequent AMA lobbying) were admirably successful in reducing and eliminating quackery. But they also effectively blocked or stunted the development of other beneficial types of health care professionals. The operative mantra is: "Only doctors can practice medicine."

There is a long-standing phenomenon in regulated industries and professions for the regulated to assert increasing control over their regulators.[2] In medicine, this has allowed the profession to lock itself into what sometimes bears a resemblance to medieval guilds. It has restricted admission, erected artificially high barriers to entry, mandated excessive and often irrelevant educational requirements,[3] enforced long and arduous apprenticeships, and maintained an often rigid resistance to changes originating from both outside and inside the profession.

It has been suggested by me and others that the medical profession is, in effect, a priesthood. "The myth we are peddling," said Dr. Stephen Baker, "is not everlasting life in heaven, but everlasting life here on earth."[4] It is no coincidence that the first hospitals were established by monastic orders as places to heal both body and soul.

Numerous examples of legitimate health care modalities are being pushed into the background by the state-empowered medical monopoly. For example, most pharmacists now receive pharmacy doctorates. They are highly trained to know much more than doctors about prescription drugs. They are also forbidden to prescribe medications or administer vaccinations for even the most straightforward conditions. There is no safety or quality reason why everyone must see and pay a doctor to prescribe generic simvastatin for high cholesterol. Pharmacists could do it for little more than the cost of the prescription itself, as they are allowed to do in the U.K. Instead, most pharmacists put their expensive and lengthy educations to work counting pills and dealing with insurance claim problems rather than counseling patients.

For many medical services, nurse practitioners (NPs) function with the effectiveness and quality of primary care physicians and of many specialty doctors.[5] Yet they are required by state laws to practice only under a supervising doctor's license—with the doctor usually billing for the services at his normal rates and pocketing the additional profits derived from much lower cost labor.

The American Medical Association is on record in opposition to NP-staffed retail clinics that offer a restricted range of competitively priced services, such as flu shots and ear infection treatment. It argues that providing such services without a doctor present puts quality at risk. The scientific evidence, however, strongly indicates that NP practice quality is equivalent to that delivered by doctors. The only significant differences are that the NPs have higher rates of patient satisfaction and lower costs. Also, most NPs in such clinics operate under a set of clinical guidelines that doctors would do well to emulate. Maybe then we would all receive the currently accepted standard of care more than half the time.

Each state licenses doctors to practice only in that state. Any doctor treating anyone who is in another state is breaking that state's law, unless the doctor has obtained licensure there as well. The educational and professional requirements for licensure are similar across all states. Only Michigan allows all-state reciprocity. All others require a laborious, expensive, and time-consuming licensing process. I'll leave it to you to conclude whether this is a legitimate quality issue or perhaps an artificial way to restrict competition.

Nobel Prize-winning economist George J. Stigler summed up the view of economists over the years who have observed the tendency of regulators to end up serving the needs of the regulated: "Regulation may be actively sought by an industry, or it may be thrust upon it...."

As a rule, regulation is acquired by the industry and is designed and operated primarily for its benefit."[6] The medical profession's attempts to control the number of doctors through restrictions on medical school enrollment and state licensure hark back at least to the founding of the American Medical Society in 1847. One of its committees reported at the time that "the very large number of physicians in the United States…has frequently been the subject of remark…. No wonder that the merest pittance in the way of remuneration is scantily doled out even to the most industrious in our ranks…. The evil must be corrected."[7] The corrections the society sought and largely achieved were the elimination of a lot of quackery—a beneficial outcome—and restrictions on the number and kinds of health care providers allowed to see to the medical needs of patients—a less salutary result.

In health care, the medical profession has been the ultimate special interest group. It has effectively enlisted the states to stifle competition despite growing evidence of high quality, low-cost alternatives.

The Hill-Burton Act

During the Great Depression and then World War II, hospital construction languished in the United States. That created serious shortages. Old facilities, improved technology, the growth of private health insurance, and many localities without hospitals led to enactment of the Hill-Burton Act in 1946.[8] The program was the first major attempt by the federal government to support medical care delivery directly.

Hill-Burton called on each state to appoint a single coordinating agency to inventory state facilities, to identify the neediest areas, and to determine the locations, size, and types of facilities that would best meet the needs of the people. The U.S. government then provided matching funds for hospital construction in those areas reporting needs. Over the course of the next three decades, the program provided money for the construction and modernization of

4,600 hospitals, of which 1,600 were rural and six hundred were built in areas that previously had none.

Many of these state-planned, federally funded hospitals were small and inefficient, reflecting the heavily politicized, Gosplan-like planning structure. Although the hospital shortage ended by 1958, Hill-Burton continued to pour funds into hospital construction until 1975, which resulted in construction of hundreds of thousands of excess beds without adequate attention to actual market demand. One of the fascinating features of the era was that Hill-Burton, a matching-funds program, actually contributed a small fraction of total hospital construction dollars during the period. Yet it had such an outsized impact on determining when, where, and how many hospitals were actually built.[9] Hill-Burton, along with Medicare, also played a major role in making hospitals the central focus of the health care delivery system, which contributed greatly to the health care cost crisis of the 1970s and beyond.

Certificate of Need Laws

The effect of Hill-Burton's hospital construction funding, combined with Medicare and Medicaid's massive infusion of patients into those hospital beds, was to create an explosion in hospital and associated doctor payments. This trend was in accord with an odd phenomenon known as the Roemer Effect, which recognizes that increased medical resource supply actually creates its own demand.

In 1974 the U.S. Congress responded to the problem by passing two major pieces of legislation, the National Health Planning and Resources Development Act and the National Health Act.[10] These laws funded and practically mandated the states to enact top-down, certificate of need (CON) controls. The purpose was to restrict construction of the very hospitals the federal government had itself been so actively promoting. CON was an attempt to reduce the total cost of health care by rationing the supply of facilities and programs.

Dutifully, by 1986 forty-two states and Washington, D.C., had enacted their own CON legislation, hired staff, and established powerful agencies and committees whose job was to review proposed construction and equipment projects of hospitals, nursing homes, and certain types of medical facilities. They also reviewed and passed judgment on new services offered by existing facilities. Even hospitals seeking to remodel existing buildings and equipment were required to first obtain a CON in some states.

Existing hospitals were allowed to be key players in the process. They worked together with the state agencies to restrict construction of new hospital beds and to divide markets among current hospitals. In effect, they became a classic cartel. Think of it as each state creating its own OPEC for health care but in the perverse hope of lowering costs. As it turned out, the impact on hospital costs was similar to that of OPEC with oil. It drove prices higher. This may help explain why hospitals were such enthusiastic supporters of CON legislation.

CON recognized the failure of market forces to balance supply and demand. Indeed, the structure of the hospital market allowed no such forces to assert themselves. The patient may have been the consumer of services, but the hospital's actual customer (the one making all the purchasing decisions) was the doctor. The third-party payer's role (whether private insurance, Medicare, or Medicaid) was to pay the bills. Since the price to doctors was zero, they neither asked nor cared about how much the hospitals charged. Actually, the price was really negative. Private insurers back then paid physicians for services they provided to hospitalized patients but not for outpatient services, which served as a powerful financial incentive for the informal medical standards that led to massive, medically unnecessary hospital utilization nationwide.

On the supply side hospitals recognized that there was no effective regulation by either markets or governments of the prices they could charge. They were paid by third parties, not the first parties—the patients. This asymmetry between "customer" perceptions of low (or negative) prices and high real prices resulted in significant demand beyond anything a normally functioning market would ever produce.

Helping drive this demand, via the Roemer Effect, had been hospital administrator access to plentiful Hill-Burton and private capital. They could spend whatever it took to attract the doctor customers, whether it was the latest, damn-the-expense medical technology, low-priced office space, or close-in doctor parking. It was a good time to be a hospital administrator. Revenues gushed in and fed healthy profits or surpluses. (What's the difference between a profit and a surplus? The former is earned by a for-profit hospital and is taxable as corporate income. The latter is earned by a not-for-profit hospital and is not taxable. The only distinction is the accounting terminology. The only difference is taxability.)

CON utterly failed to constrain hospital costs. As Patrick John McGinley discovered in his 1995 review of the scholarly CON literature, "one cannot find a single article that asserts that CON laws succeed in lowering health care costs."[11] There are, of course, studies showing that CON increased costs.[12]

The good news is that Congress recognized the CON failure rather quickly. It repealed the CON near-mandates in 1978, four years after enacting them. The bad news is that now—thirty years later—thirty-six states and the District of Columbia still have CON requirements in place. Despite no evidence of effectiveness and significant evidence of harm, the American Health Planning Association, the trade group of state health planning agencies, still maintains, "The rationale for imposing market entry controls is that regulation, grounded in community-based planning, will result in more appropriate allocation and distribution of health care resources and, thereby, help assure access to care, maintain or improve quality, and help control health care capital spending."[13] Thus, economic goods are being regulated as though they were public ones.

State Minimum Insurance Benefit Laws

Health insurance, indeed all non-federal insurance, is regulated at the state level under the provisions of the McCarran-Ferguson Act of 1945. That federal law provided limited insurance antitrust exemption for insurers in exchange for increased oversight by state insurance regulators. This is not to say there is no overriding national insurance regulation. It exists primarily in the form of the National Association of Insurance Commissioners. The organization has been very active in promoting interstate regulatory communication, common regulatory and reporting requirements, and model legislation in many different areas.

Health insurance, however, has become a political football in state legislatures. It has benefited relatively little from interstate regulatory collegiality, which has led to a balkanization of health insurance rules around rates, benefits, and underwriting rules. All fifty states have laws requiring that health insurers include coverage for specific people, benefits, or providers. No two states' requirements are the same.

The first minimum benefits law was passed by Massachusetts in 1956. It required dependent coverage for handicapped children. Since then, more than 1,900 such mandates have been enacted by the states. There are requirements for coverage of chiropractor services, social workers, massage therapists, dental anesthesia, infertility treatments, acupuncture, hairpieces, and drug and alcohol abuse treatment.

It has been estimated that mandates for nonstandard, unnecessary, or optional services have driven up the cost of health insurance by as little as 20% in some states and by more than 50% in others. Drug rehabilitation mandates, for example, drive up insurance premiums by an average of 9%. Requirements to cover psychological services drive premiums up by 12%.[14]

State legislators have been ripe targets for special interests intent on spreading the costs of narrowly defined services across entire state-insured populations. The incremental effect on premium costs of any one such proposal is often small. Few interest groups have appeared to challenge such proposals effectively. The problem shows up when you take a single mandate that increases costs by 1% and multiply it by the scores of similar mandates in a given state.

Large employers have been able to avoid these costs by self-insuring under federal ERISA rules that exempt them from such requirements. That has placed the costs of benefit mandate compliance squarely on the shoulders of small employers and individuals who have no such option. AHIP, the insurance industry association, has estimated that 20% to 25% of the forty-six million uninsured have been forced out of the market because of the excessive costs of state-mandated benefits, as I related in chapter 4 in my discussion of the uninsured.

Although recognition and concern have grown over these mandates, the number of mandates continues to grow each year. Their proliferation has further blurred any distinction between prepayment for normal consumer purchases and true insurance against unaffordable health care events that few consumers can otherwise afford. Mandates are one of the most blatant examples of unchecked government intervention in health care.

The solution, however, is not to get government completely out of the business of regulating minimum benefits. Some degree of regulation is necessary for an optimal health insurance market to function (as I will explain later), but it must include the discipline to restrain favor-seeking special interests that offer no systemic value.

State High-Risk Pools, Guaranteed-Issue, and Insurance Reform

Currently, thirty-three states offer insurance-of-last-resort through their own high-risk pools. They had total enrollments of 190,361 people at the end of 2006. Overall, the premiums collected by these programs averaged approximately half of claims expenses. Florida's high-risk pool has been closed to new applicants since 1991 and has only 320 members. Probably twenty thousand people need it. Minnesota's, arguably the most successful, has 28,500 members, with premiums capped at 125% of standard insurance rates.[15]

Most states also allow uninsured residents to first seek insurance coverage from individual (i.e., non-group) insurers that require applicants to meet medical underwriting requirements through questionnaires, personal interviews, and medical record reviews. I have previously discussed why these individual insurer requirements are necessary to screen out individuals with significant current or previous health problems. Without medical underwriting, the insurers would quickly find themselves in an endless loop of inadequate premiums to pay claims, leading to higher premiums, fewer healthy subscribers, even higher losses, yet higher premiums, and so on, until insurers eventually fail or otherwise depart from the market.

Although individual insurers provide affordable insurance to more than sixteen million people, the process of medical underwriting further funnels people with significant illness risk into the ranks of the uninsured. Such individual insurance programs siphon off the healthier individuals, leaving the state guaranteed-issue programs with adversely selected risk pools. That is why the state program premiums cover only half of their claims expense.

An interesting aspect of these pools is that though they may accept those who are uninsurable by regular insurance companies, their losses are often covered by assessments on those same commercial insurers, which constitutes a dysfunctional separation of authority (by the states to set benefits, premiums, and enrollment standards) from responsibility (of the commercial insurers to pay for them). Only the political clout of the insurers stands between the states and their ability to insure more people at the insurers' expense. A more rational system would combine the authority and the responsibility under the same insurer's roof to allow everyone to buy insurance at affordable rates, as I discuss in chapter 9–12.

A number of reform advocates have promoted the expansion of such high-risk pools as a safety valve for those unable to get insurance either through an employer or via individual health insurance. Some even support getting rid of employer insurance altogether and having everyone apply for medically underwritten individual insurance. Those rejected would get somewhat more expensive—but still money-losing—coverage through the state high-risk pools.

Interestingly, some of the advocates of this approach consider themselves free-market adherents. Yet an odd consequence of expanding such high-risk pools is that the door is opened for employers and insurers to find ways to vector their sick members into those pools. This maneuver leaves the commercial insurers with the healthy folks, but the insurance companies still have to charge higher premiums to subsidize all the sick people in the risk pools. It's that negative externality problem I described earlier that makes your head hurt as individual insurers shed their high costs onto the broader base of all insurers. Each such insurer benefits itself by doing so but not the system as a whole. That's because when *all* insurers do it, they are all harmed, but none has any incentive to stop. The ultimate, theoretical end-point is that all sick people will end up in the state-run pools, with the healthy ones keeping their conventional insurance—until they become sick. At this point, another term should be applied to the risk-pool concept—single-payer—at least at the state level, because the state has effectively become the insurer for all sick people. This is not exactly what the free market folks have in mind.

Other states have tried to address the problem of the uninsured by simply forcing commercial insurers to take all comers, thus obviating the need for separate state-run risk pools. This is usually referred to as "guaranteed-issue" insurance. In 1996 Massachusetts tried it with individual health insurance reform that set standard benefits, required guaranteed-issue to all applicants, and imposed premium restrictions. As a predictable result, approximately twenty health insurers stopped selling coverage in the state, and others ceased writing any individual policies.[16] This failed program was replaced by new reform legislation in 2006 that mandated minimum coverage for all Massachusetts residents. To date, it is the only state to mandate universal coverage although its early experience suggests it has been far more successful in expanding state-paid insurance coverage than the self-paid variety. Massachusetts has failed to do anything effectively to restrain surging health care costs.[17] Other states with guaranteed-issue requirements include Maine, Vermont, New York, and New Jersey. Several other states have enacted modified forms of guaranteed-issue (e.g., California and Washington).

Overall, high-risk pools and guaranteed-issue have not caught on, due to high premiums, adverse selection, and difficulties with keeping willing insurers. There is still the problem of separation of authority and responsibility, with the states having the authority to force insurers to accept the responsibility. That's why these much-vaunted programs have succeeded in attracting only about 0.4% of America's forty-six million people who are uninsured either out of convenience (thirty-one million) or necessity (fifteen million).

Solving the uninsured problem with either high-risk pools or guaranteed-issue is much like eliminating the obesity problem by legislating a 25% reduction in the force of gravity. Fundamental economics (and physics) still apply.

"Any-Willing-Provider" and "Freedom of Choice" Laws

Any-willing-provider (AWP) laws have been defined as any "statutory requirement, adopted in some states, for managed-care plans to accept any health care provider willing to meet the plan's terms and conditions. The requirement eliminates a managed-care plan's screening process in developing quality and cost control programs."[18]

These laws, which are on the books in at least twenty-one states, might also be characterized as "low-quality provider protection acts" or "health insurance premium inflation acts" or possibly "health care provider competition prevention acts." Such laws have emanated solely from the lobbying efforts of—you guessed it—health care providers who can't effectively compete without them.

The presumption in AWP laws is that all doctors, pharmacists, hospitals, and chiropractors are created equal. Thus, by virtue of being licensed, they must be treated the same by health insurers that might otherwise wish to offer higher volumes exclusively to a more limited number of providers that offer lower prices and higher quality than run-of-the-mill providers.

You might also call it the anti-Lake Wobegon Effect. No health plan is allowed to contract selectively with providers that are above average. In an Orwellian twist, proponents of such laws have argued that they actually want to improve quality by allowing patients greater access to doctors providing higher quality. The operative assumption is that health plans will otherwise contract with lower-quality doctors and other providers.

AWP's ugly stepsister, with similar effects, is the "Freedom of Choice" (FOC) laws, which require health plans to pay for services received by plan members from non-contracting providers.

Why should we care? Because such laws decrease competition and increase costs of health care. The Federal Trade Commission has analyzed these laws for years and stated unequivocally:

> When insurers have a credible threat to exclude providers from their networks and channel patients elsewhere, providers have a powerful incentive to bid aggressively. Inclusion in a restricted panel offers the provider the prospect of substantially increased sales opportunities. Without such credible threats, however, providers have less incentive to bid aggressively, and even managed-care organizations with large market shares may have less ability to obtain low prices.[19]

Overall, the FTC has concluded that such laws have the unwelcome consequences of limiting competition, undermining freedom of choice, and increasing health care costs. These conclusions have been borne out by various studies, including one by FTC economist Michael Vita showing that AWP and FOC laws have increased health care costs by 2% in the states that aggressively utilize them.[20] On the off chance that 2% strikes you as not worth the bother, consider that it is equal to roughly $19 billion in total waste if applied on a national scale. Legend has it that the late Senator Everett Dirksen once intoned in his mellifluous baritone, "A billion here, a billion there; pretty soon you're talking real money." Or in the words of the old soul tune, "Every little bit hurts."

Such anti-competitive laws have no place in a rational health care system.

"Corporate Practice of Medicine" Prohibitions

Many states prohibit doctors from practicing medicine as employees of corporations. There are sometimes exceptions, but only for hospitals and for professional corporations in which only doctors can own stock. Even in states without explicit laws prohibiting corporate practice, various state attorneys general have ruled it to be prohibited. Other states take similar positions via case law. Some states take a more permissive approach to doctors practicing medicine as employees of corporations as long as the corporation does not interfere with the physician's independent medical judgment. Such prohibitions arise from the concept "that individual physicians should be licensed to practice medicine not corporations.... The basic premise is the divided loyalty and impaired confidence between the interests of a corporation and the needs of a patient."[21]

In a 1992 article I described the medical profession as the last priesthood that operates according to the principles of the medieval guild.[22] The medical profession enjoys a state-enforced monopoly, requires excessively long education and apprenticeship, employs arcane language, often involves distinctive dress and accoutrements, and is ever aggressive in defending its monopoly against encroachment by other health care professions or innovative organizational structures.

This point was reinforced in a 2004 article by University of Kentucky College of Law Professor Nicole Huberfeld, who concluded that "the corporate practice of medicine doctrine is a physician-centric, guild type doctrine that is misplaced in the present incarnation of the American healthcare system and that does nothing to improve quality, efficiency, or accountability."[23] Prof. Huberfeld points out that such laws are based on outmoded conceptions of traditional physician practice, in which doctors practice autonomously, are unmotivated by financial gain, and guarantee high-quality health care.

She argues that CPOM prohibitions may indeed block genuine attempts to improve the quality of care.

CPOM restrictions also help perpetuate high medical costs by preventing innovations that may require more capital, higher doctor productivity, entrepreneurial vigor, nontraditional thinking, greater consumer choice, and greater flexibility in personnel skill sets and deployment. Harvard Business School professor Clayton Christenson has stated flatly, "The lack of business model innovation in the health-care industry—in many cases because regulators have not permitted it—is the reason health care is unaffordable.... The situation screams for business model innovation."[24] Overall, the CPOM doctrine perpetuates a romantic myth of the lone Marcus Welby-like doctor saving lives against all odds and without concern for personal financial reward or sacrifice. It may be an admirable notion, but it's hardly something to be enshrined in laws that are blind to the realities of contemporary medical practice as well as economic and moral consequences.

Speaking of being blind to economic consequences, we'll next explore the aptly-named COBRA act, which has been biting former employees and small employers since its inception more than two decades ago.

COBRA

In 1985 President Reagan signed into law the Consolidated Omnibus Reconciliation Act (COBRA) that allows terminated employees of most employers to continue their group insurance for up to eighteen months by paying the employer's group premium rate. It also allows families to continue such coverage for up to thirty-six months when death or divorce would otherwise terminate their eligibility. The law was an attempt to provide temporary insurance portability to workers and families insured through employer-sponsored health plans. There are approximately five million former employees covered by COBRA.

A 1998 analysis of the program by University of Chicago Professor Brigitte Madrian indicated that though COBRA has enabled workers to achieve improved job mobility and access to early retirement, the cost to employers—particularly small employers—has been significant.[25]

The problem lies in COBRA's strong tendency toward adverse selection. At least three factors are relevant:

1. *Big Premium Increase*: A terminated employee who opts for COBRA is required to pay 102% of the entire premium cost of his employer-sponsored health insurance. This constitutes a big increase in his premiums, since employees, on average, pay only about 25% of group insurance premiums—the employer's 75% contribution being invisible to employees until applying for COBRA.[26] Employees are usually shocked to learn how much complete coverage really costs: an average of $12,680 for families and $4,704 for individuals in 2008.[27] In February of 2009 federal economic stimulus legislation added a temporary relief program for laid-off workers by providing a federal subsidy for nine months to cover 65% of COBRA premiums.[28] Even with this limited exception, insurance prices under COBRA represent an insurmountable hurdle for most workers. That is why fewer than 10% of eligible workers opted for it during 2007, and those who did tended to do so because of family illness that makes it impossible to obtain individual insurance. Thus, COBRA inherently contributes to adverse selection.

2. *No Option for Reduced Benefits or Cost*: An employee electing COBRA can purchase only the same health plan she had at the time she left her employment, even if the employer offers other lower-cost benefit options. The 2009 economic stimulus legislation removed this limitation for COBRA-eligible workers who were laid off between September 1, 2008, and December 31, 2009. Anyone else must wait to change during the next employer open enrollment period. Normally, if a person has a particularly

expensive high-option plan, then she is much less likely to opt for it under COBRA unless she knows her health care costs will be greater than the premium. This too worsens adverse selection.

3. *Community-Rated Premiums*: The employer can charge COBRA premiums to the former employee only on the same basis it charges its workers. That means a departing twenty-two-year-old must pay the same premium as a departing sixty-four-year-old worker, despite the fact that the former can be expected to incur a small fraction of the health care expenses of the latter. This situation further increases the likelihood that only former employees who anticipate significant medical expenses will buy the coverage.

Thus younger and healthier workers are much less likely to buy COBRA coverage, opting instead for lower-cost individual insurance or no insurance at all. The result is a further skewing of the COBRA risk pool toward a higher level of risk than for the overall employer pool. According to Prof. Madrian, the costs of COBRA-coverage are 50% higher than active worker coverage

It is important to recognize that the employer is still providing the COBRA insurance. They are therefore responsible for paying any difference between the COBRA enrollee's premium payments and the employer's actual health care premiums or costs incurred under the plan. These higher costs are disproportionately borne by small employers. Just a few people with COBRA can make it impossible for a company to continue any insurance coverage for any of its workers.

COBRA has had two perverse effects:

1. *Harm to Small Employers*: COBRA has contributed to an increase in the number of small business employees who can no longer afford health insurance. Thus, it can have the effect of actually eliminating some of the insurance portability that it was designed to provide.

2. *Limited Applicability*: COBRA does not apply to workers who lose their jobs because their employers either went out of business or otherwise terminated their insurance coverage. This has become a serious issue for many of the hundreds of thousands who have lost their jobs during the economic downturn that began in late 2007.

Portability is a worthy and achievable goal of health reform. COBRA, however, is another of the many examples of legislation that too narrowly focuses on a particular issue without taking into account the unwanted negative consequences that result.

HIPAA

No, HIPAA does not stand for the Health Industry Papers America Act—although anyone who has thrown away reams of health care privacy information provided by doctors, hospitals, and pharmacies could well suspect a conspiracy to convert every tree on the planet into confetti. Instead, it is an acronym for the Health Insurance Portability and Accountability Act of 1996. Despite its title suggesting that health insurance would become portable as a result of the law (it hasn't), it is mostly known for its efforts to protect the confidential sanctity of our individual medical information.

HIPAA regulations set privacy and security standards for providers and insurers. It prescribes grievous penalties for failure to meet them. And it has terrified pine forests nationwide. The guts of the HIPAA law are contained in the virtually impenetrable Section II, called—without a whiff of intended irony—"Administrative Simplification." The public face of HIPAA is the privacy protection requirement to which most us have been exposed whenever we receive medical care.

In the highly likely case you haven't actually read these provider handouts, HIPAA requires that patients: (1) be informed about the practices for disclosing and using your protected health information (PHI); (2) give written consent for the use and disclosure of such information for treatment, payment, and healthcare operations; (3) have the right of access to their own health information and to amend this information if it is incomplete or incorrect.

HIPAA's use of the term *portability* is a misnomer. It doesn't involve anyone taking her current health insurance policy from one employer to another or from an employer into individual coverage (see COBRA discussion above). Rather, it allows certain employees and former employees to purchase new group or individual health insurance under very limited circumstances.

In the group market, certain employees who previously declined their employer's coverage are now allowed to enroll later in such coverage outside of normal employer open enrollment periods. Generally, the employee must have just lost other "creditable" coverage, exhausted previous COBRA enrollment benefits, or added new dependents within the past thirty days. HIPAA also has provisions that may limit group insurance exclusions for preexisting conditions and that prohibit discrimination based on employee or dependent health status.

The HIPAA code also includes provisions that may help people get individual insurance through a health insurance company. If you're not an attorney, you may want to skip the rest of this paragraph, although it does help clarify why laws are also called codes. Essentially, if a person who seeks health insurance *and* lacks current insurance or eligibility for coverage under an employer, COBRA, Medicare, or Medicaid plan; *and* who does not have group continuation coverage; *and* who has had employer group health coverage for at least eighteen months before applying (unless a dependent enrolled as such under a group health plan within thirty days of birth, adoption, or placement for adoption *and* has not had a significant break in coverage); *and* who didn't lose the previous coverage because of fraud or nonpayment; *and* who is requesting coverage within sixty-three days of losing his old coverage; *and* who resides in the individual insurer's network service area (if any); *then* he or she *may* be able to purchase guaranteed renewable insurance in the individual market on a guaranteed-issue basis without preexisting condition exclusions. HIPAA does *not*, however, provide portability from one individual policy to another. The code also allows states to set up alternate, less restrictive eligibility requirements.

Overall, the HIPPA group-to-individual portability rules incorporate loopholes big enough for insurers to drive a bus through to restrict or deny such coverage. One such exception is that an insurer offering health insurance only through one or more bona fide associations is not required to offer such coverage in the individual market. Since it is a common practice for individual insurers to offer coverage only through associations, it would appear that they have eliminated any need to offer coverage to HIPAA-eligible individuals. If anyone you know has actually obtained individual insurance under HIPAA, then I congratulate that person for persistence and bureaucratic navigational skills. One may legitimately wonder why HIPAA's group-to-individual portability provisions were ever enacted. Maybe it was a sop to the printers-ink special interest group.

Another significant aspect of HIPAA has received little public notice: its requirement for the standardization of all patient health, administrative, and financial data used in electronic data interchange between and among health care providers, insurers, pharmacy benefit managers, government agencies, and other users and processors of such information. The purpose is to replace the existing Babel of inconsistent data sets and formats with a single set of standards, which is supposed to reduce administrative complexity and ultimately facilitate simpler, lower-cost electronic transfer of information—i.e., a transition away from the paper-based systems that have held the health care industry in the dark ages of information processing and transmission technology.

At its best, HIPAA will help birth a new era of efficient provider reimbursement systems, ubiquitous electronic medical records, reduced administrative costs, and improved medical research. At its worst, it will perpetuate opaque medical pricing, prevent innovative pricing models, increase regulatory compliance costs, fill yet more prison cells with perpetrators of newly invented federal crimes, and further retard innovation with stultifying regulatory control in place of more flexible market mechanisms. It's still too early to tell how it will pan out.

Specialty Hospital Limitations

The subject of specialty hospitals is a convoluted one, involving issues of potential physician conflicts of interest, community hospital fears of competition, Medicare reimbursement rates, and how government, rather than the market, has become the arbiter for every player with a dog in the fight. In a more market-driven health care environment, arguably none of these issues would be relevant, either economically or politically. There would be little need for government to involve itself in what is essentially an issue of competition among health care providers.

Specialty hospitals are inpatient institutions that focus on patients who need treatment for specific medical conditions, typically cardiac, orthopedic, women's medicine, or surgical. They are usually contrasted with nonprofit community general hospitals that provide a much broader variety of health care services. Specialty hospitals are usually for-profit. They are often owned, at least in part, by physicians who refer to and work in them.

In 2003 the GAO counted one hundred specialty hospitals in twenty-seven states, with another twenty-six under development. By 2009 the number had increased to two hundred (out of six thousand total hospitals nationwide) with eighty-five in development.[29] Specialty hospitals tend to be concentrated in states without certificate of need (CON) requirements for hospital construction (see CON discussion above), largely because the nonprofit community hospitals have been able to block them under CON rules.[30]

The Controversy

The crux of the controversy surrounding specialty hospitals was summarized by the GAO in a report to Congress in 2003:

Advocates of these newer specialty hospitals contend that the focused mission and dedicated resources of specialty hospitals allow physicians to treat more patients needing the same specialty services than they could in general hospitals and that, through such specialization and economies of scale, the potential exists to improve quality and reduce costs. In contrast, critics are concerned that specialty hospitals may concentrate on the most profitable procedures and serve patients that have fewer complicating conditions—leaving general hospitals with a sicker, higher-cost patient population. They contend that this practice of drawing away a more favorable selection of patients makes it more financially difficult for general hospitals to fulfill their broad mission to serve all of a community's needs, including charity care, emergency services, and stand-by capacity to respond to community wide disasters. Critics have also raised concerns that physician ownership of specialty hospitals creates financial incentives that could inappropriately affect physicians' clinical and referral behavior.[31]

The issue of whether specialty hospitals reduce costs for customers is largely moot for now. Hospital pricing to third-party payers, especially Medicare and Medicaid, is usually set by the payer without regard to a particular hospital's cost structure or posted pricing (which is almost completely irrelevant to anything). Because of that, hospitals rarely compete on the basis of price. Thus, any cost reductions achieved by a specialty hospital may certainly improve its bottom line but not its competitive standing.

It's certainly possible for such a hospital to negotiate a lower reimbursement rate with private payers, especially if it gives the hospital a preferred position in the payer's provider network against competing community hospitals. That is difficult to do in many communities and impossible in the states with any-willing-provider laws. In general, the cost savings argument, though having a lot of potential in a market-driven, price-competitive health care system, doesn't hold much water under the current system of payer-fixed reimbursements.

On the quality front, specialty hospital proponents argue that the increased volume of a limited number of specialty procedures improves quality, lowers complication rates, reduces infection rates, and lowers return-to-surgery rates. Opponents point to the lack of emergency treatment facilities or on-site doctors at all hours. It is noteworthy that general hospitals, despite heavy quality regulation by government and private organizations (e.g., the Joint Commission), have hardly covered themselves in glory on the quality front. Their medical errors cause ninety-eight thousand deaths a year—more than caused by AIDS, breast cancer, or car accidents.[32]

Comparing specialty and general hospitals, *Forbes* magazine cited a University of Iowa study showing that specialty hospital patients have experienced 40% lower complication rates for hip and knee surgeries than similar patients in community hospitals.[33] *Forbes* also reported on a 2006 Medicare-funded study finding that orthopedic patients were four times as likely to die at a community hospital as in a specialty hospital and that a HealthGrades top-ten quality ranking included three specialty hospitals in South Dakota, Indiana, and Texas.

The cherry-picking argument is that specialty hospitals, by focusing only on the most profitable services, skim off such business from the community general hospitals. The latter need those profits to subsidize their money-losing services, such as emergency rooms and charity care. In a market-based health care economy, this problem would be largely nonexistent or irrelevant. It would be like criticizing BMW for skimming the high-margin end of the car market and thus depriving GM of the Cadillac sales necessary to subsidize its money-losing Pontiac division.

What we really have here is a failure of pricing and cost accounting. If a specialty heart hospital offers a lower price than a community hospital (assuming equal quality), then shouldn't that be where people get their heart surgery? If that means the community hospital has to lower its prices, become more efficient, and strive for better quality, isn't that a good thing? Not—according to the critics—if the community hospital is now forced to lose money on its emergency room and thus risk having to shut it down—or, worse, having the hospital go out of business.

Under a market-based system, a money-losing emergency room is really either under-pricing its services or being inefficient in providing those services—or both. These are problems that any competent firm in a competitive market knows how to deal with. They require management action, perhaps to increase prices and to improve productivity. That could include the judicious application of process reengineering, employee training and redeployment, product redesign, and prudent capital investment. This approach could be especially useful in, for example, triaging non-emergent patients into less-intensive and less-expensive urgent care treatment facilities, which could reduce ER demand and allow services to become better focused, more efficient, and more appropriately priced.

Today, the obvious barrier to such a management approach is that hospitals have a very limited ability to set their own prices. CMS simply tells hospitals how much it will pay them for various services that CMS alone decides. Thus, the profitability of a given hospital service is determined not by the hospital's ability to succeed in a competitive environment but by the arcana of CMS's pricing rules. Without the ability to set prices according to market conditions, general hospitals are understandably upset about having their most profitable services siphoned off by specialty hospitals. Absent a market solution, they see their only rational response as opposing such facilities through political and bureaucratic channels.

The anti-specialty hospital forces have been remarkably successful at enlisting government to their cause. Specialty hospitals have been almost completely stonewalled in the certificate of need states. Opponents were also successful in pushing through an amendment to the Medicare Modernization Act of 2003 (MMA) that actually banned new physician-owned specialty hospital construction for eighteen months on a nationwide basis.[34] In April 2008 pro-specialty hospital forces were barely able to block congressional legislation included in, of all places, the massive Farm Bill. It would have ended the ability of physicians to refer patients to specialty hospitals that they own. Both sides will doubtless continue their efforts.

Specialty hospitals do indeed offer the promise of better quality and lower cost that can result from high-volume specialization. (For two brilliant discussions of the promise of such "focused factories," I recommend Regina Herzlinger's *Market-Driven Health Care: Who Wins, Who Loses in the Transformation of America's Largest Service Industry* and Clayton Christensen's *The Innovator's Prescription*.) Unfortunately, the current government-dominated health care payment system precludes ever seeing that promise fulfilled. Since specialty hospitals cannot compete for patients on price or quality, they have had to rely on an alternate method of ensuring a steady stream of patients, most of whom would otherwise flow to the competing community hospitals.

The marketing mechanism specialty hospitals have most commonly chosen is the offer of lucrative low-cost ownership positions to the doctors they depend on for their patient admissions. Such arrangements are allowed under a specific exception to federal law—the so-called Stark II law—which otherwise prohibits many physician self-dealing practices. The exception allows a doctor to own a hospital stake if she has privileges to practice at that facility, but not if she doesn't. I know, it doesn't make any sense to me either.

There may yet be isolated holdouts somewhere in this country who still believe that doctors' self-abnegating ethical principles prevent them from admitting patients to one hospital over another because of personal financial gain. Nonetheless, specialty hospital entrepreneurs have discovered the value of offering dedicated, high-quality, specialized facilities to admitting physicians who want an excellent operating environment, dedicated staff, and a Mercedes SL600.

There is nothing inherently bad about people owning stakes in businesses in which they work. If there were, then every independent retail store and restaurant owner in America would have a serious conflict of interest. The reason they aren't a problem is that their customers are spending their own money to meet their own needs. They are able to decide whether the offered wares and meals represent acceptable values.

The problem with physician-owned hospitals is that their consumers don't give a whit about how much money the hospitals charge their insurance companies. Consumers also have no standing to demand information on hospital quality. The result: Consumers have no say in the value proposition offered by hospitals. That leaves the door wide open for the hospitals' doctors and owners to spend a lot more of insurers' money than they could if their patients had the incentives and the clout to demand accountability on quality and price. I realize that many people will view such thinking as bizarre, but that just attests to the degree to which they have come to accept the current system as the natural order of things. It's not.

Nonprofit community hospitals are quick to cry foul when for-profit specialty hospitals invade their turf. The specialty hospitals counter that they have to pay taxes on their profits and real estate, but the community hospitals get an unfair advantage from not having to pay them at all. The community hospitals are increasingly vulnerable on this count.

Nonprofit hospitals account for 77% of all private community hospitals.[35] According to a report in *The Wall Street Journal*,[36] nonprofit hospitals receive $12.6 billion in annual tax exemptions, enough to pay for a lot of indigent care and to cover a lot of emergency room losses. That is on top of a CBO estimate of $32 billion in other hospital industry subsidies from federal, state, and local sources.[37] Until the 1960s the IRS held nonprofit hospitals to the "charity care" standard that required a hospital to provide free services to those unable to pay to the extent of its financial ability. Since then, the IRS has applied the rather nebulous "community benefit" standard, requiring only that a tax-exempt hospital must promote health for the benefit of the community—arguably a barrier that any hospital can surmount, regardless of how niggardly it might be in providing free care to indigent patients.

Many nonprofit hospitals have been criticized for acting like their for-profit cousins. Some have moved to the suburbs, away from their inner city roots. They pay executive compensation exceeding $1 million a year in many cases. Perhaps a more level playing field between them and their for-profit specialty competitors might include some sort of tax equity.

The long-term solutions to the issues of skimming, quality, and conflicts of interest lie not in increased government regulation and prohibition. They must emerge from a functioning hospital market system that eliminates the deadweight costs of legislative favor seeking by rationalizing prices, encouraging quality measurement (and improvement), and rendering self-dealing practices uncompetitively expensive by engaging value-conscious consumers.

A major problem now is that hospitals either don't have or don't apply sophisticated cost-accounting processes that would allow them to more rationally price the various services they provide. There would be little point under current reimbursement rules. Market-based pricing, however, would allow them to establish pricing regimes to incorporate actual service costs, patient value, competitors' pricing, and process-improvement strategies. These measures would work wonders to end the current micro-socialism of having a few highly profitable services underwrite the unprofitable ones.

Instead, each hospital service would float on its own financial bottom. Community hospitals would no longer need nor want to provide some services if the specialty "focused factory" hospitals[38] advocated by Regina Herzlinger could sell the same services with better quality and lower prices.

Money-losing ER services would be reengineered and repriced to eliminate losses. Hospitals would certainly be under the gun to achieve improved efficiencies of operation. But consumers and insurers may have no choice but to pay higher prices. This assumes, of course, that other services prices would also fall.

Alternatively, Clayton Christensen, in his book *The Innovator's Prescription*, suggests another pricing approach. He argues that "solution shops," like diagnosis-focused community hospitals, should be able to charge on the basis of the cost of their inputs. At the same time, "value added process shops," like the specialty hospitals, should charge prices according to the value of their outputs.[39]

Whatever pricing methodology proves best, it makes no sense to restrict the growth of innovative providers just because they force legacy providers to change how they do business. We need a system that allows both to flourish by finding their own niches in a rational health care financing and delivery system that optimizes the use of scarce resources to meet the medical needs of all Americans.

EMTALA Patient Anti-Dumping Statute

In 1986 President Reagan signed into law the Emergency Medical Treatment and Active Labor Act (EMTALA). It requires all hospitals participating in Medicare or Medicaid to provide emergency medical services to any individual who requests emergency or outpatient department assistance, regardless of ability to pay. Required services include appropriate medical screening to determine whether an emergency condition exists, stabilization of the emergency condition, and transfer to other facilities as necessary to achieve stabilization. Failure to do so can result in heavy civil penalties and damages against both hospitals and doctors. Flagrant failures can cause a hospital to be excluded from the Medicare and Medicaid programs.

Christopher Conover and Emily Zeitler of Duke University have estimated that EMTALA has increased total hospital costs by $4.4 billion per year while generating benefits of $2.1 billion, resulting in a net program cost of $2.3 billion. The benefits of EMTALA are at least theoretically achieved by reducing avoidable deaths and disabilities and by expanding access to care for individuals who would otherwise not be allowed to use emergency facilities. Since EMTALA is an unfunded mandate, this cost must ultimately be borne by American consumers in the form of higher insurance premiums, copayments, and payroll and income taxes.[40] Put another way, EMTALA has been an additional source of provider cost-shifting imposed on the public by the government. Under a market-based system, the universal availability of affordable health insurance and enhanced charity care requirements for nonprofit hospitals offer a more rational approach.

The above programs hardly constitute a comprehensive reckoning of governments' sometime misguided, always piecemeal efforts to fix health care. There are many more, such as the Stark anti-kickback laws, the Veterans Administration medical system, the TRICARE program for veterans and military dependents, and our tort system that constitutes the worst, most inefficient quality-assurance program imaginable.

Yet, arguably, all of these government laws, programs, restrictions, and unfunded mandates have resulted from well-intentioned legislative, common law, and administrative efforts to address real human needs and problems. Lacking in the process has been any sort of overarching economic philosophy within which these programs are required to mesh and against which they can be evaluated and improved. The result is this Frankenstein monster of a system that we wistfully characterize as "the best medical care in the world." Lost in a legislative process that only the Johnsonville Sausage company could love is any effective political application of Hippocrates' medical advice "to tell the antecedents, know the present, and foretell the future…and have two special objects in view…namely, to do good or to do no harm."[41]

To move forward, we much accept that what the government has wrought isn't working for us. More of the same incremental law-smithing won't improve matters. At the same time, government must have a role in the process. Therein lies the conundrum. How do we establish a proper government role to restrain what needs to be restrained in the private sector but without causing it to suffer from undue government interference and endless congressional tinkering afterward?

Federal Reserve Chairman Benjamin Bernanke has suggested two possible alternatives for tackling this problem.[42] The first would be for Congress to enact something along the lines of the military base closure process. An independent commission would make recommendations that the Congress must either accept or reject without amendment. The second option would be to establish an independent Federal Reserve-like commission to set health policy. Like the Fed, it would have a high degree of independence from Congress.

Both ideas have the advantage of insulating the Congress from the kind of special interest favor seeking to which it has become so vulnerable, although, as Michael Cannon has observed,[43] the insulation is far from perfect. Under such a regime, Congress's role would be limited to legislating a new system, turning over regulation to a quasi-independent body, and then deciding on annual appropriations to fund the various safety net provisions under reformed Medicare, Medicaid, SCHIP, TRICARE, and veterans programs.

Whatever the process, we must reform and rationalize health care around principles that incorporate the essential government role of regulation and social support while maximizing the self-organizing forces of market capitalism to enable every American to obtain affordable, accessible, high-quality health care. Such a system is not only possible but can be done in a manner consistent with America's democratic principles of freedom of choice and social justice. Our country needs it, and the world could learn from it.

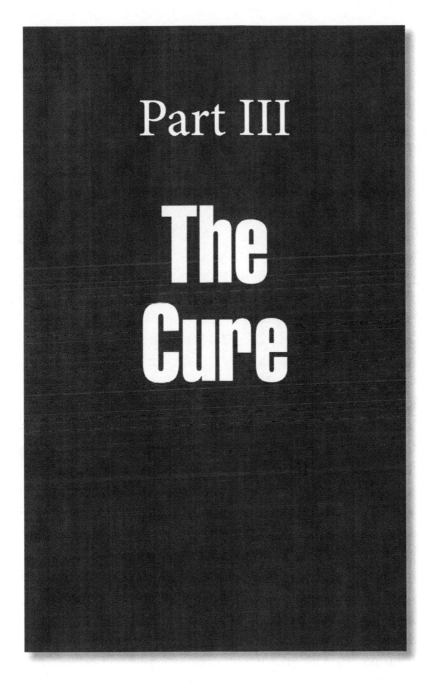

Part III

The Cure

PART III—THE CURE

I have discussed at length how and why the nation's health care spending has grown at a substantially faster rate than inflation over the past forty years and how this dynamic has shown no sign of abating. I've also discussed the reasons why that dynamic is unlikely to change as long as we maintain anything like the current structure of our health care financing and delivery system. Still, if we're willing to assume that our economy will attain similar growth rates over the coming decades as it has during the past six, it appears that the country will actually be able to afford many more years of this economic imbalance before the point at which the *dollar* growth in annual health care spending exceeds the *dollar* growth in the economy. At that point, our national standard of living will begin to decline. For the sake of brevity, let's call it the "Reinhardt Point" after the principal author of the article that laid out this scenario and that I delved into in chapter 2.[1]

The Reinhardt Point is the clear, algebraic result of a linear projection of recent trends into the future. What is not so clear is how much longer we will be able to tolerate the current health care growth rate *at the margin*, as more and more workers are driven out of conventional private insurance and into whatever inflationary band-aid programs (if any) are erected by the Obama-led government and as Medicare's unfunded liabilities begin to have real-world ramifications outside of the dry, largely unread reports of the Medicare trust fund.[2] I suspect there will be a tipping point long before the Reinhardt Point arrives. Let's call it the Arthur Point after the economist who coined the term "complexity economics," an emerging theory of economies as nonlinear complex adaptive systems.[3] When we reach the Arthur Point, all bets are off. That's when the current health care system simply and suddenly breaks down, whether economically, socially, politically, or name-your-poison-ally. When (or if) the Arthur Point will arrive is, by definition, objectively unpredictable, as were the late twentieth century demise of the Soviet Empire and the early twenty-first century economic meltdown in the United States.

A key question is whether we will have the political will to make the necessary changes to our health care financing and delivery system soon enough to preclude the Arthur Point altogether. Either we will or we won't, but either way we will be faced with having to make major structural changes to health care as we know it. The question is whether we will do that in the midst of crisis or in a more orderly manner with attendant research, debate, and clearheaded thinking. I won't guess which way it will go—although I am not optimistic.

In my view, when we do make the necessary changes, they will flow from our having made a national choice of moving in one of two more or less opposite directions. One direction will take us on the well-worn path blazed by countries like Canada, Sweden, and the United Kingdom that leads to some sort of government-run system. The purest form of such a system is commonly called "single payer," meaning that the government disburses all the funds from a fixed annual budget to pay for all its citizens' essential, permitted health care services. The single-payer approach has one major advantage over the market-based approach: It has been shown to work—albeit not under conditions that are necessarily consistent with the rights and civil liberties—or the economic principles—traditional to the United States. The U.K.'s National Health Service has been functioning more or less acceptably for British subjects since 1948, with Sweden's and Canada's programs being somewhat younger.

The second direction will require us to blaze our own trail, leading us to create a market-based system, albeit under the rule of law in the form of a much lighter government role of social safety nets and of regulation to ensure that the market operates within parameters established to meet our health care goals. Comprehensive market-based systems don't exist in any advanced country that I know of. To the extent that market principles are observed at all, they appear as bits and pieces within largely government-dominated systems, such as those in Switzerland, France, Singapore,[4] and the United States. To assemble the parts of a comprehensive, market-based system, one has to seek out these often-isolated pieces and assemble them into an appropriately regulated but definitely market-based health care financing and delivery system. There are no existing models. Perhaps that is why so much of the debate about national health reform in the United States has focused on the pros and cons of various government-dominated approaches rather than on the relative merits of two fully-formed, competing economic concepts: government-dominated plans on one side and market-directed ones on the other.

I like to think I am not inherently biased against a single-payer system and that my opposition to it is founded on facts and principles that have demonstrable truthfulness about them. But I'm not going to tell you I'm unbiased because (1) you wouldn't believe me, and (2) it's undoubtedly not true. Thus, the concluding chapters of this book are not evenly weighted between single-payer and market-based systems. Chapter 8 is my take on the issues of adopting a single-payer system in the United States. I've tried to keep it factual, leaving my more trenchant thoughts to myself. Chapters 9 through 12, as well as the conclusion, are the point of this entire book: how to engineer the necessary, diverse, and often tried-and-true components of a market-based health care system into one that will achieve the eight ambitious goals I laid out in chapter 1.

My hope is that when we finally achieve (or have thrust upon us) the political will to accept the challenge of revolutionizing our health care financing and delivery system, we will then make our decisions based on a vigorous debate about credible, workable alternatives on both the government-run and market-based sides of the question.

CHAPTER 8

Why Not Single Payer?

*"If you think health care is expensive now, wait until
you see how much it costs when it's free."*
—P.J. O'ROURKE

U nder most single-payer proposals the U.S. Government would
replace all health insurance companies, HMOs, and managed-
care organizations with a single, Medicare-like payment mechanism.
Some proposals are even simpler—to have Medicare take over the
entire job of paying for all health care for all Americans, much like
the United Kingdom's National Health Service or Canada's Medicare
system.

Congressman Pete Stark, an adherent of Medicare for All (MFA),
has written:

> To maximize profits and shareholder confidence, insurance
> companies, health care providers and drug companies have
> manipulated the system beyond comprehension.... Thank-
> fully, the cure is not nearly as complicated as the disease.
> There is a road map laid out for us: a program that already
> delivers universal healthcare to nearly 42 million Ameri-
> cans. And it is simple: Workers pay into the system while
> they're young, and when they turn 65 the government pays
> their health insurance.... Medicare has lower administrative
> costs than any private plan on the market. It enjoys one of
> the highest approval ratings of any government program. But
> the most important reason Medicare is the best model for an

expansion of healthcare benefits is that the program focuses on patients, not profits.[1]

Congressman John Conyers says that MFA would cover

all medically necessary services, including primary care, inpatient care, outpatient care, emergency care, prescription drugs, durable medical equipment, hearing services, long-term care, mental health services, dentistry, eye care, chiropractic, and substance abuse treatment. Patients have their choice of physicians, providers, hospitals, clinics, and practices. No co-pays or deductibles are permissible under this act.

Rep. Conyers claims that his plan would save $387 billion per year while reducing long-term inflation "from reduced administration, bulk purchasing, and coordination among providers."[2] *New York Times* columnist, self-professed liberal, and economics Nobel laureate Paul Krugman claims, "In purely economic terms, single-payer is clearly the way to go. A single-payer system, with its low administrative costs and strong ability to bargain over prices, would deliver more health care, at lower cost, than the alternatives."[3]

Most adherents of MFA or other single-payer approaches assert the following benefits:

1. *A single, comprehensive benefit plan for all*: This would be the ultimate in benefit simplicity, with no more of the thousands of confusing benefit plans, insurance company fine print, hidden exclusions, inter-company benefit variations, individual company interpretations, arguments over what is covered, or the Byzantine billing and collection activities that one authority claims "consume as much as 31 cents of every health care dollar."[4] Everyone would be included, eliminating the need for costly eligibility determinations by Medicaid, SCHIP, and medical providers. There would be one well-defined benefit plan for all.

2. *Administrative simplicity and efficiency*: It is often claimed that the Medicare program consumes only 2% of each health care dollar in administrative, marketing, and overhead costs, as opposed to insurance company rates of 20–25%.[5] Since Medicare denies far fewer claims than do private insurers, there would be no more ever-escalating games between providers trying to maximize re-imbursements and insurers trying to minimize them. Reduced claims delays and denials would result from standard rules for all rather than the Babel of conflicting policies, procedures, and computer systems in the current system. Proponents claim total administrative savings would be in the neighborhood of $400 billion per year, about 17% of total health care costs.

3. *MFA would expand an existing program*: There would be no need to create new agencies or payment mechanisms. Medicare has been in business providing for Americans' health care needs since the 1960s. It has an efficient, popular, well-run administrative and financial structure.

4. *Universal coverage* would eliminate all forty-six million uninsured at the stroke of a pen, with much of the added cost being covered by administrative savings and efficiencies.

5. *Consistent provider payment schedules and procedures*: Cost-shifting by hospitals and doctors among different payers would be eliminated since there would be only one payer. Providers would save billions on the personnel and the computer systems now needed to juggle the different reimbursement rules and requirements of many different insurers. Instead, they would submit all bills to Medicare and its single, well-defined set of administrative procedures and reimbursement rates.

6. *Electronic medical record savings*: A single-payer system accompanied by government assistance and mandates to require doctors and hospitals to replace outmoded paper-based medical records with electronic records would generate many billions in additional savings.

7. *Well-established international precedents*: Virtually every other major industrialized country in the world has a government-run system that works, including Canada, the United Kingdom, and France. In the U.K. and Canada everyone gets great, high-quality health care for free—everyone.

At least on the surface, such arguments are compelling. If you don't believe me, you haven't seen the movie *Sicko*, with its effective use of selective facts and anecdotes that push all the right emotional buttons in support of a single-payer system. Actually, I have to admit I didn't see it all, having dozed off during Michael Moore's paean to the Cuban health care system (even my dedication to intellectually honest research can stand only so much). But I still found the movie emotionally powerful at the same time that my rational, reasonably objective side knew it was sheep-dip (and I mean that in the most unbiased way possible).

Let's look at these arguments more closely:

A Government-Mandated Benefit Plan

Perhaps the most puzzling claim is that MFA would be simple. Medicare may be many things, but simple is not one of them. In 1998 a bipartisan commission reported that there were more than 100,000 pages of Medicare regulations and supporting documents.[6] Regulations just on health care providers published between 1982 and 1998 covered thirty-four thousand pages.[7] And that doesn't include the masses of guidelines, proposed regulations, manuals, forms, brochures, and other documents required by the system.

A quick survey of Medicare's history in the decade since that study suggests that these numbers have not since declined. Health care providers live in continual fear of running afoul of Medicare's rules, which can transform a civil infraction into a criminal infarction. Because Medicare's top-down rules replace any normal market functioning, they are necessarily complex to an almost unimaginable extent. They are often ambiguous, internally inconsistent, subject to different administrative interpretations, and continually changing to deal with the unintended consequences that have arisen therefrom. Simplicity is no hallmark of Medicare.

Even so, at least a single set of benefits under MFA would be simpler than the current profusion of private insurance coverages. But is that a good thing? American consumers, long accustomed to making their own consumption choices, may not adjust well to a one-size-fits-all health insurance program any more than they want the government making them all buy identical automobiles. It is in the nature of market-enabled consumers that they want to choose products and services that best meet their own needs. They don't like paying for things they don't want. They like even less being told they have to have something they don't need or that they can't have something they want just because some bureaucrat says it's not "approved." Having an employer force them to accept arbitrary benefits is hard enough, but having the government do it may be something else again. Employers are at least held to some competitive standards, however imperfect, in deciding what to offer their employees. Government is not.

In response, MFA proponents might well argue that consumers have so little choice now in their health benefits that converting them all to a government-run system won't be a big transition. And we certainly don't see our current Medicare beneficiaries marching in the streets demanding more choice and personal responsibility.

If there is a significant difference between Medicare as we know it and MFA, it may be the prospect of outright rationing of expensive care—services now covered by Medicare and private insurance—that would no longer be allowed under a government-run fixed-budget system. That might start with excluding expensive acute care for the elderly or new therapies that may be considered too pricey, despite their effectiveness, as the British agency NICE is now doing. I wonder if Americans will accept such restrictions *en masse,* even though our British and Canadian cousins have.

Also, the idea that the government would establish and provide a single, stable array of benefits would seem unlikely. It could certainly try—and in the process risk further suppressing entrepreneurial and technological innovation. But it would inevitably be faced with demands from special interests to improve coverage for the providers and patient groups they represent.

In the absence of price-mediated supply/demand balancing, the inevitable result of MFA would be increased non-price rationing amid perpetual attempts to adjust payments and coverages to plug holes in the financial dike. Ultimately, that dam won't hold. Even the established single-payer countries with rigid budget controls are facing increasing inflationary pressures in their programs. But it could take decades of wasted effort, money, and lives before the government would be forced to acknowledge its failure.

Administrative Efficiency

The claim that Medicare administration accounts for only 2% of costs versus private payers' 20–25% does not withstand close inspection. Mark Litow of the actuarial firm Milliman conducted an apples-to-apples comparison of the two. He concluded that Medicare's actual administrative cost figure is 5.2% when costs otherwise hidden by government accounting are factored in.[8] Even that number understates reality when you realize that the average aged or disabled Medicare beneficiary incurs much higher costs than the average private insured consumer. When normalized for that factor, Medicare's administrative costs are closer to 6–8%, and that still doesn't take into account the government's costs of collecting the operating funds necessary to run the program. Private payer administrative costs, on the other hand, average 8.9% before commissions, premium taxes, and profits are included. By adding another 7.8% for those costs incurred by private insurers—but not Medicare—we find that total private insurer costs of sales, administration, and profits run 16.7%, rather than the 20–25% often quoted. That's still more than double Medicare's costs, but there are additional factors that temper that difference considerably.

First, there's strong evidence that Medicare's administrative costs are actually too low. Medicare has suffered a widespread failure to detect fraudulent, inappropriate, erroneous, unnecessary, and excessive claims before paying them. The more scrupulous Medicare might be in policing these issues, the higher would be its administrative costs *and* the lower would be the claims paid. But that would cause significantly higher administrative costs on *a percentage basis*, since we've increased the numerator (administrative costs) *and* decreased the denominator (claims payments). Perversely, the less Medicare does in this regard, the better its administrative costs appear as a percentage of total expenditures. Thus, it can improve its administrative cost ratio by allowing its claims costs to soar while minimizing its cost of scrutinizing those claims. Medicare's historical approach to inappropriate claims is to try to catch them after the fact as part of a fraud detection program. Private payers focus on concurrent detection systems to stop inappropriate payments in the first place, which costs the private insurers more but reduces total claims liabilities. In effect, Medicare relies more on SWAT-like audit tactics to try to control inappropriate charges than it does on the kinds of internal operational controls commonly used by private insurers.

According to a General Accounting Office report, controls on Medicare's extensive home health care benefits are "virtually nonexistent," and "few home health claims are subject to medical review and most claims are paid without question." Home health care has been the nation's fastest growing health care industry, with Medicare claims tripling in only five years.

In 1992 the GAO estimated that fraud and abuse accounted for 10% of all Medicare benefits. Malcolm Sparrow, a Harvard University expert on public management controls, thinks this estimate is much too low.[9] The Insurance Information Institute estimates that "$1 out of every $7" is lost on fraud and abuse.[10] Medicare's operational controls have been so weak for so long that the GAO has listed the program "at high risk for fraud, waste, abuse, and mismanagement" every year since 1990. If you add these costs to the adjusted administrative costs calculated by Mr. Litow, then the argument for Medicare's much-vaunted reputation for efficiency crumbles even further.

Private insurers' greater care in claims scrutiny has exposed them to a triple PR whammy caused by: (1) higher administrative costs; (2) lower claims payments (both making the administrative percentage even higher); and (3) the unpopularity resulting from members with justifiably denied claims.

One of the reasons Medicare is so popular among its beneficiaries is that they are seldom bothered by claims denials. Medicare is far more likely to pay them than are private payers, no matter how inappropriate the claim. If low administration costs were the main test of insurance efficiency, then an insurer would be better off allowing providers simply to debit funds directly from the insurer's bank account without any scrutiny at all, which would result in a terrific administrative cost percentage of approximately zero. Claims payments might soar past absurd levels, but that's not important if your focus is on the administrative cost ratio.

HMOs used to get a lot of criticism for high administration costs because they spent so much money on making sure unnecessary hospitalizations were prevented. Those expenditures were probably among the most cost-effective in the history of health care, since they single-handedly reduced the health care inflation rate through the mid-1990s. But simple measures by uninformed critics made HMOs look bad. Increasingly, states are responding to this misunderstood issue by enacting limits on insurer administrative costs and profits as a percentage of total premiums. These measures may play well to the populist crowd, but they ignore the most important number: total cost.

Does this mean that private insurance is a model of administration efficiency? Hardly. The entire billing and collection system is draconian and an order of magnitude or two more expensive and inefficient that it would be under a competitive market-driven system. But such a remedy is virtually prohibited by current government-mandated rules. (See Appendix: "Who Wants to Be a Trillionaire?")

Savings with Electronic Medical Records (EMR)

Many people see EMR as a Holy Grail that will take health care into a new age of seamless, integrated health care with improved quality and lower cost. Estimates of savings from EMR replacement of current paper-based medical records range from a high of $165 billion (Sen. Hillary Clinton)[11] to the RAND Corporation's $77 billion to former Congressional Budget Office (and current OMB) Director Peter Orszag's conclusion that EMR alone is "generally not sufficient" to reduce costs.[12]

We should always be wary of believing predictions of how computer technology will improve efficiency and lower costs. In 1987 Nobel economist Robert Solow memorably observed, "You can see the computer age everywhere but in the productivity statistics."[13] Indeed, the highly lauded computer revolution has enabled us to do things never before imagined, but it did not save us any money, at least until very late in the twentieth century.

From 1948 to 1973 (before computers were so widely adopted) overall U.S. productivity increases averaged 1.9% per year and labor productivity increased by 2.9% per year. From 1973 until the late 1990s— the full bloom of the computer age—these productivity growth rates had actually declined to only 0.2% and 1.1%, respectively.[14] Although the first decade of the new century has finally begun to produce evidence of computer-enhanced productivity, it is clear that any financial returns from such high-tech investments have been very, very sluggish.[15] Electronic medical records may indeed expand our knowledge and our capabilities, but we shouldn't expect any payoff in cost savings for decades to come.

Regardless of its promise and prospects, EMR is anyway a separate issue from that of single payer. EMR's purported savings are usually trotted out by single-payer proponents as a major source of available money to help finance the massive increase in government expenditures that MFA would require. If EMR is such a wonderful innovation, then it will be so regardless of whether we have MFA or something else. It is a red herring with respect to the single-payer discussion.

Health Care Industry Profits

Let's take a look at the excessive health care industry profits that MFA would save us. The discussion above notes that an average of 7.8% of premiums goes for insurance company commissions, premium taxes, and profits. The profit component is, therefore, less than 7.8%—much less when you consider that premium taxes and broker commissions are often considerable expenses. But even if all 7.8% went to insurance company profits, it would still be below the 8.3% average profit margin for all American corporations over the past twenty-five years.[16]

Reported profit margins for publicly held insurers for the twelve months ending 7/31/07 ranged from a low of 2.52% (Humana) to a high of 6.87% (Aetna), not exactly headline news.[17] By early 2009 they had fallen considerably, owing to the economic downturn and the cyclical nature of the health insurance industry. Hospital profit margins have been running from a low of 3.54% (UCI Medical Affiliates, Inc.) to a high of 8.25% (Amsurg Corp). Again, these are below the long-term average for all corporations.[18]

Brand-name drug companies have enjoyed profit margins well above the average for all companies. In 2002 the drug manufacturers in the Fortune 500 earned 17% on sales.[19] Profits have been dropping significantly of late, however, as blockbuster brand-name drugs are losing patent protection and getting cut-throat competition from generics. There are widespread concerns that the glory days of Big Pharma may be over.

Those who have read my book *Prescription Drugs for Half Price or Less* (Bantam Dell, 2006) know that I am no fan of drug company pricing practices. Nonetheless, those practices are consistent with the perverse incentives laid down by our highly distorted health care marketplace. Big Pharma has been able to prosper by taking maximum advantage of consumer and doctor indifference to drug prices, primarily due to the fixed-dollar copayments incorporated in most health benefit plans. This lack of price sensitivity has allowed drug manufacturers to heavily advertise drugs such as Nexium, which sells for $170 per month, even though the virtually identical Prilosec OTC is available for $20 per month and without a doctor's prescription. A more market-based health care economy would rein in such nonsense very quickly and would allow Big Pharma to earn respectable profits—but only by continuing to bring true product innovations to market and at competitive prices. With a single-payer program like MFA, there would be no market price whatever upon which to base government payments. Instead, the government would be in a position to dictate prices. The problem with this is the danger that MFA, under pressure to restrain expenditures, could starve the necessary drug company R&D and profit incentives necessary to generate future drug innovations.

Why do people think health care companies are making so much money when most are actually earning less than the average for all other companies? Maybe it's because of critics like Congressman Stark who publicly lambaste health industry profits as unreasonable, albeit with little apparent evidence. Media coverage may be another reason. For example, here's a headline from *The New York Times* of February 10, 2006: "Profit at Aetna Increased 41% in 4th Quarter."[20] However welcome this news was for Aetna, it could leave the impression in readers' minds of excessive profiteering on the backs of America's beleaguered health care consumers. If you had looked below the headlines, though, you would have seen that Aetna actually earned $423 million on total revenues of $5.9 billion. My calculator says that this is equal to a profit margin of 7.2% (up from 5.8% the year previously), which is still well below the 8.3% average profit margin for all American corporations.[21] From that perspective, it is difficult to condemn sub-performing insurers like Aetna as profiteers.

Medicare's Looming Funding Crisis

This all leads us to the biggest problem with Medicare. It has completely failed to contain health care costs. And it's not just a matter of paying too many fraudulent claims. Anything more than a cursory inspection will reveal that Medicare, rather than offering a solution, is a major part of the problem. Since its inception, Medicare has driven massive health care inflation, imposed ever-greater administrative burdens on providers, driven up private insurer costs, and required tax increases far beyond anything predicted when the program was legislated during the Lyndon Johnson administration. Under MFA, the only one of the effects that would go away would be the driving up of private insurer costs since there would no longer be any.

The Medicare Hospital Insurance Trust Fund is currently projected to run entirely out of funds in 2017.[22] Even worse, Medicare's total unfunded liabilities now exceed $70 trillion.[23] On that basis alone, it is difficult to see expanding Medicare from its current forty-four million beneficiaries to cover the United States' entire population of more than 300 million.

Also of concern is the fact that Medicare currently doesn't pay its proportional share of hospital and doctor costs for its beneficiaries now. Instead, it has shifted a large and rapidly growing portion of those costs onto private insurers in the process called cost-shifting that I previously discussed. Health providers, unable to collect sufficient revenue from Medicare (and Medicaid/SCHIP), have to make up the shortfall by charging more to private payers. This cost-shifting has been rising at an alarming rate as Congress has further ratcheted down Medicare's budget for provider payments. Since Medicare for All would presumably end cost-shifting (not even government accounting can let it shift costs from itself to itself), the program would find itself in an even more untenable financial situation than it is today.

MFA would either have to increase its provider reimbursement rates substantially, cut benefits, or watch as providers are forced to cut back services or face bankruptcy. *De facto* rationing of care would inevitably result, with long lines for an increasing number of services rendered non-economic and unaffordable.

Medicare, despite its ability to control the prices it pays, has contributed greatly to out-of-control health care costs. MFA will do nothing to change that without engaging in further price controls and rationing of care. The humorist P.J. O'Rourke, commenting on proposals for Medicare to negotiate drug prices, has said, "If the government shows the same hard-headed, tight-fisted bargaining savvy negotiating drug prices that it shows negotiating defense contracts, Preparation H will cost $400."[24]

MFA proponents refer to the $300 million in cost reductions they say we would see from eliminating all that wasteful private insurance administrative paperwork. For the sake of argument, let us assume that MFA would actually achieve that level of savings—unlikely as that may be since Medicare's own pricing methods are a major cause of that waste. We would, therefore, see a one-time reduction in total health expenditures of about 13% of our current $2.3 trillion total national health expenditures. That is not an inconsiderable sum but is equivalent to less than two years of medical cost inflation at recent rates.

So after that, what? Without some mechanism to restrain medical care costs on an ongoing basis, we'll be no better off than we were after HMOs succeeded in reducing spending on hospitals by two-thirds during the last three decades of the twentieth century. After that silver bullet was fired we were once again stuck with rampant inflation. So would we be with Medicare for All, absent direct rationing or price-control-driven reductions in provider supply.

In industries driven by market economics, the interaction of buyers and sellers controls overall costs. But with a government monopsony (a single buyer, a monopoly being a single seller) like MFA, there are only two methods of containing costs—price controls and non-price rationing, which is indeed what every other country in the world with single payer has had to resort to. I don't know that

American doctors and consumers would take as kindly to such Old World measures, especially if they knew there were better alternatives available.

Single Payer in Other Countries

Single-payer advocates often rely heavily on their versions of how well government-controlled systems work in other countries, particularly Canada, the U.K., and France. They point to statistics proving that people in these countries enjoy longer life expectancies, fewer infant deaths, better access to primary care, and reductions in expensive, inappropriate, and uncompensated emergency room care. In addition, these countries perform all these wonders at far lower per-capita costs than in the United States. Before betting the fate of our $2.3 trillion health care system on these claims, though, deeper scrutiny is in order.

Take life expectancy, for example. On average, Americans live 75.3 years whereas Canadians live 77.3 years, and the French live 76.6 years. In fact, all countries in Western Europe, except Portugal, have longer life expectancies than the United States.[25] The availability of health care is undoubtedly a factor, although many health experts argue that life expectancy improvements owe more to advancements in public health than in medicine.[26] Indeed, in the case of life expectancy in the advanced countries, it turns out that any medical effect is greatly overshadowed by other factors, such as lifestyle, cultural differences, diet, alcohol consumption, drunk driving, drug abuse, exercise, accident rates, and homicides.

Obesity, for example, is a significant contributor to health problems, such as diabetes and heart disease. Americans, on average, are considerably fatter than Canadians, with 31% of American men and 33% of women having body mass indices (BMIs) at or above 30, the threshold for obesity.[27] The Canadian numbers are 17% and 19%, respectively. The Japanese, with the longest life expectancy of all major countries, have an obesity rate of 3%.[28] Obesity is not caused by lack of access to health care.

America isn't just fat but violent as well. Its homicide rate is ten to twelve times greater than in the U.K. and Japan and eight times that of France. The death rate from car and transportation accidents in the U.S. is three times higher than in Sweden or the U.K., and 1.5 to two times greater than in Australia, Canada, Denmark, Germany, or Japan.[29] In their book *The Business of Health*, Robert Ohsfeldt and John Schneider factored out such non-medical-care related death causes and found that Americans who don't die in accidents, suicides, or homicides actually live *longer* than people in any other OECD (Organisation for Economic Co-Operation and Development) country, including the overall record holders of Japan, Iceland, and Sweden.[30] As the noted economist and former Chairman of the President's Council of Economic Advisors Gregory Mankiw has said in referring to a different study with similar results, "Maybe these differences have lessons for traffic laws and gun control, but they teach us nothing about our system of health care."[31]

Let's now look at infant mortality rates. In the United States, at 6.8 per one thousand live births, infant mortality is 28% higher than Canada's 5.3. Here again, social factors other than the quality of health care are major contributors to the difference. Mankiw says that the incidence of high-risk, low-birth-weight babies due to teenage pregnancy is 32% higher in the United States than in Canada. The mortality rate for low birth weight babies in both nations is more than ten times that of larger babies. America's health care system actually gives its low birth-weight babies a better chance of survival than Canada's. But the fact that it has so many more of them results in a higher overall infant mortality rate in the United States.

Ohsfeldt and Schneider also point out that different countries use different measures for infant mortality. The United States, for example, counts a premature birth accompanied by almost instantaneous death as a live birth and infant death. Other countries count it as a fetal death not included in either live birth (the denominator) or infant death (the numerator) statistics.

To correct for such cross-national distortions, they point to the alternative health metric of perinatal mortality, which includes both late fetal deaths and neonatal infant deaths. With a rate of 7.2 (per one thousand live births and fetal deaths), the United States compares favorably with the U.K. (7.9) but not with Canada, Germany, Japan, and Sweden (6.5–7.0). But again, there is the low–birth–weight baby problem clouding the comparison. The differences are less pronounced, however, than those comparing raw infant mortality rates. Buried within the United States' 7.2 perinatal mortality figure is a white population rate of 6.2 (better than all the above countries) and a black population rate of 13.1. This latter figure is an unconscionable national tragedy, but it does not point to a problem with health insurance availability. To the extent that the high rate of perinatal mortality relates to expectant black mothers living in poverty, Medicaid coverage is specifically available for all of them, with Medicaid/SCHIP also covering their newborns. The problem is more likely to result from cultural, educational, and other issues relating to poverty—such as a lack of awareness of the need for prenatal care—than it is to the availability of health insurance or the quality of medical care itself. Although there are many things to criticize in the reality behind this statistic, access to or coverage of medical care is not one of them.[32]

Canada

Dr. David Gratzer, in his book on American health care reform, *The Cure—How Capitalism Can Save American Health Care*, writes:

> A survey in 2000 involving 1,500 people suggested that a full eight out of ten [people] consider their health-care system to be "in crisis." Since then, polls consistently show health care as the top concern of voters. Medicare is the issue that dominates talk radio debates, peppers newspaper headlines, and colors election campaigns from coast to coast.[33]

There is nothing particularly remarkable about this passage, except that Dr. Gratzer was referring to a survey of *Canadians* about the *Canadian* health care system, also called Medicare. Anyone who saw Michael Moore's *Sicko* would be surprised to hear that the oft-trumpeted Canadian single-payer system is caught in dire straits at least as serious as in the United States. The Canadian problem is not lack of insurance coverage—everyone has it—but rather rationed care. Canadians have learned that universal coverage does not mean universal access to timely medical care.

Canada does not actually have a national single-payer program but rather a collection of thirteen provincial and territorial health plans that all follow national requirements. The guidelines of the Canada Health Act state:

> Canada's health care system is best described as a collection of plans administered by the 10 provinces and 3 territories, each differing from the others in some respects but similarly structured to meet the federal conditions for funding. The simplicity of the five federal conditions...are the provision of all medically necessary services (defined as most physician and hospital services), the public administration of the system, the portability of coverage throughout Canada, the universal coverage of all citizens and residents, and the absence of user charges at the point of care for core medical and hospital services.[34]

Within these defining constraints, each province and territory uses different methods of financing its share of the health insurance plan, including premiums, payroll taxes, other provincial or territorial revenues, or a combination of methods. Premiums are allowed as long as they do not result in denied coverage for low-income Canadians. A survey of the literature indicates a wide variation from province to province in patient access, availability of health care resources, quality outcomes, and patient satisfaction.

The biggest problem with Canada's universal, government-run health care system has for many years been lack of timely access to care due to rationing by the government. Dr. David Gratzer became concerned about his native country's health care system during his medical school days. Since then, he has actively surveyed the Canadian and other systems. What he has reported in his books and articles[35] is hardly complimentary. Here are some of his findings:

- A Winnipeg hospital emergency room crowded with elderly patients, some of whom had waited five days for treatment. "The air stank with sweat and urine." Crowded ERs constitute a persistent problem in Canada.

- A man with persistent hernia post-operative pain who was referred to a pain clinic that had a three-year waiting list.

- A woman who faced a two-year delay to receive a sleep study to diagnose possible sleep apnea.

- A woman with breast cancer who had to wait four months for radiation therapy. The standard of care was four weeks.

- Serious doctor shortages. More than 1.5 million Ontarians (or 12 percent of the population) were unable to find family physicians. Health officials in one Nova Scotia community held a lottery to determine who'd get a doctor's appointment.

- M.D. Anderson in Texas, a single prominent cancer treatment organization, spends more on research than Canada does.

- Increasing newspaper headlines such as, "Vow Broken On Cancer Wait Times: Most Hospitals Across Canada Fail to Meet Ottawa's Four-Week Guideline for Radiation," "Patients Wait As P.E.T. Scans Used In Animal Experiments," "Back Patients Waiting Years For Treatment: Study," "The Doctor Is…Out."

As alarming as these reports are, they are mostly anecdotal. We could undoubtedly find equally scary horror stories in our own country. So what about some actual statistics? According to data from the Canadian Institute for Health Information, many Canadians during recent years have faced long wait times and difficulty in accessing care:

- 1.2 million Canadian adults were unable to find a family doctor in 2003 (Canada's total population was less than thirty-two million).
- 50% of Canadians wait 1–4 months for specialist visits.
- 50% of knee replacements (from specialist to surgery) take 7 to 21 months.
- 50% of hip replacements (from specialist to surgery) take 4.5 to 14 months.
- 50% of non-emergency MRI/CT/Angiographies take 3 to 13 weeks.
- One out of six Canadians had trouble getting routine health care.
- Same-day appointments for needed medical care occur less frequently in Canada (27%) than in the U.S. (33%).
- A higher percentage of Canadians (18%) than Americans (16%) use emergency rooms because regular doctors were unavailable.
- 25% waited six or more days to see a doctor when sick.
- 50% waited one to six months or more for non-emergency surgery.
- A lower percentage of Canadians (11%) than Americans (13%) report unmet health care needs.
    - Canadians report "waiting for care" as their most frequent problem.
    - Americans report "Cost" as their most frequent problem.[36]

In Dr. Gratzer's words, "At a time when Canada's population was aging and needed more care, not less, cost-crunching bureaucrats had reduced the size of medical school classes, shuttered hospitals, and capped physician fees, resulting in hundreds of thousands of patients waiting for needed treatment—patients who suffered and, in some cases, died from the delays."[37] Fortunately, because of a growing realization of Canada's shortcomings, few serious United States health care policy analysts are now promoting it as a model. Besides, if the United States adopted a single-payer system, where would Canadians go for medical care?

Europe

European countries also have a wide variety of national health care programs. Many pundits point there, as well, for particularly worthy paradigms for U.S. health reform, even though they all suffer from their own serious problems.

For example, the United States has higher per capita organ transplantation rates and better outcomes than single-payer countries such as the U.K., despite the fact that we tend to transplant to much sicker patients. In the other countries, many acutely ill patients can't get on the transplant waiting lists because of rationing-based triage rules. According to former FDA Deputy Commissioner Scott Gottlieb, M.D., such patients simply "don't pass go" in the U.K. Innovations in organ transplantation techniques, such as living-related-donor procedures developed in the United States, have been slower to appear in these other countries, as well. Also, despite former Sen. John Edwards' publicizing of a single case where a U.S. transplant candidate apparently died because of a delay in insurance coverage, most U.S. patients are transplanted before the doctors and hospitals even know whether insurance will cover them. Finance here is normally trumped by the immediacy of need and the availability of donor organs.[38]

The Wall Street Journal has reported that European health care services have been reluctant to pay for new, expensive drugs that are commonly covered in the United States, such as the blood-cancer drug Velcade.[39] The U.K.'s National Health Service has declined to pay for kidney cancer drugs that are commonly prescribed in the U.S. because they cost more than $60,000 per quality-adjusted life year (QALY).[40] A friend of mine attending the London School of

Economics recently chipped a tooth and went to his student health service. He was told he could get it treated by a National Health Service dentist in two years or he could go to a private dentist and have it done right away.

Much worse is the CNN story reporting that 6% of surveyed Brits admitted to pulling their own teeth with pliers or repairing crowns with glue. They were unable to find NHS dentists willing to take them. One woman told British television she had used her husband's pliers to remove seven of her teeth. She said the first extraction was "excruciatingly painful" but that it was the only way to end her unbearable toothache.[41] Americans complain about how they are rushed through their doctor visits, but a much greater percentage of U.S. patients spend more than twenty minutes with their doctors than do British patients.[42]

Cancer survival and mortality rates are far better in the United States than in Europe. The American five-year survival rate for leukemia is almost 50% whereas the European rate is 35%. Esophageal carcinoma survival is 12% in the United States and 6% in Europe. Prostate cancer survival rates are 81.2% in the United States, 61.7% in France, and 44.3% in England.[43] Women with breast cancer in the U.K. die at almost twice the rate of those in the United States. The U.S. also has the lowest breast cancer mortality rate among New Zealand, the U.K., France, Germany, Canada, and Australia.[44] These variations may explain why the United States is such a popular cancer treatment destination for many foreigners who can afford it.

The rate of dialysis for kidney failure in the United States is more than three times the rate in the U.K. and almost twice the rate in Canada. Even so, an American friend who was on dialysis before receiving a kidney transplant maintains that (U.S.) Medicare's limitations on the permitted frequency of dialysis are arbitrary and inadequate. Patients with occluded coronary arteries in the United States have far more access to bypass surgery and angioplasty than in either the U.K. or Canada. Coronary bypass rates per 100,000 population in the United States exceed two hundred per year while the

U.K.'s is forty-five and Canada's is about eighty. American balloon angioplasty rates are nearly four hundred per year, the U.K.'s fifty, and Canada's eighty.[45] Admittedly, some of the U.S. statistics likely reflect medically unnecessary overutilization of such procedures. Still, the five- to eight-fold differences suggest access restrictions in the two other countries.

These are not isolated statistics, but just a few examples of Nobel economist Milton Friedman's observation that "once the bulk of costs have been taken over by government...the political entrepreneur has no additional groups to attract, and attention turns to holding down costs."[46] One method of holding down health care costs in single-payer systems has been to avoid or delay technological improvements in care. That is why medical advances have overwhelmingly come from the United States and why their spread to other parts of the world has been slow.

Sweden has had a single-payer system for more than fifty years. As with other single-payer countries, Sweden has dealt with out-of-control health care costs by rationing medical care, primarily with waiting lists. During the 1990s Sweden experimented with limited market reforms, which temporarily reduced health care costs and waiting times. But the reforms were uneven, lacked comprehensiveness, and still preserved the single-payer system. The result has been a resurgence of both rising costs and lengthening waiting lists.[47]

Among the many universal health care systems in the developed world, that of France is generally acknowledged as having avoided most of the problems that have afflicted single-payer systems in other countries. Michael Tanner of the Cato Institute, who produced an overview of the French system in a recent policy paper, has concluded that much of this success results from regulatory limitations and market innovations that most single-payer advocates consider undesirable. Even so, the system does not appear to be financially stable and, according to Tanner, "is the largest single factor driving France's overall budget deficit...threatening France's ability to meet the Maastricht criteria for participation in the Eurozone."[48]

Actually, France doesn't have a single-payer system but rather a series of heavily regulated, largely employment-funded, semi-private health insurance pools. French workers' employers are required to pay almost 19% of their income into these funds. In addition, most government-mandated services require 10–40% copayments, equivalent to about 13% of health care costs (roughly the same as in the United States). Although rationing has not been a significant problem, the government controls access to new technology. And there are increasing signs of access issues for patients. Since government-mandated benefits are limited and don't cover many medical services, more than 92% of the French buy complementary private insurance from 118 different carriers. French doctors are not required to abide by government fee schedules and a third don't, charging patients the difference.

The inflexible and heavily regulated nature of French health care has been blamed for problems in treating victims of a 2003 heat wave that caused the deaths of fifteen thousand people. The French government blamed the national health care system in part for allowing doctors and nurses to leave for their normal lengthy August vacations during the crisis.[49]

Interestingly, the private insurance aspects of the French system offer hints of how a successful market-based health care system might work. Overall, however, it seems hardly a model worthy of emulation. The French people would seem to agree, with 65% of them opining that the need for reform is "urgent."[50]

Single Payer Is Not Necessary

Overall, the single-payer and heavily regulated national systems have problems that appear to be at least as serious as ours. Where our system has gaps in insurance coverage, single-payer countries have inadequate provider resources, rationed care, and health outcomes that are not as good as the United States'. There is also the common problem of costs rising unsustainably faster than inflation in virtually all these countries—ours and theirs. Replacing one problem-ridden system with another is hardly a recipe for success.

Another aspect of single-payer systems is worth noting. Although all were created for the purpose of providing uniform health care to all, they have actually created two-tier systems. The poor and middle class have to settle for the government plans while those with higher incomes are able to purchase better, more comprehensive, and more immediate care. Single payer is increasingly becoming a class-based system.

Americans have long had an almost visceral antipathy for monopolies, whether private or public, and with good reason. As Sir William Wells, a senior British health official who is quite familiar with single-payer health care, has concluded, "The big trouble with a state monopoly is that it builds in massive inefficiencies and inward-looking culture."[51] We should expect no better from such a system in the United States.

Based on the above factors, Medicare for All and its international single-payer siblings don't look promising. Probably the best argument against such an approach is that it's not necessary. I will explore another alternative in the next three chapters to enlist the power of regulated market forces to bring to health care the same benefits we see in virtually every other industry that serves our needs. We have an unparalleled opportunity to apply uniquely American solutions to the serious American problem of health care.

CHAPTER 9

The American Choice Health Plan

"We cannot solve the problems that we have created with the same thinking that created them."
—ALBERT EINSTEIN

So how can we fix the system? First, let me once more review the eight goals I propose to achieve a fair, efficient, and effective health care system. All are achievable under a properly regulated, market-based health care financing and delivery system.

1. *Universal Insurance Access*: Everyone in America should be able to obtain health insurance, regardless of individual health status, history, genetic predisposition, or financial circumstance. High-quality medical care is a basic need—on a par with food, clothing, housing, and transportation. It is the only one of these that requires insurance to enable everyone to consume the full range of necessary services.

2. *Sustainable Value and Affordability*: Whatever we do with health care reform, we must include mechanisms that will get spending under control while encouraging innovation and better quality. We must reverse the trend toward increased unaffordability and levels of quality that represent poor value. Our goal should be for health insurance and medical care to become affordable for everyone, whether through personal resources or safety net assistance that the government can afford to provide.

3. *Free Rider Prevention*: Universal insurance access must be accompanied by mechanisms to prevent people from gaming the

system to its detriment. We must prevent people from forgoing or delaying insurance purchases until they become ill and know they will receive more in benefits than they pay in premiums. The cost of any such gaming should be removed from the system and placed on the gamers themselves—not the insurance risk pools.

4. *Voluntary Participation*: Many advocates of insurance reform believe it is necessary to require everyone to purchase health insurance in order to keep adverse selection from destroying universal availability. It's not. Others believe that everyone should be required to purchase insurance because it is good for them. That is arrant paternalism that runs afoul of essential American values. No one has ever been required to purchase anything from a private or governmental third party as a condition of American residence. It is important to make insurance purchases a voluntary process while preventing adverse selection and enabling social and economic safety nets to assist the elderly, the poor, and the disabled to participate.

5. *Financial Protection*: Health insurance should first and foremost protect people against the unaffordable costs of involuntary and largely unpredictable adverse health events. It should not be required to pay for consumer purchases of normally affordable medical care.

6. *Choice of Insurance and Providers*: Consumers should have the right to determine how they live their lives, how they set their health care priorities, and how they meet their own medical consumption needs. In choosing insurance and provider services, consumers should determine what they need to buy, who they will buy it from, and how much they are willing to pay. They should be able to choose insurers and providers on the basis of quality and price—that is, value. Only with choices can they meet their own wants and needs within their own priorities and resources.

7. *Portability*: Each person should be able to choose and own her health insurance policy, regardless of who she works for and whether she is unemployed, retired, eligible for government-sponsored coverage, or just taking a long sabbatical. This goal is necessary to remove today's major gaps in insurance access caused by eligibility restrictions tied to employment, individual insurability, and eligibility for government coverage.

8. *Personal Responsibility for Prevention*: Health insurance should avoid creating or continuing moral hazard that subsidizes unhealthy personal behavior. Instead, it should provide incentives for people to manage their own individually controllable health risks.

Not everyone will agree with these goals, particularly those who believe that health care should be treated as a public good best provided by a government single-payer system. I don't believe those views hold water economically, philosophically, or psychologically for the American people. I have presented my reasoning elsewhere in this book. Except for those irrevocably inclined toward single-payer or equivalent approaches, most people, I believe, will essentially agree with these eight goals—albeit with a likely dose of incredulity that they can all be accomplished. I invite and look forward to an ongoing debate and discussion about these goals and the means to accomplish them.

Starting with these goals, I propose to craft a set of basic rules under which the health insurance and medical delivery system can achieve them. It is my contention that all of them can be met through a single, congressionally-established regulatory mechanism that I call the American Choice Health Plan.

American Choice consists of seven essential, interdependent features. Why seven? Albert Einstein once said that we should, "make everything as simple as possible, but not simpler." While different descriptive approaches to American Choice might revise the number of key features, it does appear that removing or substantially degrading any of the following functions will substantially degrade or even destroy the power of the whole. They interlock to create the essentials for an internally consistent, self-sustaining regulated market for health insurance that will accomplish the above eight goals:

1. *Universal annual open enrollment periods will allow all American residents to purchase health insurance from a choice of voluntarily participating individual health insurance plans.* During an open enrollment period once each year, every American resident will have the opportunity to purchase health insurance from any qualifying insurer, managed-care company, or integrated health care organization that operates in his area of residence. Anyone will be able to change from his current plan to any other plan during subsequent open enrollment periods. Neither insurance availability nor prices will be dependent upon anyone's health status, history, or genetic makeup. Premium adjustments, however, will be allowed for individually controllable health risk factors, as I will explain in detail in chapter 11.

2. *Private insurers, managed-care organizations, and integrated health care delivery systems will provide all American Choice insurance coverage in a new, competitive, regulated insurance market.* Each such participating insurer will offer its own choice(s) of health benefit plans, subject only to national rules on minimum coverage requirements and premium rating principles. It is important to note that the minimum coverage rules will permit, *but not require*, the inclusion of primary and preventive health care services in any and all health insurance plans. The only required medical services will be those that are both medically necessary and generally unaffordable for most consumers.

   All current health benefit programs provided or operated by employers, individual-insurance companies, and federal or state governments will cease to enroll new members, and all will cease altogether over time. Those that continue will give all their existing members the opportunity to opt out and participate in

American Choice. The intent will be a complete sunset for all such existing programs in the shortest practicable time. I will discuss this later in more detail.

Employer and government insurance coverage originally arose because of a failure of self-organizing insurance markets to extend affordable individual coverage to everyone. Later cast in place by federal tax rules, this system is now on the brink of collapse. American Choice corrects that market failure. It establishes a regulated market for health insurance with availability for all. It will make every insurer primarily and directly responsible to its members rather than to the vagaries of employers, the Congress, or bureaucrats of either public or private ilk.

3. *Conversion from defined benefits to defined contributions is a central feature of American Choice.* The role of employers, Medicare, Medicaid, SCHIP, and TRICARE will shift from directly providing health insurance and benefits to one of funding their respective constituents to buy their own insurance and medical services in the American Choice marketplace. With limited exceptions for any grandfathered members of employer and government health plans, all such organizations will entirely exit the health benefits and insurance business, thus converting from a system of defined benefits to defined contributions.

All health insurance regulatory functions of these organizations will also cease. Those functions will become the responsibility of a new independent government agency empowered to establish and enforce a consistent set of regulations embodying American Choice's principles. Some insurance regulatory functions will continue to be delegated to the states.

This change will allow consumers to make their own decisions about how much of their total funds they will spend on health insurance and how much to retain in cash to pay for normal consumer purchases of medical services. Providers will become directly answerable to their patients. They will have to compete for their business on the basis of objective, demonstrable quality of care. They will have to make a revolutionary shift to competing on the basis of price, but only with the removal of the industry price regulation currently controlled by the Center for Medicare and Medicaid Services (CMS). No longer will the system be able to tolerate a value-subtracting reimbursement system that consumes up to thirty-one cents of every health care dollar in administrative costs. Consumers will become the locus of authority, responsibility, and accountability for their own money and their own health.

This creation of a consumer market for insurance and medical services will result in the rationalization of the entire delivery system. It can double the quality and halve the price. The available data says that these levels of improvement are certainly available. American Choice creates the mechanism for this to occur.

4. *Individual participation will be voluntary.* I have discussed the numerous reasons why health insurance must not be mandatory. No one will be required to participate in the American Choice Health Plan. A decision to participate late or not at all will, though, carry significant limitations, responsibilities, risks, and penalties, thus the requirement for item number 5.

5. *Enrollment limitations to prevent adverse selection*: Any health insurance that is both universally available and voluntary on an individual basis must include rules to prevent the kinds of gamesmanship that can lead to adverse selection and the ultimate failure to achieve a financially self-sustaining system. Among these rules will be all or various combinations of the following:
   - Annual open enrollment periods
   - Continuous creditable coverage requirement
   - Penalties and restrictions for late enrollment
   - Provider requirements for ability to pay
   - Personal bankruptcy risk

Whatever their reasons for non-timely participation—except for poverty and disability—non-participants will bear the full financial consequences of their inaction—rather than those who participate. Although this principle may initially appear harsh to some observers, similar rules have long applied to Medicare and to employer-based insurance. Such participation rules are inherently fair, as I will address later.

6. *HFA-funded*: All health care funds to pay for insurance premiums and out-of-pocket medical costs will flow through each individual's (or family's) tax-free health funding account, up to annual legal contribution limits. There will be no maximum limits on accumulations within an HFA. The HFA is similar in concept to its antecedent MSAs, HRAs, and HSAs but will correct the substantial legislative and regulatory limitations of each.

7. *BAGLE premium pricing*: All insurance premiums will be established by insurers under a uniform set of regulatory principles that will be blind to medical condition, history, or genetic makeup. At the same time, these principles will allow "BAGLE" adjustments for member Behavior, Age, Gender, Location, and Employment/Extracurricular risks.

There will be no regulatory determination of whether premiums are excessive, leaving that function to the market. State regulators of fiscal soundness will, however, be allowed to intervene if they determine premiums to be financially inadequate.

BAGLE pricing has multiple benefits. It eliminates current employer discrimination against younger workers while ensuring adequate funding for older ones. It encourages the emergence of niche insurers that focus on the differing health and prevention needs of women, men, the young, the elderly, and other population segments. It ends the subsidization of those choosing certain unhealthy behaviors by those with healthy lifestyles, but does not affect coverage for treatment of the medical conditions that may result from such behavior.

It provides strong financial incentives to stop smoking, abusing alcohol, being obese, and allowing uncontrolled blood pressure, cholesterol, and blood sugar to continue. It doesn't require anyone to do anything about such conditions if they choose not to or even to disclose that they have them. They will need to disclose only those conditions for which they are in compliance in order to receive premium discounts. In other words, the burden of proof will be on the individual to show her insurer when she does comply with any or all risk factor standards. Otherwise, the insurer will assume noncompliance and assess higher premiums. I will discuss this more fully in the next chapter. The important feature to note is that this provision fairly assesses the financial responsibility to those whose behaviors predictably lead to increased sickness.

These seven necessary, interlocking provisions that constitute the American Choice Health Plan will achieve all eight of the goals listed above. The following table summarizes how each provision supports the various goals. The goals are listed in the vertical column and the American Choice components across the top row. The Xs indicate

	1 Open Enrollment	2 Private Insurers	3 Defined Contrib.	4 Voluntary Particip.	5 Enrollment Limitations	6 HFA Funding	7 BAGLE Pricing
1. Universal access	X	X					
2. Value/ affordability	X	X	X	X	X	X	X
3. Anti-adverse selection	X				X		X
4. Voluntary participation				X			
5. Financial protection	X	X				X	X
6. Consumer choice	X	X		X		X	X
7. Portability of coverage	X		X			X	
8. Prevention incentives						X	X

each American Choice component that directly contributes to the achievement of each goal.

Some of these features of American Choice could be enacted by individual states for their own residents, but in the absence of a national program to enact key components of federal legislation regarding income and payroll taxes, ERISA, Medicaid, TRICARE, SCHIP, and particularly Medicare, no state plan can be comprehensive and will risk continued problems of fragmented risk pooling and the negative consequences that inevitably follow.

Fundamental, Comprehensive Reform

American Choice offers fundamental, comprehensive reform that counteracts past problems by enabling regulated market forces to assert themselves to provide universal, affordable, effective health care for anyone who wants it and who has the reasonable resources to afford it. With the improved ability of government to provide more rational safety nets, there will be few financial reasons for anyone not to participate.

I have emphasized throughout this book how American Choice asserts that the only way to achieve the above eight major goals will be to have a system that encourages—even requires—prospective patients to ask for and act on the answers to two questions:

1. For my medical needs and personal circumstances, which health care providers, procedures, services, and products offer me the highest quality, most beneficial outcomes?

2. Of those high-quality treatment options, which ones are the least expensive?

Enabling consumers to ask and to receive answers to these questions means doing something almost unthinkable according to today's health care debate: giving consumers the control of all the money necessary to purchase their own health insurance and all of their medical and health care services. Only this step can make both insurers and providers directly answerable to the consumers using their services.

Armed with this new authority, consumers will be in an unprecedented position to demand information on price and quality—not to mention customer service. This will allow consumers to make judgments about the value of competing offerings and to decide which ones to buy. Insurers and providers that can't answer these questions will soon find themselves losing customers and patients to those that can. Competition for consumers' dollars will become a powerful motivator.

Both of these questions are the same we as consumers ask about virtually everything else we buy. That's how we figure out which cars, MP3 players, clothes, groceries, books, Elmo dolls, and houses to buy, lease, or rent. You can name virtually any product and then find information on its proper use, the standards under which it was produced, its reliability, the customer service policies of its vendors, its quality assessments and ratings, its appropriateness for your use, and, of course, its price. As perhaps the best trained, most experienced experts on personal consumption the world has ever seen, Americans know how to get what they need and want.

Of course, not everyone is equally adept or capable. None of us makes rational decisions 100% of the time. Yet our entire market capitalist economy is based on the premise that most consumers (and investors and governments and lenders and manufacturers) make mostly rational decisions often enough to beat out any other known system of economic organization—over time, perhaps, but every time so far. Gary Marcus, NYU psychology professor and author of *Kluge: The Haphazard Construction of the Human Mind,* has written: "Evolution equipped us not with fool-proof, steel-trap rational minds, but something more like a 'kluge,' a clumsy and inelegant mental patchwork that is good enough to get the job done, but far from perfect."[1] Getting the job done has brought us economic growth and increased prosperity throughout America's history. When our collective mental inelegance has occasionally gone awry, we've gotten manias, panics, crashes, economic dislocations, bubbles, busts, recessions, and the rare depression. Fortunately, economic growth has always outweighed the contractions over time. History tells us it will most likely continue to do so.

American Choice Regulatory Reform and the Role of Government

Creating American Choice will require radical reform by the federal government in three areas: taxes, health insurance, and safety nets. American Choice also requires radical reform of health care providers, but that will spontaneously emerge as a result of the market forces enabled by these three reforms. Here's a summary list of the three reforms:

1. *Tax reform* will grant the tax treatment to all individuals now enjoyed by only those who have employer-based insurance. A detailed discussion follows below.

2. *Insurance reform* will enact all key features of American Choice and override all state and federal laws that conflict with them. Further discussion follows tax reform below.

3. *Safety net reform* will transform the roles of Medicare, Medicaid, SCHIP, and TRICARE from defined-benefit insurance providers to defined-contribution contributors to their constituent members and beneficiaries. The funding aspects of safety-net reform are included in the insurance reform discussion below. How American Choice will affect the poor and the Medicaid/SCHIP programs is discussed in chapter 12.

The provider reform necessary for the achievement of the eight goals will follow as the direct result of these reforms to cause providers actively to compete for patients on the basis of value, quality, and price. I will discuss provider reform in chapter 12.

Tax Reform and HFA Funding

The American Choice Health Plan will replace all current insurance and health benefit plans with individually purchased insurance. To enable that change to take place, American Choice will offer all individuals the same tax benefits now given only to people with employer- or government-sponsored insurance. The mechanism to accomplish this will be a new type of individually owned funding account called the health funding account, or HFA.

All health care funds to pay for insurance premiums and out-of-pocket medical costs will flow through each individual's tax-exempt health funding account, up to annual contribution limits established by law and updated periodically by the IRS. There will be no maximum limits on accumulations within any HFA.

The purpose of HFAs is to put American Choice members on a level income-tax playing field with the current employer-based health insurance system. An alternative might be to level the field by simply eliminating all health benefit tax exclusions, but that would invite too many opportunities for legislative mischief, economic disruption, and other unintended consequences, which I discuss below under the heading "Why Not Just Abolish the Tax Exclusion?"

The HFA is similar in concept to its antecedent MSAs, HRAs, and HSAs but will correct the substantial limitations of each. Existing legislation severely limits annual HSA contributions and allows funds to be used only for the payment of health care products and services and not for insurance premiums (with the limited exceptions of Medicare premiums and health insurance premiums during limited periods of individual unemployment). Also, no contributions can now be made unless the individual or family has health insurance that meets certain minimum deductible and maximum out-of-pocket expenditure standards. Current tax law does not similarly limit employer-based insurance as to either the amount or form of tax-exempt health benefits an employee may receive.

The proposed HFA mechanism will correct this inequity while placing an upper limit on tax-exempt benefits to prevent high-income individuals from exploiting a new, unlimited tax shelter for current income.

Families could decide to establish a single family HFA for parents and dependent children, or they could set up separate HFAs for each family member, with funds transfers being freely allowed between family member HFAs without tax penalty.

HFAs will provide tax neutrality by the following process:

1. *Converting existing MSA and HSA accounts into HFAs* will transfer all existing savings into the new, more flexible funding mechanism.

2. *Eliminating other tax-advantaged medical spending accounts* will recognize that there will no longer be a need for separately funded HRAs by employers or the medical expense aspects of FSAs by employees. These functions will be incorporated into the new HFA allowances.

3. *Annual contributions to HFAs* will be subject to the same exemptions from FICA/Medicare payroll taxes and state/federal income taxes that employer group members enjoy currently.

4. *Higher contribution limits than currently allowed for HSAs* will provide individual tax exclusions for all HFA contributions necessary to fund reasonable levels of both insurance and qualified out-of-pocket health care costs.

5. *Annual changes to contribution limits* will be indexed to the health care component of the CPI, which should begin to fall below the overall CPI itself.

6. *Insurance premiums* will be payable from HFA funds, thus removing current restrictions on HSAs and MSAs.

7. *HFA payments for American Choice insurance premiums and qualified health and medical expenses* will not be subject to taxes, other than possible state sales taxes.

8. *HFA eligibility standards* will remove current HSA requirements for minimum insurance deductibles and out-of-pocket spend-

ing limits. All American residents will be allowed to establish an HFA, whether they actually use it to purchase health insurance or not.

9. *HFAs for children* will allow separate HFAs for residents below the current HSA minimum age of eighteen.
10. *HFA investment proceeds* will be exempt from income and payroll taxes.

Under American Choice, participating health insurance companies, managed-care organizations, and integrated health delivery systems will offer an array of qualified health insurance choices to everyone in their chosen market areas. Each will be required to certify that its health insurance plans sold under American Choice meet minimum regulatory requirements for continuous creditable coverage (see discussion in chapter 10).

Each consumer will be free to choose one such plan for the coming year. Some consumers might opt for richer benefit plans with higher premiums, leaving less in their HFAs for out-of-pocket medical expenses or end-of-year rollovers for investment and future use. Others will choose high-deductible, high-coinsurance, lower-option plans with lower premiums and, thus, more remaining HFA funds for out-of-pocket expenses and future investment growth.

Each consumer will pay all insurance premiums and out-of-pocket health care costs directly from her health funding account. The HFA will be hers to open, maintain, and control at a bank or other financial institution. She could also choose to purchase no health insurance at all, leaving HFA funds intact against future medical expenses. That, however, would involve significant risks and penalties for anyone experiencing catastrophic health problems or wanting to purchase insurance later, which I discuss below under Access and Adverse Selection in chapter 10.

Any HFA balance remaining at the end of any year will remain in the consumer's HFA to be invested and to pay for future insurance premiums and health expenses. As currently permitted with HSAs,

HFA funds could also be used for retirement expenses at age sixty-five, after the payment of normal income taxes on any withdrawals for non-health purposes. Also, as with HSAs, there will be significant penalties and tax recapture for any use of HFA funds for purposes not allowed by the American Choice legislation.

In the event that HFA funds are ever insufficient to cover an insured member's health care costs, she might have to pay from her own after-tax resources. This will provide an incentive for consumers to fund their HFAs to their maximum abilities, to purchase at least catastrophic insurance coverage and to pursue healthy lifestyles.

Instead of employers and governments paying insurers or providers under their current defined-benefit programs, they will, under American Choice, make defined-contribution payments into their constituents' HFAs. The payments will be in whatever amounts the contributors deem necessary and appropriate. The payments will be apportioned, however, to each payee according to the AGL aspects of BAGLE rating. That is, each employee will receive funds based on age, gender, and residence location according to adjustment factors contained in approved actuarial tables.

The premiums that the recipients will then pay for insurance will be based on similar—but not necessarily identical—adjustment factors. This approach will be the fairest for apportioning contribution disbursements. Otherwise, AGL premium adjustments are very similar to those now used by insurers of both individual and group business.

As for the B part of BAGLE rating (Behavior), all employer and government program HFA contributions should be blind to the individual behavior-based risk factors of the recipients, even though the premiums they will pay are not (see the full discussion of BAGLE rating in chapter 11). There are two reasons for this. First, it would be unwise to allocate higher contributions to people with unhealthy behaviors as that would perpetuate subsidies for such counterproductive habits. It would also punish those who pursue healthy behaviors. Second, not adjusting employer contributions for behavior will allow behavior-based premium incentives to be most effective. The rewards for healthy behavior will be equally available to everyone but enjoyed only by those who actually meet the requirements.

American Choice Separates Functions for Funding, Insuring, and Regulating

Changing the role of employers and government agencies to that of funding contributors is a key feature of American Choice. It will effectively separate the functions of funding, insuring, and regulating, assigning each to its most appropriate operators.

- *The Funding Function*: Employers, Medicare, Medicaid, SCHIP, and TRICARE will be involved only in determining eligibility for and the amounts of their funding support for their respective constituents. They will no longer have any role in setting or approving insurance benefits, premiums, or provider reimbursement rates—with only minimally necessary exceptions to support any grandfathering of current members in legacy programs until they all finally sunset.

- *The Insuring Function*: Private insurers, managed-care companies, and integrated health care companies will entirely assume the insuring function in a highly competitive marketplace. With only two exceptions, no employer or government agency will be allowed to offer health insurance or self-funded health benefits. The first exception would be for limited grandfathering of some current participants in employer and government legacy programs. The second exception would be only for any areas of the country in which no private insurer chooses to operate. (This is extremely unlikely. It is virtually certain that nationwide companies will offer nationwide plans, just as they do with Medicare Part D and FEHBP.)

- *The Regulatory Function*: A single federal agency, preferably one with Federal Reserve-like independence, will take over all federal regulation relevant to the American Choice Health Plan, which will include all determinations relating to continuous creditable coverage, third-party HFA contributions, and BAGLE rating requirements. It will engage in a regulatory hands-off policy with respect to any other aspects of insurance premiums, benefits, and provider reimbursement rates and prices. Such unified and independent regulatory authority is critical for American Choice's success. It will ensure consistent application of uniform rules to all American residents, insurers, employers, and government funding agencies. State insurance commissioners will continue to have authority over the financial viability of insurers operating in their states.

Employer HFA Funding

Employers will continue to provide financial health care support to their employees for the same reason they do now—to remain competitive in labor markets. Large employers could continue to pay the large sums they do now. But they will pay them to the employees themselves on a fully disclosed basis. This, by itself, will be a revolutionary change from today's system. Employees are now completely in the dark about how much their employers actually pay on their behalf for their health insurance.

Smaller employers will no longer be faced with an all-or-nothing health benefits option. They will now be able to offer fixed contribution amounts to their employees' HFAs, based on each employer's economic circumstances and need to be competitive in its labor markets. Even more important, employees of small firms will no longer be penalized for working for such employers. Instead, each will now have exactly the same health plan options at exactly the same prices as employees of the largest employers.

Most employers will welcome American Choice as a way to get out from under the increasing burden of managing health insurance benefits. They will instead be able to contribute the health benefit portion of total compensation in much more transparent, predictable, budgetable amounts. That's exactly what they do now with wages, salaries, payroll taxes, and 401(k) contributions.

All companies will be able to get out of performing a health benefits function they do poorly. They can focus on the key business drivers of their respective competitive business strategies. They will give up these health plan management functions with full knowledge that their employees will have access to better, lower-cost options than any employer could ever have provided on its own.

I've repeatedly derided the reverse-age discrimination embalmed in today's employer practice of community rating employees' health insurance contributions. I propose to remedy that with the age-adjustment feature of BAGLE rating, but let's look more closely at the older workers who currently have employer-sponsored insurance and who now pay the same amount for it as their younger coworkers. American Choice, with its age-adjusted BAGLE rating, will certainly remove the price discrimination burden from young workers, but that means the older ones will be required to pay more as a direct result. That may be a fairer way to allocate health care costs, but won't the changeover to American Choice hit older workers in their pocketbooks? Won't their premiums become unaffordable if they have to pay their full freight from now on?

The answer is no. Let's see why.

According to one set of actuarial tables I consulted, a sixty-year-old non-smoking man incurs health care expenses at about 3.3 times the rate of a twenty-two-year-old non-smoking man. It is important to realize that the sixty-year-old's employer is already paying his total premium at that higher rate. It is just the employee's portion that is not being similarly allocated. That is why the sixty-year-old pays the same amount as the twenty-two-year-old in the form of payroll deductions.

Under American Choice, the employer will now recalculate its share of the contribution based on the employee's age, gender, and location. In other words, the employer will pay approximately 3.3

times as much into the sixty-year-old's HFA than it will to the twenty-two-year-old's HFA.

To match the amount of money that was previously being paid for his health insurance, the older worker will have to contribute more into his HFA than he did for his contribution to the old employer's plan. Likewise, the twenty-two-year-old will now be contributing significantly less into his HFA because he will no longer be subsidizing his older colleague. Several aspects of American Choice, however, will significantly dampen or even reduce the older worker's necessary HFA contributions, which I will address later.

Government HFA Funding

Similarly, the relevant government agencies will make defined, tax-exempt HFA contributions to their respective constituents. Medicare will thus fulfill its obligations to America's retired and disabled. Medicaid and SCHIP will meet their safety-net obligations to the poor and near-poor, and in a far more dignified and economically supportive manner. The Veterans Administration will help pay our debt to our veterans, although American Choice could be optional for veterans. And TRICARE will meet our national obligations to our military dependents and retired military personnel. Even the unemployment compensation system could join the ranks of contributors by making defined contributions to their beneficiaries' HFAs, which could help the temporarily unemployed maintain their fully portable American Choice coverage until they regain employment.

Retirement Health Benefits Funding

The funding, or more appropriately, the gross under-funding of defined-benefit retiree health plans has become a major issue in recent years, both for industry and state-local governments. *Business Week* reported in 2006 that the companies in the S&P 500-stock index owed $442 billion more in retiree benefits than they had funded. All companies were estimated to understate their retiree health and pension obligations on their balance sheets by $1 trillion.[2] *USA Today* reported in 2009 that state and local governments have more than $1 trillion in unfunded retiree medical benefit obligations.[3]

Soaring costs and straitened resources have caused more and more employers to drop or severely cut retirement health benefits. American Choice's defined-contribution feature, linked to the HFA mechanism, will offer a dual solution to this problem. First, defined-contributions, combined with American Choice's market mechanisms to lower costs, will allow employers to predict their employees' future needs more accurately for retirement health spending, which will greatly increase the likelihood they will be able to fund and honor their long-term commitments while their employees are still working. Second, the HFA feature will allow younger employees to fund their own future retirement health costs, much as they do now by making pretax contributions to their 401(k) accounts for retirement income.

Future retirees will become much less subject to the goodwill and financial fortunes of their previous employers. They will be able to put aside the necessary funds for retirement health care over the decades of their working lives via their HFAs, which could similarly help reduce future Medicare funding requirements.

One problem with personal 401(k) retirement accounts has been that employee 401(k) contributions and overall savings rates in recent years have not been adequate to support many Americans during their retirement years. One reason is that all such employee contributions are entirely voluntary. HFAs would be different, however, since employers would be able to fund them directly, regardless of whether employees provide additional contributions of their own. Some critics might argue that employers should simply increase their employees' salary compensation and let them make their own decisions about whether and how much to fund their HFAs, just as they make their own decisions about how much to spend for food, clothing, housing and their other wants and needs. I believe there is a strong argument to be made, however, that employers have a direct financial interest in their employee's health, as I related in my earlier discussion of Maslow's hierarchy of needs. Thus, it would not seem unreasonable for employers to be allowed to fund their employees' HFAs directly in order to ensure that employees can pay for their health care needs.

It would still be the employees' money, which would even be available for retirement income later in life.

Consumer HFA Funding

Consumers and self-employed individuals will be allowed to contribute to their HFAs, topping off the contributions of other contributors, if any, up to the legal maximum annual amounts. In total, each person's HFA funding could come from a combination of sources, depending on the employment and economic circumstances of the individual consumer. These sources could include employers, government agencies (Medicare, Medicaid, SCHIP, TRICARE, unemployment insurance), friends and family members, charitable institutions, and consumers themselves.

You may be wondering how low-income consumers, especially those not eligible for Medicaid, will cope with American Choice. Many of them now work for employers that don't provide group health plans, especially for low-paid, part-time, and temporary workers. At least two funding mechanisms will enable them to fare much better under American Choice than they do now.

The first will be to convert Medicaid/SCHIP to a sliding scale, defined-contribution plan to replace the all-or-nothing defined-benefit arrangements they have today. This will allow the Medicaid/SCHIP state agencies to provide progressively lower HFA contributions to low-income workers as they ascend the income scale while continuing to provide full support to the truly poor. This end to the "cliff-effect" will have significant advantages I will discuss further under Medicaid and SCHIP Reform in chapter 12.

The second mechanism would be to extend refundable tax-credit payments by the IRS to low-income workers' HFAs, thus providing a wad of cash each year for these consumers to use for health benefits.

Note that all such HFA contributions could be used only for purchasing health insurance and services by their recipients, much like food stamps can be redeemed only for food.

Both of these funding methods for the poor and near-poor will dramatically improve the ability of low-income workers to afford health insurance and necessary medical services. Initially, such programs will likely increase the overall level of government transfer payments to extend these new benefits. The significant decline in health care costs and insurance premiums over ensuing years, however, would more than make up for such short-term adjustments. Also, the sliding-scale nature of Medicaid's defined contribution will allow fine-tuning of benefits according to recipient income, which could effectively stretch scarce Medicaid funds well beyond today's inefficient system.

Under American Choice, each consumer will, for the first time, learn the real price of both her health insurance and all health and medical services she purchases—whether paid by her insurer or from her own funds. This will have a transformative effect on behavior. Consumers will become value-conscious buyers, demanding the answers to questions about insurers' and providers' quality and price. All such vendors will become active competitors. Consumers, by controlling the purse strings, will have the power they now lack to demand convenience, quality, price, value, and respect.

Why Not Tax Credits?

Some health reform advocates have proposed to replace the current employee tax exemption for employer-provided health insurance with tax credits. The purpose would be to put everyone on a new, level playing field. Presidential candidate John McCain proposed in 2008 an annual $2,500 annual tax credit for individuals and $5,000 for families. American Choice, on the other hand, proposes to level the field by extending the current tax exclusion to all Americans, not just those with employer-based insurance. The American Choice approach to tax reform is the better one.

To explain, let's take a look at how health benefits would have been taxed by the IRS under Senator McCain's tax credit proposal. We'll start with two people. One is Arthur, a sixty-year-old single man. The other is his son Brad, who is twenty and single. We'll assume that Arthur and Brad both work for the Baseline Company, which provides an employee group health insurance plan. The total monthly cost of the plan is $600 per employee. Baseline pays $350/month, so employees pay only $250, or $3,000 per year.

Under Senator McCain's proposal, the entire $600 per month will become fully taxable to each man. (Note: Currently, neither the employer nor employee's health insurance payments had been taxable to the employee.) At the end of the first year of taxability of such benefits, the company reports to each worker and to the IRS the average taxable health benefit of $600 per person per month, or $7,200 for the year. Accordingly, each will report $7,200 in new income on his tax return.

Arthur is a senior executive and in the top 35% income tax bracket, so he will have to pay $2,520 in new taxes for his health benefits. Brad works on the assembly line and is in the 25% marginal bracket, so he'll pay an additional $1,800 in taxes. (Note: Each man will also have to pay additional FICA and Medicare payroll taxes on his newly recognized $7,200 income under the McCain plan, but I've left those out of this example.) Each man also gets the McCain $2,500 tax credit, leaving Arthur with a net tax increase of $20 whereas Brad reduces his total taxes by $700. Arthur thinks the change to tax credit is no big deal. Brad is overjoyed.

Unfortunately, Baseline Company had its entire investment portfolio invested with Bernie Madoff and is forced to shut down and fire all its employees. Because of Baseline's shuttering, neither Arthur nor Brad is eligible for COBRA. Each applies instead for individual coverage from private insurers. Fortunately, both men are healthy enough to be accepted. Because of his age, Arthur is charged a premium of $700 per month or $8,400 per year. Brad pays only $200/month or $2,400 per year, which is less than his contribution alone to Baseline's plan. That's because individual insurance pricing is based on the applicant's age. The younger you are, the lower the price. Employers, on the other hand, just look at the average cost per employee, regardless of age, when assessing employee contributions to health insurance.

On their tax returns for the following year, neither Arthur nor Brad reports any taxable health benefit income. But because they both have insurance, they can claim their respective $2,500 tax credits. Brad's $2,400 insurance cost is completely offset by his tax credit, and he pockets a net savings of $100, so now he's even happier about the tax credit.

Arthur, on the other hand, is able to offset his new $8,400 premium expense by only the $2,500 tax credit, leaving him $5,900 in the hole. This upsets him, but he becomes even angrier when Brad tells him how well he came out. "I've been screwed," Arthur wails, vowing never to vote Republican again. You may not be sympathizing with wealthy Arthur's plight, but the same thing would be happening to the poor sixty-year-old janitor laid off by Baseline.

The reality is that Arthur is, indeed, suddenly being discriminated against by the tax credit. But Brad has a different take on it. "Dad," he says, "I now know that I was the one being screwed all those years working for Baseline. It charged me the same premium contribution as you—$250 a month. I had been paying *more than my entire premium cost* at Baseline while the company was paying a very high percentage of yours." What is particularly striking about this reverse-age discrimination is that Arthur had been making far more money than Brad. When the men figured all this out, it became obvious why so many of Brad's young coworkers had chosen not to buy into Baseline's insurance plan at all. For them, it had been grossly overpriced.

The tax credit is highly discriminatory against older workers because it is not based on the men's ages, even though their premiums now are. It would have worked okay for them if they still worked for Baseline, but it completely broke down with individual insurance, which was what Senator McCain was proposing that a lot more people would buy under his health reform program.

Besides the fact that a tax credit will do nothing to reduce medical inflation, it would require automatic cost-of-living adjustments, based not on the CPI but the health care component of the CPI. Without that, Congress would need to address the issue annually, with uncertain political outcomes every time. Otherwise, continued high health care inflation would eat away at the value of the tax credit, becoming a backdoor way of raising taxes.

The fundamental problem with replacing the tax exclusion with a tax credit is that it is an attempt to solve a complex problem with an overly simplistic solution. For tax equity, credits are a blunt instrument that fails to recognize the realities of how things really work with health insurance.

Why Not Just Abolish the Tax Exclusion?

The current employee tax exclusion's existence is a historical accident, dating back to problems unique to the WWII labor market when wage and price controls prevented employers from competing for labor on any basis other than the amount of fringe benefits offered—such as health care, which the IRS ruled to be nontaxable to workers. Wouldn't it be a more rational tax policy simply to make everyone pay for their health care on an after-tax basis? Wouldn't that level the playing field for everyone just as effectively as extending the tax exclusion to everyone?

Well, yes, removing all tax advantages from health care benefits would indeed be another way to equalize the tax impact of health insurance for everyone. Unfortunately, all else being equal, it would also dramatically increase the cost of health care for the majority of Americans who now receive the tax benefits.

Although it may have been a mistake for the government to have sheltered employer medical benefits two-thirds of a century ago, the fact is that our entire system is now based on it, and we're accustomed to it. That in itself is hardly a reason for keeping it. But the real question is whether it would be better to reform both health care *and* a major part of the income tax code simultaneously or just to confine ourselves *only* to fixing health care for now.

Wall Street Journal columnist Jason Zweig has wrapped himself in the mantle of Truth by saying, "Of all the decrees that come spewing continually out of Washington, there is only one that works every time: the law of unintended consequences."[4] Accordingly, I acknowledge that no matter how closely Congress might someday hew to my prescriptions for American Choice, there will still be unintended consequences to deal with. I believe they will be far fewer and of far less magnitude than we've seen from our current system. But they will be there, nonetheless.

Perhaps only someone wanting to kill the whole American Choice endeavor before it starts will propose a wholesale change in tax policy at the same time. For one thing, removing the current tax exclusion by itself would constitute a massive tax increase. It would also push many workers into higher marginal tax brackets, which would obviously increase their health care costs, counter to the goal we've established for the system. I suppose Congress could rejigger tax rates, credits, deductions, and other aspects of the tax law to limit this penalty. But then we'd just be replacing one set of anomalous tax policies with another—but with untold consequences beyond anyone's ability to predict. On balance, the negative consequences of such a dramatic federal tax change would most likely be far more problematic than simply extending current tax treatment of health benefits to the small minority of Americans who currently don't receive it.

It would indeed be wonderful to have a fairer, simpler, and easy-to-navigate tax code. But that's an issue best separated in concept and in time from health reform. Extending the tax exclusion will spread both the tax benefits and the tax burden more equitably. And it will enable the health reforms we need now.

Insurance Reform

Health insurance regulation is now a patchwork of inconsistent and conflicting state and federal rules that produce all manner of negative consequences, not the least of which is driving up health care costs. Federal legislation to enable American Choice will sweep away these conflicts and inconsistencies with a single set of overarching rules aimed at achieving the eight goals described above. They will do this by establishing nationwide regulations within which the new health insurance system will operate. Such legislation will end, for example, many of the health insurance aspects of the McCarran-Ferguson Act of 1945, which granted regulatory powers to the states for all non-federal insurance.[5] A panoply of restrictions on and requirements for minimum benefits, underwriting procedures, high-risk pools, pay-or-play requirements, rating methodologies, underwriting rules, employer mandates, group insurance, and individual insurance will be eliminated and replaced by a remarkably simple set of uniform rules that will apply to everyone—consumers, insurers, employers, government agencies, state legislatures, and regulators. I realize that states'-rights advocates may not like this idea, because the federal centralization of regulatory authority would be at the obvious expense of state authority. Whatever the constitutional issues may be, it seems clear that the current Babel of conflicting federal and state health insurance regulations has created a major problem for the entire country. I suspect there is some sort of jurisdictional solution that can be achieved, perhaps along lines similar to those that enabled federal ERISA and HMO rules to trump state insurance regulation.

In any event, states should continue to regulate the financial soundness of insurers and their adherence to non-preempted state laws. They seem to have the necessary mechanisms and experience.

Allowing everyone to purchase individual insurance will require legislation to replace most existing forms of federal, state, individual, and employer-based health benefit programs (including FEHBP) with a nationwide program of individual, private health insurance. There will be some exceptions. These include active duty military personnel and prison inmates. Eligible veterans could opt to use the VA health care system in lieu of an American Choice health plan without losing eligibility for American Choice. Likewise, Native Americans could opt out of the Indian Health Service to participate in American Choice.

Limited ERISA Grandfather Provisions

Employers' self-funded ERISA programs could be grandfathered and permitted to continue, although I wonder why any employers would want to. Employers will not, however, be allowed to enroll new employees in those legacy programs, thus ensuring their eventual sunset. Employers will also be required to allow all current employees to opt out of legacy coverage to purchase any American Choice health insurance policy during an annual open enrollment period. The employer will be required to contribute the same amount to such an employee's HFA as it would contribute to his self-funded plan, taking into account the employee's age, gender, and location factors consistent with American Choice's BAGLE rating requirements.

For an employee to continue to have the annual choice to opt out of his employer's plan, the employer will need to ensure that its plan meets American Choice's continuous creditable coverage requirement and to disclose any failure to do so in time for employees to switch to American Choice without penalty. Otherwise, the risk of adverse selection to American Choice would be unacceptable.

New self-funded employer plans will not be permitted, unless both employers and their employees are willing to give up any future right to participation in American Choice without having to pay late enrollment penalties and to accept other enrollment limitations. In any event, it is likely that very few grandfathered employers will choose to continue their self-funded plans for long because of American Choice's administrative simplicity and its superior choices, prices, and cost-control features.

Government Program Grandfathering and Alternatives

Concerns, some legitimate, will arise about the ability of some Medicare, Medicaid, and other government program constituents to leave their current defined-benefit programs and choose from the plethora of benefit and price choices thrust upon them by American Choice. There were similar concerns with the introduction of Medicare's Part D prescription drug benefit in 2006 although that was an entirely new benefit that had not previously existed. Even then, Medicare Part D's implementation went relatively well, even though there were many who had difficulty choosing.

Grandfathering such people to allow them to remain in their current programs could be an option; however, it should be a last resort after other options are explored, such as the following:

1. *Insurance Brokers*: American Choice will allow state-regulated insurance brokers to collect uniform commissions for providing expert, independent assistance to Medicare beneficiaries to make appropriate insurance plan choices each year. These brokers could assist any individuals needing help in navigating the new marketplace of insurers, benefits, and prices.

2. *Equivalent Health Plans*: American Choice could allow Medicare/Medicaid et al., to contract with at least one insurer in each market that will initially offer a plan identical in all key aspects to the current government program it is replacing. None of the agencies, however, will be able to dictate that any of its beneficiaries actually join such plans. Thus, a "Medicare Equivalent Plan" and a "Medicaid Equivalent Plan" could be offered by at least one insurer to allow current beneficiaries to transfer smoothly from the government program to a private one without any change in benefits. The relevant agencies would have to fund beneficiaries choosing such plans so that their personal outlays will approximate those before the change. This should be a transitional requirement only since beneficiaries, often with expert assistance from brokers and others, will become better able to

compare their current plans with competing ones that offer more personally appropriate benefits and financial advantages.

3. *Last-Resort Government Coverage*: In only one circumstance should these government programs be allowed to continue as in the past, again assuming the avoidance of wholesale grandfathering. They may continue to function in any area of the United States in which there are no American Choice offerings by private insurers. This provision would provide a safety net similar to the one included in the Medicaid Part D drug benefit law. That provision, however, was never triggered since many insurers offered nationwide Part D plans open to everyone. The same is highly likely to occur with American Choice, allowing a complete shutdown of the current government-defined benefit programs.

It would be far less desirable for the government to grandfather existing Medicare, Medicaid, SCHIP, and TRICARE programs for those beneficiaries wanting to continue with them. Such continuation could delay the achievement of American Choice's market reforms. It would also complicate the process of terminating these programs' roles in regulating benefits, provider prices, and participation rules. Even with any grandfather options, however, American Choice legislation will require all such programs to offer their participants the ability to take their benefit values as cash contributions to their HFAs. Any beneficiary could switch to American Choice's individual coverage during any open enrollment period. In any event, American Choice will require that no new eligible participants be allowed to join such grandfathered programs, thus ensuring their eventual sunsets.

An End to CMS Regulation

Under no circumstances will CMS (Centers for Medicare & Medicaid Services) be allowed to continue regulating insurance benefits, provider prices, or provider participation rules. It will no longer maintain or require the Resource Based Relative Value System (RBRVS), CPT, DRGs, ICD, HCPCs, or any other provider price-setting mechanism. Instead, providers will set their own prices subject to consumer determinations of their value—with help from their insurers.

Likewise, the government will no longer require CPT and other codes as the only basis for electronic provider billing. Such coding schemes are based on provider costs and efforts rather than consumer outcomes and value. Enacting this provision is necessary to allow other useful coding standards to emerge, which is important for enabling the private sector to evolve quickly into a market pricing system. Medicare, Medicaid, et al. will have to figure out how to adapt any grandfathered programs to the new market-based pricing regime. They must not be allowed to engage in any further gerrymandering of prices and cost-shifting to other payers. Their roles will be only to determine beneficiary eligibility, to provide funds to their beneficiaries' HFAs, and perhaps to provide outreach to help them become more savvy consumers.

Other than any grandfathered programs, all employers and government agencies will cease dictating health insurance benefits and premiums for their constituents. They will no longer negotiate or set provider reimbursable rates and prices. They will stop contracting with or paying providers. These functions will be decided among consumers, insurers, and providers, each acting independently to maximize his or her own self-interest under the competitive dynamics of regulated market capitalism. The only government regulatory roles in this regard will be over continuous creditable coverage for benefits and BAGLE rating rules for premiums, and those will be made by an new federal agency that is independent from any of the funding contributor agencies.

Under American Choice, the roles of the federal government will be critical, but significantly reduced to these two functions:

- *Regulation* to establish and enforce the essential insurance and HFA ground rules necessary to create a level playing field for all consumers and insurers.

313

- *Financial support* to make contributory funding payments to the individual HFAs of those covered by Medicare, Medicaid, SCHIP, FEHBP, and TRICARE—that is, the aged, the disabled, the impoverished, government employees, and the military's civilian dependents.

Probably the most difficult government task will be to restrain itself from interfering further with the newly formed insurance market and the self-emerging medical care market. But that forbearance is an absolute necessity for achieving American Choice's goals.

Availability and Freedom of Choice

Each individual, family, or family member will decide which of perhaps seventy-five to one hundred or more individual health plan choices to purchase each year. Family members could all choose the same plan. Innovative insurers could specialize in various categories of members, such as children, women, and men by offering benefits and services to meet the specific needs of each category. Thus, each family member might choose a different health plan.

Making these decisions for the first time will involve the most difficulty. It will be like buying a car but with a deadline and without the eager anticipation of the end result. Alas, I doubt anyone will ever see owning health insurance as evidence of one's sexuality, affluence, taste, or class. American Choice can accomplish only so much.

Fortunately, every health insurance broker in America will have the opportunity to retool herself as an expert in her locality's specific insurance offerings. She will earn commissions by helping her clients choose the best plans for themselves and their families. Brokers will offer personal counseling, seminars, and personalized, easy-to-navigate websites to help each client narrow his choices to the best plan, based on benefits, premiums, insurer reputation, provider selection, and additional features, such as multi-year rate guarantees and rebates for healthy behavior and risk factor control.

Broker websites could link consumers to independent measures of each insurer's financial strength, reliability, call center responsiveness, claims payment promptness, member retention rates, and member satisfaction rankings. Brokers will retain clients year after year by offering service upgrades, such as secure websites that maintain client information on family demographics, preferences, previous choices, and even confidential medical claims and expense histories. As each new open enrollment period rolls around, a broker could use specialized software to provide up-to-date recommendations to each client on new and better options for coverage.

Insurers will no longer be able to hold on to their clients by making nice with HR managers. They will have to continuously improve their products, services, prices, customer responsiveness, warranties (yes, warranties!), and convenience. It will be a whole new ball game, with a lot of new players. As we saw with traditional players during the advent of HMOs, we'd probably see many of the old ones leaving the field.

Portability

American Choice provides complete health insurance portability for every American resident. Each will have his own individually purchased, universally available health insurance that is paid for with pre-tax income. Like owning a car, you won't lose your insurance just because you change or lost your job or become ineligible for government support. You will be able to take it with you if you move, as long as your insurer offers a plan in your new residential market. If it doesn't, you'd be able to change immediately to a new plan there with equal or lesser coverage. You will continue to pay your insurance premiums from your HFA, and if your finances change, you can buy up or down during the next open enrollment period. Actually, American Choice's underwriting rules could allow any member to buy down to a less comprehensive policy at any time. Buying up to more comprehensiveness will be allowed only during open enrollment periods to prevent adverse selection.

Your available annual choices of health plans during open enrollment will be the same as everyone else's living in your area. The only factor that could force you to drop your coverage would be the inability to pay for it. That should become increasingly rare because of the availability of a wide range of insurance policy options and prices; declining health care and insurance costs; an emerging cultural phenomenon of people saving money against future medical costs; and the availability of last-resort safety nets. Under American Choice no one will be uninsurable, thus obviating the need for any state to continue operating its special high-risk insurance pools. Indeed, a key tenet of American Choice is that there will no longer be *any* government-operated health insurance programs.

Insurance Transparency and Access Reform

Transparency of employer/government contributions, insurer and medical provider prices, and provider quality is essential to consumer-empowered health care reform. Proponents of heavier government involvement in health insurance now point to the lack of such information as a key reason why such consumer empowerment won't work. That's a lot like predicting the failure of the automobile in 1905 because of a lack of paved roads. One of the most powerful features of American Choice is that every consumer will, for the first time, have the standing and the financial clout to know three critical things:

1. *Employer and government contribution amounts of funds for each person to purchase health insurance and medical services* will become completely transparent to each person.

2. *Total health insurance premiums* will be known by each person, because he will be paying for them each month from his HFA.

3. *Medical service prices and rates for every service* will be known upfront by each individual because he will be the one approving each purchase as well as the price, whether from his own funds or from insurance coverage. Insurers will create further incentives for their members to seek the highest quality care at the lowest price, thus benefiting both.

The key to enabling consumers to demand high quality and low price will come from their knowing how much money they have at their disposal, where it came from, and how it can be spent.

Under American Choice, any employer's HFA contributions will become completely transparent to each employee receiving them. Any employee's share that might have previously been deducted from his paycheck may now be paid directly into his HFA, along with any additional personal contributions up to the maximum allowed by law. In all cases, these will be actual cash payments into 100% employee-owned savings accounts in financial institutions completely separate from the employer or insurer. Each employee will now know exactly how much his employer paid him in total compensation, and employers will begin to compete for labor with the relative generosity of their tax-free HFA contributions alongside the pre-tax salaries and wages—that is, with the entire *amount* of the compensation package.

Independent rating services will expand and emerge to crunch both objective and subjective data on each insurer and publicly rank it according to such measures as quality; cost-effectiveness of its provider networks; claims payment and denial practices; history of premium stability; disease and prevention management assistance programs; ease of claims submission and payment; provider satisfaction with the insurer; number of customer appeals and how resolved; complaints to state insurance commissioners; effectiveness in assisting insureds to navigate the health care delivery system; and satisfaction survey rankings of their insureds on ease of use, consumer service, benefit clarity, and overall satisfaction with the company.

Insurers could be independently ranked from one to five stars on objective measures and consumer experiences by such organizations as Consumer Reports, J.D. Power, and Zagat. Before making an annual insurance choice, each consumer would be able to consult this and other information directly. Or she could seek the assistance of an insurance broker, who could help her navigate the plethora of offerings to find the optimal plan for each member of her family.

Any individual who becomes dissatisfied with his insurer will be able to leave it for a better choice during the next annual open enrollment period. Smart insurers will become adept at focusing on delivering value and member satisfaction.

Likewise, providers will make available their electronic medical record data on patients' diagnoses, treatments, and outcomes (stripped of patient identification data, of course) to third-party rating agencies, which will publish quality ratings, also perhaps on a five-star rating system much like HealthGrades.com does now.

Initially, such information will likely be derived from electronic invoice data. In time, consumers will learn that the longitudinal granularity of data from electronic medical records produces much more accurate, useful ratings. Increasingly, the doctors and hospitals that use electronic medical records will have a competitive advantage for attracting patients. Their paper-bound competitors will show up as "unrated" on the quality reporting websites. This dynamic will lead providers to incorporate electronic medical records proactively into their practices, which will obviate any need for the various regulatory mechanisms currently being discussed to incentivize, subsidize, or force providers to adopt them.

CHAPTER 10

Free Rider Prevention and Insurance Company Regulation

O ffering individual insurance is, inherently, a very risky business. It requires strict adherence to underwriting principles that prevent adverse selection and fiscal instability. Most state attempts to guarantee individual access to insurance plans have either established externally subsidized high-risk insurance pools or required insurers to accept all individual comers under guaranteed-issue rules and rates that never cover the costs of those who sign up. All such mechanisms are deeply flawed and completely unnecessary for American Choice.

Access and Adverse Selection

Allowing uninsured individuals to sign up for coverage only when they know they will incur more health expenses than they pay in premiums has the perverse but predictable effect of making the coverage too expensive for the healthy and for many of the sick. Such programs inevitably become subsidized payers of last resort for the unhealthy uninsured. The following American Choice rules will inherently deal with this problem without the use of special high-risk pools, guaranteed-issue rules, or mandates that everyone buy insurance.

1. *Annual open enrollment periods*: Every eligible United States resident will be able to choose any qualified health plan offered in his residential market by any insurer licensed in any state *but only* during an annual thirty to forty-five-day open enrollment

period. There will be exceptions only for: (1) newborns and recent immigrants who could become eligible for health insurance upon initial appearance; (2) people who move and need to change plans midyear; (3) consumers who may have opted for multi-year benefit and premium plans from their current insurers; (4) recently unemployed or financially strapped consumers who will be allowed to switch to lower cost, less comprehensive insurance; (5) any individual wishing to "buy down" to a lower benefit health plan; and (6) "orphaned" members of insurers that have been shut down by state regulators for fiscal soundness or other reasons.

The purpose of the open enrollment limitation is to remove the ability of anyone to buy insurance whenever they decide they need it. Any consumer who fails to purchase insurance during his first eligible open enrollment period will be unable to do so until the following year.

Limited open enrollment periods will present reluctant consumers with the risk of going without insurance and then incurring catastrophic medical expenses during the interim period. With no access to insurance, they will be faced with the prospect of exhausting their own and their family's assets and resources to pay medical bills. Open enrollment periods have successfully been in use for many years by employer-based group insurance plans and by Medicare for coverage under Parts B (for non-hospital-based benefits) and D (for drugs). They have long served as effective tools for controlling adverse selection.

2. *Continuous creditable coverage*: Each insurer qualified to sell American Choice health plans will offer its own choice(s) of medical benefits in its chosen market areas, but each benefit package will have to meet minimum federal standards for continuous creditable coverage (CCC). Done properly, CCC will have a double impact on reducing adverse selection.

First, it will eliminate all extraneous, optional, and medically unnecessary benefit mandates currently required by federal and state governments. In its place will be a consistent definition of minimally necessary coverage, which will immediately reduce health insurance premiums in every state. Lower premiums have the advantage of further reducing the risk of adverse selection. Fewer healthy people will avoid paying them.

The second and larger impact of CCC on adverse selection will be the elimination of any risk of an insurer race-to-the-bottom with minimed-style benefit coverage. This is a critical feature of American Choice to prevent healthy consumers from buying cheap placeholder coverage with few benefits and then buying up to comprehensive coverage when faced with catastrophic medical expenses. These and other aspects of CCC are discussed more fully in the section, "Reform of Minimum Benefits Requirements," below.

3. *Penalties and restrictions for late enrollment*: Those enrolling (a) after failing to do so during their first eligible open enrollment period or (b) after having let their coverage lapse for more than a very brief period will be required to pay lifetime insurance premium penalties.

This is a key provision of American Choice to prevent adverse selection and is intended to place the costs of free-riding gamesmanship squarely on the gamesmen to prevent them from damaging the system with adverse selection. It is based on Medicare's long-standing practice of doing the same thing for its voluntary Part B program and its Part D drug program.

Anyone who waits one or several years without buying insurance will still find it available. He will, however, find the price to be considerably higher than it would have been had he joined the system and maintained continuous coverage from his first eligible open enrollment period. That's because each of the insurers' actuaries will calculate the cost of such adverse selection as permanent premium surcharges that could run anywhere from 12–50% above the standard rates—or higher. Anyone unable to afford these higher rates may find himself having to forgo other lifestyle priorities just to afford insurance coverage. Exceptions might be allowed to lower (but probably not eliminate) the penalties (a) with proof of insurability (under a process similar to today's medically-underwritten individual insurance) and/or (b) by allowing insurers to exclude coverage of preexisting conditions for a period of years.

The only exception to the late-enrollment penalties will be for newly minted adults at age eighteen, whose parents may have forgone health insurance for them during their childhood. It would be unfair to burden them with late enrollment penalties because of their parents' decisions. Besides, any liabilities accrued by them during their childhood will be obligations of their parents, not themselves. Anyone attaining age eighteen will become immediately eligible to participate in American Choice without regard to previous participation. Because of the other mechanisms in place, there is little adverse selection risk inherent in this approach.

To avoid adverse selection risk among children, all penalties for late enrollment will apply to their premiums after their parents' failure to enroll them upon their first eligibility, but only until they attain the age of eighteen. Again, the parents will bear any resulting liability, not the children.

Some might argue that children should be required to have insurance, but that is not necessary. Children tend to require much less than adults in the way of health care expense, and none can be turned away from emergency care, either now or under American Choice. Low-income children will have funds paid into their HFAs by Medicaid or SCHIP. That money could be used only for health insurance and medical expenses, so there will be no financial reason for nonparticipation.

In the case of actual parental child abuse or neglect, society already has mechanisms, however imperfect, to remove children from their homes to state protective custody and foster homes. The services available to such children could include establishment of their own HFAs and enrollment in an American Choice–qualified insurance plan—perhaps under a Medicaid/SCHIP John/Jane Doe policy or optional mechanisms to avoid late enrollment penalties (discussed below).

In any event, with children's premiums based on the BAGLE rating, they will tend to be so inexpensive that no responsible parents should ever fail to enroll their children even if they themselves abstain.

4. *Provider requirements for ability to pay*: Medical providers will be allowed, even encouraged, to deny or restrict non-emergent care to anyone without the ability to pay. Although the lack of insurance alone will not be grounds to deny care, lack of ability to pay provider bills will be.

Going even further, wage garnishments and asset seizures will be encouraged for unpaid medical debts. Currently, such attempts by hospitals, particularly not-for-profit hospitals, are often met by adverse publicity and social opprobrium. The distaste is understandable when those being pursued have no access to health insurance. Under American Choice, however, the universal availability of affordable coverage will turn the tables. Aggressive debt-collection activities will serve the positive purpose of reducing the moral hazard inherent in consumers' circumventing participation by expecting free care from providers. Another mechanism that has been suggested will be for providers to file IRS Form 1099's for the market value of any free services provided to indigent patients. That would make it taxable income subject to IRS enforcement.

I recognize this approach constitutes a major cultural shift away from longstanding practices by many providers to forgive payment by those unable to pay. These changes will be justified on the basis that, with American Choice and improved government safety nets, there will be few valid excuses for anyone not to purchase insurance against otherwise unaffordable medical expenses. Doctors and hospitals, as suppliers of economic goods, will thus begin to behave the same way that vendors of other goods and services do. Cash and carry will become the rule for health services, just as it has for an even more essential commodity—food.

Hospitals with emergency departments could still be required to provide emergency care to anyone regardless of ability to pay as they do now under the EMTALA law of 1986. American Choice, however, will ensure that the amount of free care should decline dramatically from today's levels. This much-reduced burden could then be more reasonably absorbed via modest price increases to the hospitals' other customers—a vestigial version of today's cost-shifting.

An even better approach might be a return to the pre-1960s "charity care" standard by the IRS. That required tax-exempt not-for-profit hospitals to provide free care to those unable to pay, to the extent of their financial ability. The "extent of their ability" could even be measured as the amount of federal and state corporate income taxes forgone. This rule would make such costs an issue of operating surplus allocation rather than of increasing prices.

5. *Individual bankruptcy risk*: Because of the universal availability of health insurance *and* the presence of safety net funding, individuals who fail to acquire adequate coverage or who lack independent means of paying could be subject to losing all their non-exempt assets in personal bankruptcy proceedings.

Currently, medical debt is the primary cause in about 17% of bankruptcies (not the more commonly cited 50% or so).[1] American Choice will effectively remove financial reasons for most Americans to forgo health insurance and face such a public fate.

People without appreciable personal assets might not be motivated to purchase insurance for fear of bankruptcy, although they will probably have a higher likelihood of qualifying for safety-net assistance. The goal of American Choice is not to demand complete universality of health insurance coverage. As Voltaire is supposed to have observed, "The perfect is the enemy of the good." The risk of bankruptcy may not deter everyone, but most people will continue to avoid it to protect their families, reputations, and credit ratings.

These rules might seem overly harsh to many advocates of health reform. But I will argue that they are inherently fair. Remember, they will exist only within the context of universally available, affordable health insurance. People will certainly have the personal freedom to abstain, but they should not be able to do so at the expense of those who responsibly participate.

I hasten to add that there will be those who fail to apply for government safety-net assistance because of economic, social, or disability barriers. In those cases, there should be exception mechanisms to allow them to enroll late and without penalty while protecting the viability of the system. Two options will be John/Jane Doe policies and Assured Enrollment Options, which I will discuss later.

Widespread public advertising and publicity about the importance of buying health insurance will not be heeded by everyone. Although their plights might be alleviated by charitable family members, friends, and church bake sales, relatively few will rationally decide to go that route. And the few who do will not be appreciably worse off than those who now have no insurance. The difference is that, though they do not currently have access to affordable insurance, under American Choice they will.

Overall, these mechanisms will minimize or negate adverse selection and allow American Choice Health Plan to be both universally available and voluntary.

Luck-of-the-Draw Adverse Selection

Even with precautions, some insurers will inevitably suffer unexpectedly high costs from too many sick members. It's virtually a statistical certainty for some of the smaller insurers that lack the normal bell-curve distribution of health risks enjoyed by their larger competitors. Even large insurers, though, can suffer from the phe-nomenon if they fail to properly balance their benefits and premiums against the realities of their competitors' offerings.

Some health reform advocates have argued that government reg-ulators should directly deal with such events. They have proposed various mechanisms to redirect a portion of premium payments to insurers that end up with a disproportionate share of sick members. They would obtain this money by taking it away from the insurers with healthier, lower-risk populations.

There is a fundamental problem with this approach. Insurance markets already deal with it through an effective market mechanism. It's called reinsurance, and it spreads such risks across many insur-ers. It pays off in the event one of them experiences unexpectedly high levels of catastrophic claims. Thus, an insurer may decide to purchase reinsurance against individual member costs exceeding, for example, $100,000 in a given year. That can protect the insurer in the event it gets an unexpectedly high volume of such claims.

Reinsurance strategy has long been an essential element of sound financial management by insurers and managed-care companies. When I was the federal government's chief HMO financial regula-tor more than thirty years ago, the prudent use of reinsurance was always a key element in our assessments of HMO fiscal soundness. Numerous insurance carriers have offered it. American Choice will likely generate expanded interest in the business. This is one of the few aspects of contemporary health insurance that ain't broke, so there's really no need to fix it.

Reinsurance should be any insurer's last-ditch defense against adverse selection, however. It is expensive and hardly a substitute for sound management. Under American Choice—or any other insurance system—every insurer will have to balance the desire for enrollment growth with the need to attract no more than a normal share of high-risk members. That will require a level of actuarial and underwriting sophistication (that is, management) that takes into account such factors as competing insurer benefits and prices, government-mandated continuous creditable coverage benefit requirements, provider pricing, the use of best-practice providers, accurate utilization and unit cost projections, optimal BAGLE premium adjustment factors, member incentives for savvy provider shopping and utilization, programs for member information and guidance, and the availability of effective disease management programs.

Juggling all these factors to maintain profitable growth—while having to accept all comers—will present a new challenge to insurers unaccustomed to competing for individual customers. Some will adjust and thrive, but others—as we saw with indemnity insurers during the HMO onslaught of the last three decades of the twentieth century—will prudently leave the business. Others will simply fail and be taken over by state insurance regulators, with the members being protected by the insurers' remaining claims reserves, statutory risk-based capital, and state-wide reserve pools.

In all likelihood, the most successful insurers—as we saw during the HMO era—will be entrepreneurial ventures untainted by obsolete attitudes about consumers and providers. These insurers will approach the business of insurance as one of empowering consumers and facilitating their access to the best providers offering the best prices and customer service. This is a challenging problem, but an eminently tractable one for well-run insurers.

If we were to follow the advice of those health reformers and institute the mandatory reallocation of premiums to insurers with higher claims, we would be creating moral hazard that would remove much of the incentives for sound management. Poorly run insurers would lack the incentives to change, knowing they would be bailed out by the well-run ones. That's not a good idea.

Individual Predictive Risk Modeling

Some health reform proponents who argue for such premium reallocations do so based on the use of objective individual member health assessments. These would supposedly allow regulators to discern justified versus unjustified cost differences between members in deciding how to reallocate premiums. With predictive risk modeling, an underwriter would—initially, and periodically thereafter—scrutinize each insured person's health status and predict his medical care needs. This could require a comprehensive member questionnaire, accessing and reviewing the member's medical record, requiring the member to undergo a medical examination, and engaging in an extensive interview with any member who had more than minor medical conditions. Or it might involve no more than a review of each member's recent claims history to assess risk. The process would also factor in each member's age, gender, and regional variations in medical costs and then attempt to predict his medical claims. Then, any insurer with a higher percentage of healthy members would be required to surrender a portion of its premium revenue to insurers with a greater proportion of sick members.

The biggest problem with this approach is that no one knows how to make sufficiently accurate individual predictions to allow such a system to work, no matter how fine-grained the assessment. Current medical underwriting practices by individual coverage insurers are nowhere near sophisticated enough to predict a person's health care experience with the precision needed. Even the most sophisticated predictive models are, at best, only about 20% accurate.[2] Any one individual's demand for, and outcomes from, health services are rarely predictable. Each assessment will require a significant dose of judgment on the part of a medical underwriter, which will necessarily vary from one underwriter to another, no matter how thick the underwriting manual. Even if this approach could work, it could be expensive and time-consuming, and it would not remove the moral hazard enabling ineffectively run insurers to be bailed out by their more enlightened peers.

It would also constitute invasion of personal privacy. Under a system of individually risk-adjusted underwriting, anyone wanting health insurance could be forced to divulge his or her own health history and genetic information in minute detail to private and/or government bureaucrats, which could invite mischief by employers and agencies wanting to manage other risks or to otherwise intervene for beneficial or nefarious purposes. Only one's health care providers—and perhaps life insurers—have a legitimate need for such information.

Individual risk assessments for setting premiums or reallocating them to other insurers is neither desirable nor necessary. It is a solution without a problem.

Another variation on the risk assessment theme is to let everyone apply for individual insurance under current rules that require acceptance based on medical status and history. Such proposals were made by Senator McCain and various policy advisers. Their approach recognizes the obvious problem of people who are unable to pass medical muster for private insurance. Their solution is to require some form of government-operated risk pools as the insurers of last resort for these people.

Unfortunately, this approach is little more than a creeping single-payer plan. It would systematically funnel the sick into subsidized government insurance. Even people accepted for individual insurance and who subsequently become ill could find themselves sluiced into the government programs, which would be unsustainable without massive subsidies from taxpayers or other external sources.

To demonstrate, let's look at two fictional insurers operating under this approach. Oldco is an individual insurance company that has been in business for many years. Although all of its members originally passed underwriting muster before joining, many are now older and have gotten progressively sicker and more expensive to service. Newco is a newly formed insurer with no such legacy morbidity. All of their members have recently undergone medical underwriting and are almost uniformly healthy. Both Oldco's and Newco's rejected applicants were all directed into the government's "Pool of Last Resort."

Because Oldco's overall risk profile has reverted to the mean (become less healthy), Oldco's premiums have increased much faster than medical inflation and are now a lot higher than Newco's. This has not been lost on Oldco's remaining healthy members. Increasingly, they have discovered they can successfully undergo fresh underwriting with Newco and pay lower rates for identical coverage.

Oldco's sicker members have no such option. They have to stay where they are, paying ever higher premiums as their healthier compatriots depart. Thus, the 80/20 Rule has become the 70/20 Rule, as Bruce Pyenson termed it. Oldco is getting more and more adverse selection while Newco is prospering.

As the cycle tightens, Oldco is finally forced to exit the business. Its now uninsurable former members have no alternative but the "Pool of Last Resort," which is becoming indistinguishable from an entitlement program for sick people. Newco is sitting pretty for the time being, until, to paraphrase The Who, "Meet the Newco, same as the Oldco." Thus continues the inexorable progression of all the sick people into the Pool of Last Resort. Taking this example to its logical extreme, healthy people will be better off not buying any insurance at all. Instead, they should bypass all that extra hassle and insurance overhead and just pay their own medical bills as long as they can afford them. When they become too high, they should simply join the Pool of Last Resort. Thus it would become what its proponents had originally hoped to avoid—a single-payer program. Bad idea.

The more you move toward charging or allocating insurance premiums based on individual health status, the more you're actually moving away from the concept of insurance. The whole idea of insurance is to have as many people as possible sharing the financial risk of unaffordable medical problems. That way, those who suffer from them won't be bankrupted or denied necessary services. When we start making underwriting allowances based on the actual conditions you're trying to insure against, you're removing some of the protection you seek to achieve.

Under American Choice, no one will be uninsurable by private insurers, so there will be no need for any segregated high-risk pools. Insurers will all be protected from adverse selection by a combination of prudent management, American Choice's rules against consumer gamesmanship, and reinsurance.

Oddly, programs like the Pool of Last Resort tend to be proposed by advocates of free markets. Their goal is to preserve the supposedly market-oriented parts of the current system they like (individual insurance as they know it) while doing away with the more socialized, bureaucratic parts they don't (government and employer group insurance programs). Unfortunately, their health reform proposals, like so many others, are low-altitude solutions to a high-altitude problem. No amount of tinkering around the edges of the current system is going to fix it. It's time for a wholesale fix.

Transition Adverse Selection

Some critics might argue that American Choice will initially provide an unfair benefit to current free riders who have forgone buying health insurance and accumulated a list of dire conditions through poor personal choices. Those who now lack insurance will receive a windfall by joining American Choice and immediately receive far more in expensive medical services than they'll pay in premiums. This will indeed be an unavoidable effect of American Choice. Fortunately, it appears that the uninsured, *en masse*, are not any sicker than the insured population. Given the current preponderance of young people without insurance, American Choice might even enjoy a better risk profile overall than the current insured population. In any event, getting virtually all of the uninsured into the pool shouldn't have a negative net effect on the pool's average morbidity risk.

Also, any such windfall for those with unhealthy lifestyles will be attenuated by the inherent BAGLE premium adjustments for controllable health risk factors. Someone with smoking-induced lung cancer will get immediate, expensive treatments. But those costs will be paid by all the other smokers, just as their costs will be subsequently covered by their fellow puffers. In the longer term, cradle-to-grave coverage under American Choice will virtually eliminate such free riders. That's because any smoker will have a choice. As I explain below in chapter 11, he can either pay higher premiums over his lifetime to cover the full average cost of his smoke-induced illnesses, or he can stop smoking and pay nothing to treat smoking-related diseases. A fair choice for everyone, but one currently illegal under HIPAA rules.

Reform of Minimum Benefits Requirements

Under American Choice, each insurance company will decide how many different benefit plans to offer in each market and what benefits to offer with each plan. These could also include plans in which consumers will agree to multi-year commitments that forgo interim open-enrollment options. All American Choice health plans, though, will be required to meet federal minimum benefit requirements for continuous creditable coverage (CCC).

Why will any minimum benefit requirements be necessary? Haven't such mandates in states such as Minnesota, Massachusetts, New York, and New Jersey driven up health insurance costs by as much as 50%?[3] Why can't we simply eliminate all benefit mandates and just let consumers and insurers decide among themselves in a free, price-mediated marketplace? Wouldn't that be more consistent with the goal of maximizing market forces and minimizing intrusive government regulation?

To explore the answer, let's take a hypothetical example of an American Choice Health Plan with no CCC requirement. I'll call it American Freeride.

Bob is a healthy thirty-two-year-old Wyoming cattle feedlot foreman. When American Freeride debuted in 2012 offering him fifty-seven different health plans, his employer, the Lazy H Feed Lot, told him they would contribute $7,000 a year to Bob's HFA to help him buy insurance and pay for out-of-pocket medical costs. The federal legislation creating American Freeride had established a limit on annual HFA contributions to $15,000 for individuals. Bob thought about it and prudently decided to contribute an additional $3,000 per year from his own pay.

Then Bob had to choose to sign up for one of the fifty-seven available health plans during the November 1 and December 15, 2011, open enrollment period for his 2012 coverage. He was healthy and didn't anticipate needing medical services in the coming year. In fact, with $10,000 in total annual contributions to his HFA bank account, he had plenty for a rainy-day fund if he got sick and needed care. As he scanned the Internet list of plans being offered in his area, he saw a very rich benefit plan offered by a Minnesota insurer that cost $1,500 per month. It had no deductible, covered unlimited hospital days with no out-of-pocket cost, and unlimited doctor visits with only $15 copayments. But when he saw a plan for only $200 per month, Bob got interested. It was the Less Health for Less Plan offered by Mo's Health Insurance and Storm Door Company in Boise, Idaho. It didn't cover much—no more than five doctor visits per year, a maximum of $25,000 of inpatient hospital services to a maximum of $300 per day, $1,000 for emergency care, $1,000 for doctor and outpatient care, and a total maximum annual benefit of only $50,000. But the price was right, so Bob signed up.

Bob was able to buy such bare bones coverage because the congressional legislation enacting American Freeride had required that no state or federal agency could mandate any minimum benefit levels for health plans. Congress had decided to let the market set all benefits and prices.

For the next two years Bob stayed with Less Health for Less and had only four doctor visits the entire time. At the end of the two years he had more than $15,000 in his HFA. But thirty years of wearing high-heeled, pointed-toe cowboy boots had given him foot problems. His podiatrist told him he needed $10,000 worth of bunion surgery. Also, Bob had been a rodeo bull rider in his youth, and all those falls had added up to a torn ACL in his right knee and increasing lower back pain. His orthopedic surgeon told him he should have the ACL repaired ($10,000) and a spine implant ($125,000). Otherwise, he would experience increased difficulty walking and working.

Bob instantly realized that his current limited insurance coverage would wipe out his HFA and leave him deep in debt. Fortunately for Bob, the American Freeride open enrollment period for 2014 had just begun, so he started looking for better insurance coverage. He found it in another Idaho insurer, American Liberty Life and Health Insurance Company, which offered a plan called Comprehensive Plus. It had a deductible that required members to pay the first $5,000 of expenses but then covered 100% of doctor and hospital expenses up to a $3 million lifetime limit. That coverage was priced at $1,000 per month. The $5,000 deductible, plus the $12,000 for a year's premium, was more than the $10,000 Bob and his employer would contribute to his HFA that year, but the improved coverage and his current $15,000+ HFA balance would allow him to get the surgeries and still end the year with an HFA balance of around $8,000. Moreover, Bob knew that after he had all his surgeries and recovery taken care of, he could go back to a low-priced health plan.

Bob signed up for Comprehensive Plus, and all went well. He had the surgeries and made a full recovery. He was still a healthy non-smoking man and had no fear of falling ill and needing more medical services. So when the open enrollment for 2015 began, Bob went back to the Less Health for Less coverage. It now cost $240/month. Over the next several years, Bob piled up HFA balances and started investing part of it in no-load long-term equity funds in anticipation of his ultimate retirement. But as he signed up the second time for Less Health for Less, he noticed that the 2015 monthly premium for the Comprehensive Plus plan he was dropping had more than doubled in a single year from $1,000 to $2,200. "What a rip-off," he muttered. He filled out the paperwork to return to the low-cost plan.

In truth, there was a rip-off, but it was from people like Bob gaming a flawed system that permitted low-ball minimed benefit plans to siphon off the good risks until they became bad risks. The flaw was in allowing insurers to cap benefits at extremely low levels and not provide the catastrophic insurance that is essential for American Choice or any other universally available insurance system to function.

Bob and others like him, when healthy, could avoid contributing to the larger risk pool that is essential to sustain the costs of those relatively few who incur major medical expenses. The huge increase in the Comprehensive Plus premium in one year was not insurer profiteering but the inevitable result of people like Bob cherry-picking their benefits (adversely selecting them) from year to year.

When low, non-catastrophic-level benefit caps are permitted, insurers that offer plans with truly catastrophic caps will get the worst risks. That leaves them with three choices: (1) raise premiums to cover the additional claims; (2) reduce their own benefit caps; or (3) exit the market. Raising premiums to compensate for adverse selection is a losing strategy. It chases out any remaining low and moderate risks, leaving an even more concentrated pool of high-cost members. Unless the insurer cuts benefits, it will experience a death spiral of ever-increasing costs followed by higher premiums followed by higher costs, etc., until forced to leave the market entirely. The end result is a race to the bottom to see who can offer the lowest benefit caps—thus creating an "insurance" system consisting of prepaid primary care and little or nothing in the way of financial protection against financial hardship or catastrophe.

Artificially low benefit maximums, like those in Bob's Less Health for Less Plan, are exactly the opposite of what a consumer needs. Minimed "insurance" products are available now, and they are a pox on the system. It's not the cheap stuff that needs to be insured against. It's the expensive stuff.

Carefully crafted, CCC actually encourages greater participation by insurers, lower premiums for consumers, and wider access to competitive insurance plans for all Americans. The key is for the regulators to strike a balance between making minimum benefit limits high enough to prevent such gaming and low enough to offer affordable coverage to everyone.

American Choice's CCC rules will prevent renegade insurers from avoiding or failing to meet the needs of their sickest members. No insurer will be allowed to cherry-pick its members by excluding any necessary and expensive medical services. Each insurer, knowing that it will be enrolling some high-cost individuals no matter what, will have a strong incentive to promote high-quality, effective, innovative, low-cost provider solutions to meet their needs.

Providers, knowing that funds are available for these services, will compete aggressively to provide the most cost-effective care to these members, which will attract the business of both the members and their insurers.

Under American Choice, there will doubtless be some insurers that will try to drive off their sickest members by delaying claims, denying services, and generally being jerks. But any such abuse will be largely self-correcting. The abused sick members will certainly leave such insurers for better plans at their earliest opportunities. But so will droves of the healthy ones as word gets around—and it will—that they can expect no better when they need care.

People rarely buy any kind of product or service from companies they don't expect to honor their commitments. It will be just as easy for the healthy to leave a bad insurer as it will for the sick—during the next open enrollment period. Remember, no insurer will have a lock on any of its members, unlike the current system of individual, government, and employer-sponsored coverage in which a person's ability to change insurers is too often not an option.

There will be numerous other remedies for such tactics—many present in the current system—including appeals procedures, public exposure, regulatory sanctions and penalties, and, ultimately, disqualification from offering American Choice coverage. The most effective corrective will be each consumer's ability to vote with his feet. To paraphrase the old movie mogul Samuel Goldwyn, "If people don't want to sign up with a bad insurer, nobody can stop them." Consumer markets deal harshly with customer abuse.

As for the problem of state-mandated benefits driving up insurance costs, all such mandates will be abolished by American Choice's federal enabling legislation. Thus, the purpose of CCC is *not* to pander to the special interests who want coverage for non-standard, unsafe, unproven, low-cost or unnecessary medical services that fall outside the realm of necessary, unaffordable medical care. Instead, each insurance company will be allowed to decide what benefits to offer in its benefit packages, and any insurer will be able to offer more than one plan in any market area, all, of course, subject to CCC.

Setting CCC Limits

In establishing CCC's regulatory requirements for minimum benefits under American Choice, five issues should be taken into account by the regulators who oversee the system:

1. *Catastrophic Benefit Caps:* This is a primary requirement of CCC. Every American Choice insurer will be required to offer plans that provide effective coverage for a large portion of the costs of the most expensive medical care that most consumers are likely to find necessary. This requirement concentrates on benefit caps at the catastrophic end of coverage, not on low-end first-dollar coverage. That means that rules for CCC high-end coverage will specify the lowest maximum benefit limits or caps that an insurer could place on any insurance plan.

   How much should American Choice require for such a minimum benefit cap? This requires more analysis and debate by actuaries, providers, and legislators, but it is likely that a minimum benefit cap of $3,000,000 or so will currently provide adequate catastrophic coverage for the vast majority of Americans.

   Should benefit caps be prohibited altogether? I suggest not. I am aware of at least one credible story of a hospital's "valiant" fight years ago to keep a patient technically alive but with no chance of her ever regaining physical or cognitive function. The effort was continued until the poor woman's insurance benefits ran out. At that point the hospital summoned its medical ethics committee to review the case. The hospital administrators recommended that the patient's relatives be counseled as to the hopelessness of the patient's condition. The ethicists agreed. Very soon thereafter, the family had the patient taken off her respirator, and she promptly died. Had there been no benefit cap at all, I fear they would still be keeping her "alive" and driving the medical bills up by millions more.

The point is not that benefit caps should determine when patients be allowed to die. The two issues should be completely divorced from each other, but the story points out the moral hazard implicit in giving health care providers a blank check, even to the potential detriment of the patient.

2. *Continuous Coverage*: After American Choice's inaugural open enrollment period, eligibility for normal coverage and premiums must be dependent upon each participant having continuous coverage. Otherwise, they will be subject to penalties, limitations, and surcharges. Although short gaps may be permitted (Medicare allows a maximum of sixty-three days), the risk of adverse selection is otherwise too great.

3. *CCC Requirements for Services That Must Be Covered*:
If the answer to *either* of the two following questions is no, then American Choice's regulators should not require any given medical service to be included as a minimum CCC requirement:

   a. Is it medically necessary?
   b. Is it expensive?

In other words, does it fit into the upper right quadrant of this 2x2 table?

	Low Cost Care	High Cost Care
Necessary Care	Insurance Coverage Unnecessary	Insurance Coverage Necessary
Unnecessary Care	Insurance Coverage Unnecessary	Insurance Coverage Unnecessary

Low-Cost, Necessary Care. The upper-left quadrant includes necessary care, but that which would be normally affordable as a consumer purchase. This would include primary care (including minor doctor office visits, laboratory tests, and most medical imaging), preventive care, and most prescription drugs. Insurers would certainly be allowed to cover such services, but they should never be required to do so for CCC. We don't buy car insurance to cover oil changes, tires, gasoline, or battery replacement. These are all normal consumer purchases that competition keeps affordable. Likewise, health insurance should not be required to cover any care that is readily affordable by all but our poorest citizens.

Buying such services through an insurer can often double the cost. The primary and preventive care component of insurance premiums typically includes 15–45% for insurer overhead and profit, plus higher medical reimbursements to pay providers for their top-heavy billing and collection systems. To this you can add several more percentage points for excess utilization by people who don't really need care but get it anyway. That's because current benefit copayments make it appear to be less expensive than it really is. If consumers could cut out the insurance middleman and buy primary care directly from providers, it would cost much less than it does now.

Dr. Benjamin Brewer, a family practice doctor who writes a column for *The Wall Street Journal*, has said:

> What's missing in the debate over our nation's health-care crisis is that primary care is cheap. Cheaper than your cell phone bill. Cheaper than a tank of gas. Cheaper than dinner and a movie. It's so cheap the average person doesn't value it properly. I could have covered my salary for 2007 and the costs of all my staff and overhead *for less than $20 per patient per month*, including maternity and hospital care. My practice covers 80% to 90% of what the average person will ever need a doctor for. Compare that to what you or your employer is paying for health coverage, and you'll find that the high costs are due largely to catastrophic illnesses, hospital charges and money going to middlemen.[4] [emphasis added]

There should, however, be no prohibition on coverage for such services. Some organizations, such as the Kaiser Foundation Health Plans, provide them efficiently without incurring most of the additional overhead faced by traditional insurers. And because Kaiser pays its contracted physicians on a capitation basis, it forgoes the burdens inflicted by the toxic provider billing and collection systems.

Insurers should remain free to continue offering primary and preventive care coverage alongside expensive acute care; however, relatively few consumers are likely to find it worth the price, unless it comes from a Kaiser or similar plan. Most will choose instead to buy it directly from doctors and nurse practitioners, either on a fee-for-service, prepayment, or other basis. It will be a lot cheaper overall, with competitive, transparent prices.

Still, there will likely be people who have become so accustomed to insurance coverage for such services that they will be willing to pay outsized premiums in order to continue them.

Some may fret that, though positive financial incentives are fine, forcing people into high-deductible health insurance plans will provide an equally effective financial incentive *not* to seek care. They will now have to pay for their own primary and preventive care out of their own pockets. American Choice will likely encourage high-deductible catastrophic insurance and more personal responsibility for primary care expenses. Nothing, though, will prevent health care providers from attracting patients by offering low-cost prepaid and fee-for-service primary care and better, lower cost solutions for long-term chronic disease management. Indeed, such solutions would be far more likely to find a ready market under American Choice than they do now.

Under American Choice, consumers will be demanding low-cost services that provide continual assistance to people for preventing and treating chronic (and acute) diseases. Such services are hard to find today because most insurers simply won't pay for them. But with financially enabled consumers with the money and the motivation to pay, innovative entrepreneurs will emerge to serve them in ways we cannot even imagine now. Even today, the Joslin Diabetes Center in Boston has a program costing about $75/month that has dramatically lowered patients' blood sugars to healthy levels on an ongoing basis. Nonetheless, it is struggling because of lack of insurance coverage to pay for it.

Although most medical prevention has not been cost-effective for insurers, prevention based on personal lifestyle improvement—and assisted by medical intervention—can greatly enhance *individual* financial, physical, and emotional well-being. Under American Choice, the vast majority of Americans will find themselves able to purchase the products and services that will enable them to prevent and manage their diseases. Cost-effectiveness will be based on each individual's assessment of value across the full range of his life's capabilities and activities rather than on narrow insurance company measurements.

We must reject the chronic, paternalistic myth that, absent free primary care, people won't buy it. Most people want to take care of themselves and, armed with the money and information on price and quality to take action, they will. Enlightened self-interest will accomplish what paternalism hasn't.

Low-Cost, Optional Care. The lower-left quadrant includes those medical products and services that are both optional (i.e., not medically necessary) and affordable as consumer purchases. These might include Botox treatments and recreational use of erectile dysfunction drugs. None is appropriate for required CCC.

High-Cost, Optional Care. The lower-right quadrant contains all the high-cost, optional medical procedures. Breast augmentation/reduction procedures, facelifts, Lasik eye surgery, and most bariatric surgery for weight loss would be included here. Mandatory CCC insurance coverage is not appropriate.

High-Cost, Necessary Care. The lone upper-right quadrant includes all high-cost (normally nonaffordable) necessary health care services that constitute the proper universe of minimum allowed CCC requirements. In general, it includes proven, non-experimental, medically necessary services to preserve life, to restore necessary body function, and to alleviate pain and suffering. There should be no coverage requirement for any provider category for which there is no independent literature based on scientifically-controlled studies of their medical efficacy. Necessary services include those for which there are established medical treatment standards, preferably nationally recognized. Absent such standards, medically necessary services will include those required for treatments for which there is adequate scientific evidence of effectiveness for the patient. Examples of covered services include necessary hospitalizations and inpatient surgeries; many medically necessary outpatient surgical procedures; and expensive drug, biological, and chemotherapy treatments.

4. *Out-of-Pocket Spending Limits*: In general, CCC requirements for consumer out-of-pocket payments for deductibles, coinsurance, balance billing, and copayments should be reasonably affordable for the insured members. They should not be abused by insurers as a way to offer low premiums and seemingly rich benefits when in fact the consumer is left with an empty HFA, personal debt, and needing better coverage during the next open enrollment period.

A significant complicating factor is that different consumers will have different perceptions of what constitutes affordable out-of-pocket payments. For example, someone who has maintained a healthy lifestyle and built up a substantial HFA balance of, say, $100,000, might well afford a $25,000 or $30,000 annual deductible. A person recovering from serious cancer treatment or suffering from uncontrolled chronic disease may not have that option.

It is generally in the public interest for each consumer to accept the highest out-of-pocket payment responsibility that she can reasonably afford. Properly structured, we should seek to create a virtuous cycle of prudent purchasing and healthy living, which leads to lower insurance requirements, which leads to greater HFA savings, which leads to greater individual financial responsibility and incentives, which leads to greater health provider competition on price and quality, which leads to healthier living, and so on.

As long as catastrophic benefit caps are kept appropriately high, it will be feasible to allow consumers to choose levels of first-dollar deductibles and continuing coinsurance on the basis of their personal ability to pay them. One approach might be to establish maximum annual consumer out-of-pocket exposure each year at the higher of $5,000 per person or 25% of the beginning balance in a person's HFA, which will create an additional incentive for healthy behavior, savvy health care purchasing, and maximized HFA savings. There will be no need, however, to require minimum deductible levels, such as those now imposed for the high deductible health plans people need to open HSAs.

5. *Closed Provider Networks*: Insurers should not be allowed to promise coverage for comprehensive cardiac care while offering too few available cardiologists or cardiac surgeons in their provider networks, if they have networks at all. At the same time, they should be allowed to exclude low-quality or inefficient providers or others that don't fit with an insurer's preferred model. State any-willing-provider laws, enacted under pressure from favor-seeking provider interests, should be abolished. They enforce the pretense than all licensed providers are equally competent and honest. They're not. They also assume that insurers' business models don't count. They do.

Under American Choice, innovative insurers will help guide their insureds to high-value providers. Both insurers and members will share the same incentive to seek doctors and hospitals that offer the best outcomes and the lowest total short-term *and* long-term costs. Hard-of-thinking insurers that try to play the old claims-denial game and control their risk exposure by denying access to the best providers will not only be committing financial suicide from higher long-term costs but marketing suicide when the consuming public quickly learns to avoid them altogether.

Under the current system, consumers are locked into their insurers, allowing some companies to succumb to the temptation to play games with provider access, prior-authorization requirements, and claims denials without fear of consumer retribution. That cannot continue with American Choice. Every consumer will demand value from his insurer. He will take his business elsewhere if he doesn't believe he'll get it when the chips are down.

Regulating Insurer Participation

The question arises as to the extent to which the American Choice regulatory function should limit insurer participation. Currently, analogous regulators of the Federal Employee Health Benefit Program (FEHBP) and the Massachusetts Connector take an active role in vetting insurers before allowing them to offer their wares. Such regulators, when so empowered, seem to inevitably tend toward "improving" on legislative intent by assuming an unwanted, often paternalistic role that ends up arbitrarily limiting the number of insurers offered.

Under American Choice, it should be sufficient for each participating insurer to certify periodically that each of its participating health plans meets all CCC, BAGLE-rating, and other regulatory requirements. Certifications by properly licensed insurers should be on a file-and-use basis. Regulators should not require application and approval before properly licensed insurers could offer benefits and rates. Regulators must have no authority over rates it might consider excessive (other than in cases of insurer collusion), leaving that determination to consumers. The only regulatory oversight of benefits will be with respect to enforcement of minimum CCC requirements.

All insured members should be legally entitled to assert regulatory definitions and interpretations of CCC in claiming coverage—regardless of actual policy language or other insurer limitations to the contrary. Self-certification of CCC by insurers will be subject to member complaints and regulatory investigation and enforcement. There should be no official government certification process, common market, "connector," or other government-regulated gateway mechanism to limit market access by participating insurers.

American Choice insurers should be subject to their respective domicile state's fiscal soundness regulations and triennial examinations. American Choice could delegate to the states the requirement to review and confirm insurer compliance with its requirements.

A Uniform Benefit Plan for All?

Shouldn't the government eliminate the whole body of CCC rules with the simple expedient of a single standard for insurance benefits, with everyone buying the same plan? The answer is unequivocally no. That would be shooting a rabbit with an elephant gun—you get a dead rabbit but nothing to eat.

Mandating uniform benefits is bad policy because (1) it removes any ability of consumers to select plans with benefits and prices that best meet their own needs; (2) it eliminates the ability of innovative insurers to create products, features, and value that better meet consumer needs; and (3) it similarly retards innovation in medical and other care modalities that technically fall outside the standard benefits.

Nor, for the same reasons, does it mean that the government should mandate several standard health plans as it currently does for Medicare supplements. Legislators and government employees have zero ability to move quickly to adjust offerings to meet current and anticipated consumer demand. This would be like the government mandating five standard automobiles that all car-buyers must choose from—a two-passenger coupe, a four-passenger sedan, a minivan, an SUV, and a pickup truck—with no options and no ability of car makers to innovate to address changing consumer tastes, gasoline prices, technological opportunities, or safety innovations.

The best argument against the government setting standard benefit designs is that it is unnecessary. This lesson has been abundantly demonstrated in virtually every other arena of consumer choice, whether automobiles, food, clothing, housing, or recreation.

Even in health care, the benefits of allowing the market to design its own benefit plans has been demonstrated by Medicare Part D.

A Challenge to Insurers

American Choice's flexible approach to benefits will present a definite challenge to insurance company actuaries and underwriters. They will have a much tougher time balancing their marketing departments' desire for attractive benefits with the CFOs' demand that those benefits don't attract too many high-risk members.

But making it easy for insurers is not a goal of American Choice. They will have to work harder and smarter for their profits, but the wiser, innovative ones will do just fine. This was one of the positive lessons we learned from the HMO revolution. Insurers with less wisdom exited the business or were put out of business. When that happens now, we get more uninsurable people. Under American Choice, all such orphaned members will find immediate refuge in the welcoming arms of other participating insurers.

As I expect to see with Part D, there will be some, maybe a lot of, early turmoil in the American Choice marketplace. Insurers that under-price their products will have to make adjustments to prices, benefits, or both. Insurers that fail to gain sufficient market share might have to exit the market or merge with their successful competitors. American Choice's federal regulatory body should not be as controlling as Medicare has been in restricting the plans to be offered. It should not regulate premium levels at all, only the BAGLE calculation method. This will permit innovative insurers to enter the market to provide better value and better choice than current players.

Consumers will benefit from American Choice's multiplicity of product and price offerings, but they will need to be watchful and nimble enough to make advantageous changes, possibly every year— at least until the market stabilizes. Choosing one health plan initially and then standing pat with it will not be wise for many people. This circumstance has been perhaps the biggest challenge of Medicare's Part D and federal FEHBP programs. Their members, often accustomed to a traditional benefits package in any color they want as long as it's black, must now extend the savvy consumer skills they've acquired over a lifetime to the purchase of insurance. American Choice might create initial consumer grumbling about "too many confusing choices." It could take a while for the market to settle in, but it will happen.

CHAPTER 11

Premium Reform

A necessary feature of American Choice's regulatory boundaries will be the premium rating methodologies permitted for participating insurers. In chapter 4 I discussed in some detail the various rate-setting methodologics and the relevant issues of each. I will now address my proposed BAGLE rating system.

Overall, BAGLE rating is an adjusted community rating approach. Premium adjustments for member health status, history, or genetic makeup will not be permitted. Member-specific adjustments will be permitted for the following factors:

1. Member achievement of objective personal health risk indicators (B for *behavior*)

2. Member age, gender, and residence location (AGL for *age, gender,* and *location*)

3. Member vocational and avocational risks (E for *employment/ extracurricular*)

Considering the alternatives, BAGLE rating seems to be the simplest and fairest form of premium rate setting. It will work for both insurers and insureds across large populations—indeed, the entire U.S. population. It is simple to understand, simple to administer, straightforward to regulate, and easy to adjust over time. Anyone will be able to quickly and easily determine how much his or her premiums will be for a multitude of health plan options. There will be no waiting for an underwriter's ruling or the results of some complicated, arbitrary personal health assessment. BAGLE rating requires no health questionnaires, no medical records review, no health screening, and no underwriter judgments about one's health status or history. It requires disclosure of personal health information only for people who wish to take advantage of savings from having achieved personal health-risk indicators. But even then, it does not require anyone to disclose his failure to achieve them.

BAGLE rating does not punish the sick for being sick, but it fairly assesses the costs of voluntary involvement in risky occupations or behaviors. This could virtually eliminate the moral hazard of behavioral free riders whose obesity, smoking, and other habits are currently subsidized by those with healthy lifestyles. BAGLE recognizes and assesses the inherent risks of higher morbidity and medical expense as one ages. It recognizes that women incur higher costs than men, at least at certain ages. It eliminates current discrimination against the young while providing strong savings incentives for all ages.

The age, gender, location and employment/extracurricular adjustments are the same ones in wide use today by insurers of employer groups and individuals, as well as employers that self-insure. Except for individual insurance, though, these adjustments are now used by employers and their insurers only to calculate total premiums needed to provide insurance to each group in its entirety. They are rarely used to set the premium contributions of the employees themselves. I have previously discussed the problems arising from this practice, in particular the discriminatory pricing against workers who are younger and usually lower-paid. I have also discussed the public policy implications of recognizing the inherent differences in medical costs between women and men and for people living in different parts of the country.

In correcting the reverse-age-discrimination issue, BAGLE rating will lower premiums for younger workers while increasing them for older ones. However, there are a number of key features of American Choice that should significantly soften the blow or even reduce total costs for the older workers. Here are the key ones:

1. *They Can Better Afford It*: Since they tend to earn considerably more money than the twenty-two-year-olds, the sixty-year-olds might decide just to pay the difference and be content that they were able to take advantage of their younger workers for as long as they did. Many of the elderly will likely not be so philosophical about their newfound equality, so this may not be the best lead argument on this subject. That's probably why I'm a finance geek, not a sales guru.

2. *Employer Assistance*: The sixty-year-olds and other older workers could appeal to their employers to boost their contributions to them to help defray the higher costs, at least on a temporary basis. Many employers, eager to get out from under the increasingly intractable and administratively costly burden of providing health insurance, might well agree to such petitions in order to make the transition to defined-contribution more palatable for all their workers. Employers may well consider themselves still to be better off than had they continued to pay double-digit annual premium increases under the old system.

3. *Lower Comparable Premiums*: The older workers will find that they can purchase the same level of insurance benefits for a lower price than their employers paid. This will result from the elimination of government cost-shifting to employers and from increased insurer competition for worker memberships. Employees of smaller, formerly commercially-insured firms will find even larger premium savings from the elimination of unnecessary benefit mandates and the inherent inefficiencies in small group rating. This approach will reduce their insurance costs dollar-for-dollar with such premium reductions since their employer's contributions will remain constant regardless of the plans the workers choose to buy. It should be noted that the excessive administrative and sales costs of today's most common

form of individual insurance would vanish under American Choice with the elimination of medical underwriting and high sales costs.

4. *Lower-Cost Options*: The older workers will be able to decide whether to buy lower-cost insurance with lesser benefits than their old employer plans, which could be particularly appropriate if the old plans were laden with unnecessary benefits that they didn't need anyway. This will also reduce workers' required HFA contributions on a dollar-for-dollar basis.

5. *Prevention Savings*: The older employees may be able to reduce their HFA contributions further by taking advantage of insurance premium discounts and rebates from achieving and demonstrating healthy risk indicators, such as by not smoking, not abusing alcohol, controlling their weight, and other factors.

6. *Systemic Savings*: Whether the older employees do any of the above, over time they will see their premiums and health care costs drop significantly. American Choice's market-based system will rationalize these prices in response to consumer demand for value.

Overall, the older workers may have to make more decisions about how to spend their money. But if they do it with reasonable diligence, they will end up much better off both financially and personally under American Choice than they are now.

"B" Is for Behavior

I have described how our society and our medical delivery system have failed to prevent the current epidemic of uncontrolled chronic disease that accounts for more than $1.5 trillion of our nation's $2.2 trillion in annual health care expenditures. Between at-risk Americans who fail to prevent and manage their own chronic diseases and doctors who fail to follow accepted standards of care, we have a major problem. Any attempt to reform health care must include mechanisms to alleviate it. I believe that BAGLE rating can do much in this regard.

The primary mechanism is to provide an immediate, direct financial incentive for people to identify and control their own personal behaviors that are leading to increased health risks. These incentives will result in two different behaviors. One group of at-risk people will respond by discovering and correcting their risks. They will be rewarded with lower premiums. The other group will do nothing except pay higher insurance premiums. Either way, it will be the individual's decision to make. These premium adjustments will be calculated by each insurance company's actuaries to equal the long-term expected average costs of a person's increased morbidity over his lifetime for each behavior-based risk.

To the extent such incentives are effective in motivating consumers to ask their doctors for help, it will resolve many current problems of doctors failing to detect and treat related medical problems. There is nothing more effective for getting doctors to change their behavior than patients asking them to do something to help. In my own consulting practice, I have found that providing financial motivation for patients to ask their doctors for help in saving money on their prescription medications has yielded savings of 35+% *and* an increase in the number of dispensed prescriptions. The same dynamic can be applied more broadly across the entire spectrum of health care prevention and treatment.

American Choice combines the individual's primary responsibility for disease prevention with the incentives and financial clout to demand services that support his efforts to stay healthy. The clout will come from directly controlling all the money, via his HFA. He will get to decide which health insurance plan to buy and which health products and services to purchase to meet his needs. The incentives will come from the opportunity to save a lot of money on those health insurance and medical costs.

Because of the substantial discounts involved, BAGLE can help tip the balance and lead to a critical mass of at-risk people who take better care of themselves. In the process, it can also force the transformation of the medical delivery system from a focus on episodic acute care to providing continually available chronic disease care. If this is allowed to happen, the savings in health care expenditures will be enormous, and our nation will be far healthier.

Behavior-Based Health-Risk Factor Adjustments

Under American Choice, health insurers may offer premium discounts and rebates to anyone who can demonstrate with the results of inexpensive, easily available lab tests or other certified measurements that she has met objective targets for specified health-risk indicators. For example, an insurer could allow premium discounts to anyone demonstrating that she doesn't smoke or abuse alcohol. If she couldn't show that, she would pay the full quoted premium. From a privacy standpoint, it is important to note that no one will ever have to disclose to an insurer (or anyone else) that she *has* an uncontrolled health risk factor, only that she *doesn't* if she wants to take advantage of premium discounts.

In chapter 2 I referenced the 2006 Harvard study that identified six individually controllable, objectively measurable risk factors that lead to the diseases and injuries that make the largest contribution to death throughout the United States. They are alcohol abuse, tobacco smoking, being overweight or obese, elevated blood pressure, elevated serum lipids (e.g., cholesterol), and elevated blood glucose.[1] People who successfully avoid these conditions tend to live much longer, healthier lives.

Other significant risk factors that are individually controllable include bad habits (such as failing to wear seatbelts or motorcycle helmets), dangerous pastimes (BASE jumping and aerobatic flying), and high-risk jobs (farming and construction), all of which may be priced into insurance premiums or out-of-pocket requirements according to BAGLE's employment/extracurricular risks. Each insurer will determine which risk factors to use and the various thresholds for what constitutes "normal," as well as the amount of discounts to offer for compliance. Since all such criteria and premium adjustments will be publicly disclosed, each insurer will have strong competitive incentives to set them neither too high nor too low for fear of competitors offering better, more attractive insurance policies with more accurate risk pricing.

The six risk indicators are the primary ones that lead to chronic diseases *and* that are individually controllable. Any insurer could decide to offer premium discounts for these or any other risk factors that meet the required criteria listed below. It will not be sufficient for a member to show that he is attempting to achieve a goal; he must have actually met it and provided evidence of it with certified measurements by an independent lab or other appropriate health care provider. Given the substantial risks and costs attributable to these six risk indicators, anyone who can achieve all of them will likely stand to save a lot of money. Conversely, anyone who fails to do so will pay that amount in higher insurance premiums. The additional payments will, on average, equal the lifetime incremental costs that result from the increased incidence of chronic and acute diseases caused by a person's uncontrolled health risks.

The process will start with insurers setting and publishing their BAGLE-rated insurance premiums on the presumption that everyone has *failed* to control the stated risk factors. Thus, if the Harvard factors are used, everyone is initially quoted a rate that assumes they smoke, abuse alcohol, are overweight, and have high cholesterol, high blood sugar, and high blood pressure. The initial premium quote is thus calculated by including the specific actuarial revenue requirements for each health risk, which is then added to the similarly calculated "riskless" premium for people with none of the specified health risks. An insurer's actuary might calculate the following premium to be quoted to a forty-year-old Denver man for the Silver Individual Plan. (Note: These are completely imaginary numbers for the purpose of illustration and have no actuarial basis or significance.)

Premium Category	Premium
"Riskless" Premium	$250
Risk Factor A: Smoking	100
Risk Factor B: Alcohol Abuse	75
Risk Factor C: Obesity	30
Risk Factor D: Blood Glucose	25
Risk Factor E: Hypertension	20
Risk Factor F: Cholesterol	15
Total Premium–All Risks	$515

Thus, every forty-year-old man in Denver interested in purchasing the company's Silver Individual Plan will start out being quoted a monthly premium of $515, or $6,180 per year. He will also be quoted all the above premium discounts if he objectively demonstrates via certified measurements to the insurer that he is not at risk for one or more of the specific Risk Factors A through F. For example, Risk Factor A is smoking. If a prospective insured doesn't smoke, he will be able to reduce his monthly premium by $100 by submitting test results showing the appropriate biomarkers indicating to the insurer that this is so. There are currently clinical, laboratory, and other measurement tests available for all of these risk indicators, and no insurer will be allowed to specify *any* health risk factors for which no such measurement is reasonably available. Depending on his ability to show the non-applicability of all of these risk factors, the Denver man could get his monthly premium reduced to the "Riskless" Premium of only $250, thus saving $265 per month.

This discount savings are intended to accomplish two things:

1. *Measurement*: First, the insurer will want everyone it insures to find out exactly what their personal risk factors are. Although they certainly will know whether they smoke or not, they might not know anything about their blood pressure, cholesterol, or blood sugar. Any of these can be at dangerous levels without showing any outward symptoms. Currently, an estimated 35% of

workers with hypertension, 41% of those with high cholesterol, and 41% with diabetes have not been diagnosed and are unaware they have these risks.[2]

American Choice Health Plan's health risk factor financial incentives are intended to motivate everyone to go to a health fair, clinical laboratory, health clinic, nurse practitioner, doctor, or other approved testing facility to be independently tested and measured for each risk factor. Everyone will then submit all favorable test results to their insurers and receive the appropriate premium discounts. They will not need to tell the insurer anything about their health risks that aren't under control. Only they need to know, and they can then decide what to do about them.

You may be wondering whether these tests will be expensive and who will pay for them. The answer is that there are currently low-cost lab tests or other measurements available for a wide range of health risk indicators, including these six. Given the massive demand for such measurements under American Choice, improved techniques are inevitable, and vigorous competition for consumers' business will drive prices down to trivial levels with greatly improved customer convenience. This is exactly what we have seen for improvements in diabetes blood testing as demand has increased. The cost of testing will be borne by the consumers themselves from their tax-exempt HFAs. Their returns on these investments will be the premium discounts and improved health for those who change their behaviors to get aberrant risk factors under control.

2. *Management*: The second desired outcome will be for people discovering they are at risk to get those risks under control. Let's say that a person discovers that her LDL cholesterol exceeds the threshold amount her insurer requires for a discount. She will pay a higher premium and not disclose her cholesterol level to anyone. Ideally, she will seek medical assistance. She can, perhaps, start taking a statin medication and change her dietary and exercise habits. If she succeeds in getting her LDL level below

the threshold, she will submit the test results to her insurer. The company will reward her with immediately lower premiums. Her monthly premiums will stay at the reduced level until the next certification deadline established by her insurer.

It is important to note that detecting and even disclosing one's health-risk status will not in any way affect her insurability—just her premium. The current system of individual insurance underwriting can penalize an applicant for having taken the initiative to learn and manage her health risk factors. She can be denied insurance for anything in her medical record that the underwriter considers to be a problem, such as a genetic predisposition to a disease. That can never happen under American Choice, since no one may be turned down because of health history, status, genetic predispositions, or anything else other than the inability to pay the premiums. Indeed, no health insurer will need to have any access whatever to an insured's medical record without her permission, other than to verify claims accuracy and appropriateness.

Critics might assert that charging more or less according to health risk factors will really be no different than punishing the sick. After all, making someone with high blood sugar pay more sounds no different than charging more for people with diabetes, since the presence of the former defines the latter. It's an interesting criticism, but it misses the point. Sick people will pay exactly the same premiums as healthy people as long as they succeed in controlling what they can reasonably be expected to control. Someone with diabetes will pay no higher premiums than someone without it, provided that the person with diabetes makes appropriate changes to his diet, exercise, and medication to keep his HbA1c (a multi-month blood sugar measure) below his insurer's standard. A diagnosis of diabetes will not affect his premiums. Controllable high blood sugar levels will.

BAGLE rating makes a clear distinction between actual illness and controllable risk indicators that might predict or accompany it. The goal is to control the latter without in any way penalizing the former. Under American Choice, no one need fear getting a genetic test that might confirm a high risk of developing a heritable disorder, such as cystic fibrosis or breast cancer. The test results will have no effect whatever on either her insurability or her premiums. But it could help to warn her to take early preventive and treatment actions.

Once again, each insurer will be able to use any risk factor it determines to be worth controlling and price it into the premium. No insurance policy, however, will be allowed to prohibit any legally permissible behavior or to deny any legitimate medical service. But any individually controllable factor that statistically predicts higher morbidity may be subject to such price incentives.

BASE-jumping, not wearing automobile seatbelts, motorcycle racing, and technical mountain climbing could be allowable risk factors for requiring their practitioners to pay extra to compensate for those risks. In cases like these for which there are no practical means to price such risks into insurance premiums, insurers would be allowed to, for example, double a person's deductible if he is in an automobile accident in which he was not wearing a seatbelt, assuming that can be reliably determined. In such cases, the measurement of the voluntarily controllable risk doesn't take place until it actually results in an episode of care. So does this mean a person's costs are really tied to actual illness? No, because people seriously injured without having engaged in voluntary high-risk activities would receive their full insurance coverage without any consideration of the cause or severity of the need for treatment. And only those risky behaviors specifically listed and openly disclosed to insured members in their insurance policies would be subject to such higher costs—which would also be specifically disclosed upfront to prospective new members.

Theoretically, an insurer could utilize dozens of risk-factor adjustments, but the market has a way of punishing those who make their products too complicated, unwieldy, and user-unfriendly. The desirability of pricing individual risks will need to be balanced against the countervailing needs for marketing and administrative simplicity. Insurers that fail to strike that balance will be unlikely to prosper in the American Choice marketplace.

In choosing any risk factor, insurers will be required to show that it meets four regulatory requirements. It will have to be:

1. *Measurable*: The factor must be objectively measurable with reasonable convenience and cost.

2. *Predictive*: The factor must be supported by sound evidence that it statistically predicts increased morbidity.

3. *Controllable*: The factor must be reasonably amenable to individual control, whether by individual behavior (diet, exercise, not smoking, etc.), medical intervention (medications for blood pressure, blood glucose, cholesterol, dieting, etc.), or combinations of the two.

4. *Independent of health status*: No risk factor may be defined as any health status, preexisting condition, medical history, or genetic factor.

A fifty-year-old male office worker in Syracuse suffering from diabetes and hypertension will be quoted exactly the same premiums as his fifty-year-old male coworker in perfect health. Both will be eligible for the same premium rebates and discounts if they refrain from smoking and keep their individual body mass, alcohol consumption, extracurricular behavior, blood sugar, cholesterol, and blood pressure within healthy ranges. The worker with diabetes will find it takes more effort than his colleague will to keep his blood sugar and hypertension within normal ranges. But we know that control is individually achievable for the great majority of people with sufficient determination and assistance with proper monitoring, diet, exercise, and medication. They will have a financial incentive to do it and, having earned it, will not be forced to subsidize their fellow insureds who fail to do so.

To some, this approach may seem harsh or discriminatory—even paternalistic. Others may argue that the premium discounts and rebates for healthy behavior will not be sufficient to get Americans to change their unhealthy ways. But as long as the above four criteria for establishing allowable health risk factors are followed, I believe this will be the fairest method for assessing individual accountability for the costs of preventable disease. If it incentivizes some people to take better care of themselves, both they and society will benefit. If it doesn't for others, they will have to pay for the estimated costs that follow. This helps eliminate the moral hazard from currently required subsidies from those who do take care of themselves to pay for those who don't. Rewards for good behavior are better than subsidies for bad. My guess is that there will be more than a few pack-a-day smokers who will find an average annual premium discount of $1,623—not to mention another $1,690 in cigarette cost savings—sufficient incentive to stop smoking,[3] as difficult as that may be to do.

Critics may also argue that incentives are unfair for those who, despite their best efforts, aren't able to earn them. It can be very difficult for some individuals to lose weight, control their blood sugars, or stop smoking, given a multitude of personal, social, economic and environmental variables. Nicotine is extremely addictive, and 95% of all diets fail, with dieters gaining back all the lost weight within a few months or years. Some hypertension sufferers are unable to control their blood pressure with medication alone.

But we must distinguish between what is difficult and what is impossible. There may indeed be small numbers of people for whom it is impossible to achieve healthy risk factors under any medically appropriate circumstances or with any amount of personal determination, resources, and effort. There can be carefully crafted exceptions for those situations based on sound medical and behavioral research. But the fact remains that, for the vast majority of Americans, health-risk goals are attainable, although many may find them hard to achieve.

The fact that most diets fail doesn't mean it's impossible to lose weight permanently. It means it's easier to go on a short-term crash diet and then return to old habits than to develop and maintain new, permanent eating and exercise habits. The extremely addictive nature of nicotine will probably continue to hold millions in its thrall, regardless of the incentive. Virtually anyone with high blood sugar can get it down for a day or two, but it can be much more difficult to do over a lifetime. Yet, these things are possible, and millions of people have successfully achieved control. They should not be required to subsidize those who do not.

Other critics of this financial incentive approach may point out that existing models to predict individual future health costs don't work. The best of them, as I have previously pointed out, are only about 20% accurate.[4] I am *not* proposing to adjust individual premiums based on individually predicted costs, however. The critics are correct that this doesn't work. Anyway, that would not be insurance but prepayment that would become unaffordable to anyone who becomes really sick.

The adjustments I'm proposing are *statistical* estimates based on epidemiological studies of *populations* with these and other selected characteristics. Thus, a prospective insured member presenting with a poorly controlled HbA1c blood sugar level of 12 will not be charged a faulty estimate of his future health care costs. Instead, he will pay a higher premium based on the estimated *average* higher costs incurred by *all* members with similar characteristics. These costs, statistically spread over large populations, are predictable with a relatively high degree of confidence.

It is unwise to accept an entire national health care financing and delivery system that sanctions unhealthy behavior just because it is difficult to change. It is more sensible to have a system that requires responsibility from the majority who can accept it while reserving social safety nets for those relatively few who are physically or mentally unable to cope.

The real economic power of BAGLE's health-risk premium discounts lies in the determination of which factors will be used and how they will be priced by those in the best position to measure their medical cost effectiveness: the insurers and their actuaries. They will have the financial incentives to measure the true impact on medical costs of different risk factors and to price them properly. The insurers will be the ones to benefit or suffer from their calculations. It is they who will determine the value of not smoking for people of different ages and to price that into their insurance policies. If an insurer fails to price a factor properly, then it will suffer either competitively or financially against any of its competitors that were able to calculate the price-benefit more accurately. Any insurer that overprices its coverage for smokers, for example, would be at a serious competitive disadvantage to more carefully priced competitors that actively and profitably recruit smokers to their coverage.

BAGLE rating strongly encourages insurers to seek data on any preventive measure that may be cost-effective. Of equal importance, insurers will discard health risk factors that are ineffective predictors. This will be of great benefit in identifying and promoting individually controllable health risk factors that make sense while debunking those that don't. If, as the data suggest, we're currently wasting a lot of money on prevention,[5] then BAGLE will help lead the way to reducing such waste.

Regardless of whether an insurer promotes a particular form of prevention or not, each individual member will be free to decide what preventive measures are worth taking and how much she is willing to pay for them—regardless of anyone else's analysis of cost benefit. No one will be held captive to any insurer's determination of whether a particular preventive service will be a covered benefit. Indeed, most won't be covered, leaving it up to the individual consumer to decide what is worth the expense and what is not.

Consumers will be incentivized to avoid the costs of failure to achieve healthy risk factors, but each will be able to decide the best way to do it or not to do it at all. Insurers and providers may offer assistance and promotion for their favored approaches. There will arise a plethora of consumer information and assistance services, but the ultimate decision will be up to each individual. On average, most consumer decisions will be mostly rational often enough to effect improvements in prevention and their attendant costs. But for those that aren't, at least those people will be wasting their own money—and not that of others who pursue healthy lifestyles.

In summary, there are numerous virtues to the behavior-based discount approach:

1. *Privacy*: Compliance will be purely voluntary and private. It will not force anyone to disclose any personal health or behavioral information or to change her behavior.

2. *Incentive*: There will be positive incentives for people to engage in healthy behaviors and to get measured for indicators and conditions for which they may be otherwise unaware.

3. *Responsibility and authority*: The locus of prevention responsibility will be moved from the provider to the individual consumer, with the latter then accessing the former for help—and having the financial clout to get it.

4. *Fairness*: For those consumers who fail to detect or control their own health risk factors, they alone will pay for the predicted results of that behavior over their lifetimes in the form of higher insurance premiums—not to mention less healthy lives. People who successfully pursue healthy lifestyles will no longer be required to subsidize those who don't.

5. *Innovation*: The health care delivery system will be challenged to innovate to provide the necessary support in response to enhanced, enlightened consumer demand for affordable measurement, diagnosis, and treatment. The history of market capitalism tells us that consumers with money who are ready to pay for something they want will get it.

CHAPTER 12

Toward Universal Participation, Provider Reforms, and Lower Costs

I have previously discussed the futility of expecting 100% participation in any reformed program of universally available health insurance, mandatory or otherwise. There will always be some people who just won't show up.

So how many people will enroll in the American Choice Health Plan? A lot will depend on how well the government improves its safety-net programs for those without the money to participate. Assuming that health reform makes adequate strides in that direction, then American Choice should get us as close to universal participation as any approach short of a British "you're in if you show up at the doctor's office" model.

Existing Insured Groups

American Choice will be immediately available to all participants in every current employer and government-sponsored health insurance program. They will all have funding contributors helping to pay their premiums and to fund their HFAs. They will all join American Choice, except for the few holdouts who might be permitted some sort of grandfathered coverage under their old programs.

Thus, everyone who previously had employer, individual, or government-provided health insurance will continue to have the means to participate in American Choice. Since this cohort currently accounts for about 85% of the U.S. population, its immediate participation in American Choice will provide the necessary actuarial underpinnings for a self-sustaining system.

The Uninsured

The big challenge for American Choice will be enrolling the forty-six million Americans who now don't have insurance. There are really two big questions here. The first one: Will their participation in American Choice drive up premiums for everyone else? The second: Won't they be unable to afford coverage anyway? The answer to both questions is no.

On average, the uninsured aren't any less healthy than the overall insured population. Surprisingly, 85% of them are employed, and almost 75% describe themselves as being in either excellent or very good health.[1] Thirty-seven percent live in households making more than $55,000, and 19% make more than $75,000.[2] Forty percent of them are young, between eighteen and thirty-four, but haven't found health insurance to be worth its currently inflated price. Sixty-two percent of all uninsured children and two-thirds of poor uninsured parents qualify for publicly funded health coverage programs but haven't enrolled.[3] Many of the uninsured are healthy but temporarily between jobs. Most will be back in the employed pool in less than a year.

It's worth reprising the problem of the uninsured from chapter 4, which revealed that two-thirds of the uninsured have voluntarily opted out, even though they can afford it. Also, others were forced out because they were uninsurable—even though they have the money to purchase insurance if it were available. Or they were priced out of the market by the excess costs of unnecessary benefits mandated by the states. Putting all this together, I estimated that there are currently only about six million people who might be characterized as the hardcore uninsured who currently cannot afford or find insurance on any basis. That's still a lot of people. But even if we double that estimate, it's still a tractable problem from the standpoint of reinforced safety nets.

Premiums under American Choice will be immediately lower than before its implementation:

- *No More Cost-Shifting*: Government payers will no longer be able to shift costs to employers and private payers, thus lowering premiums for them.

- *Competition*: Insurers will be more competitive on pricing.

- *No Unwanted Benefits*: Unwanted, optional, and unnecessary benefits mandates will disappear.

- *More Options*: Most people will be able to find health plans with lower premiums than they are paying now.

These and other factors will make American Choice's insurance immediately more affordable and progressively more so over time. And even though total safety net payments may increase initially, the cost control dynamics of American Choice will ensure more long-term viability of these programs than under the current system.

If American Choice is properly and fully implemented, all the significant barriers to universal participation will be demolished.

Medicaid and SCHIP Reform

How will the poor fare under American Choice? Overall, it will make their health care more available and accessible. It will also eliminate Medicaid's and SCHIP's negative incentives for its beneficiaries to achieve economic self-sufficiency.

The impact of poverty on health care status is significant and complex. We know that people living in long-term poverty have the worst overall measures for almost all health-risk factors, many of which are amenable to individual behavior change, like smoking, poor diet, being overweight, and a sedentary lifestyle. The lack of personal control of such factors helps explain why the poor are more likely to suffer from chronic illness, disability, and shorter life expectancies than higher income people. Certainly other less individually controllable factors are involved, such as poor education, substandard environmental conditions, and low awareness of needed medical care.[4]

American Choice will not solve the problem of poverty in America, especially for many who are also blind, disabled, and elderly. These individuals now account for 73% of Medicaid's expenditures. It will, however, offer new and useful tools that, tied to improved public health and outreach programs, could help bring about better health outcomes for many of the poor children and adults in that population.[5]

By converting Medicaid/SCHIP from defined-benefit to defined-contribution programs, American Choice will effect a philosophical and financial restructuring to eliminate current disincentives for work and to encourage healthy personal behavior, engaged consumerism, and personal savings. It will also remove any current provider biases against the Medicaid/SCHIP programs and their recipients. Providers will no longer know or care whether a patient's health care dollars came from Medicaid, Medicare, a private employer, or their own resources.

This defined-contribution feature will allow Medicaid and SCHIP to dispense with their current "cliff-effect" coverage. It's called that because recipients who earn even one dollar more than the eligibility cutoff now fall off the coverage cliff. They can immediately lose health benefits worth thousands of dollars. The cliff effect provides a powerful disincentive for a single mother, for example, to seek a better job if that means telling her sick child that she can no longer afford to take him to the doctor.

Under American Choice, these programs can provide means-tested, sliding-scale benefits so that a dollar of extra income will be only partially offset by a decrease in government Medicaid/SCHIP contributions. This will allow recipients to seek educational and career paths with the expectation of progressively improving income and the ability to move gradually from government support to financial self-sufficiency. In addition, Congress could extend refundable tax credits to low-income workers who are not eligible for Medicaid to provide funds to help them afford health care.

Medicaid/SCHIP beneficiaries under American Choice will be charged the same insurance premiums as everyone else *including* the built-in incentives for demonstrating compliance with personal health-risk factor control. Today, Medicaid is paying for the effects of recipients' smoking, obesity, hypertension, and uncontrolled Type II diabetes with no incentives for recipients to do otherwise.

Under American Choice, state governments' total payments could continue for these problems, but the incentives will change. Every program recipient will then have the opportunity to earn hard-dollar premium discounts by periodically demonstrating that she has a healthy body mass, has not abused alcohol, doesn't smoke, and has healthy blood levels of lipids, glucose, and pressure.

Such factors could add up to hundreds or thousands of dollars a year in additional money for the recipient's HFA funds. These incentives alone may not be enough to achieve widespread risk-factor improvement. However, they can still prove decisive for many people. This will be especially true when incentives are combined with active public health programs to provide education, training, instruction, social interaction (Biggest Loser Clubs, anyone?), and support to help recipients achieve these goals and bank the savings. There could also be provisions to allow Medicaid/SCHIP beneficiaries to use such banked discounts for things besides health care expenses, such as education, child care, and basic transportation expenses to allow recipients to improve their employment opportunities further.

With Medicaid/SCHIP paying all support funds directly into recipients' HFA accounts, every recipient will have the same responsibilities to allocate funds between insurance and health service purchases as everyone else. There will be the annual decision about which health plan to enroll in. There will be the shorter-term decisions about what health services to buy and which ones are worth the prices charged. This will impose both the responsibility and the authority on the recipient herself to spend her money wisely.

Many will require active support and counseling to be able to do this. Others will take to it naturally, having learned the hard lessons of allocating scarce financial resources to meet their personal needs. Still others will regrettably function no better under American Choice than they do now. These varying needs and responses will put a greater responsibility on assistance programs to provide recipients with active help and accurate information on what actually works and what doesn't. That means focusing on evidence-based services that are effective and that provide benefits worth the money.

Considerable precedents exist for such a move to private sector coverage of Medicaid recipients. Many Medicaid beneficiaries now belong to private managed-care organizations under the auspices of state funding. It is not a stretch to envision expanding this concept to American Choice's universal access to all participating health insurers. Those offering the lowest premiums and the greatest quantity and quality of services will gain the most market share—whether of Medicaid beneficiaries or anybody else.

A significant advantage of American Choice for Medicaid/ SCHIP is the achievement of recipient parity in being able to make the same kinds of health insurance and service choices as everyone else. By choosing their own personal American Choice health insurance policies, they will appear to their providers not as low-status, low-paying Medicaid/SCHIP recipients. They will be full-fledged participants in a class-blind system that treats everyone with equal dignity. Other than assistance program employees and the recipients themselves, no one else need ever know the source of a person's HFA funds, insurance premiums, or health service purchase dollars. Under American Choice, Medicaid/SCHIP's notoriously stingy provider reimbursement rates will vanish, replaced by market-based pricing. That will mean the end of doctors withdrawing from participation in these programs because they will no longer deal with these programs, only with patients and their commercial insurers.

All payments into Medicaid/SCHIP recipients' HFA accounts will become the recipients' money, albeit restricted to health care uses (unless, as suggested above, health risk discounts could also be applied to other uses). The less they spend on health insurance and services, the more they get to keep—to save and invest against future health care or retirement needs. Since the money in an HFA will not be available for non-medical expenditures until retirement, there should be little opportunity for recipients to favor short-term enticements over long-term health goals. Those who use their funds to enable healthy behavior and enlightened access to medical care will have the salutary effects of improved health, lower costs, and increased funds for savings. In seeking these outcomes, it will be important that Medicaid/SCHIP's means testing not include any HFA fund balances in the calculation. Otherwise, it could create negative incentives for the healthy behaviors and savings habits we want to promote.

Again, not everyone will respond positively to American Choice's incentives and personal empowerment. Our goal, however, will be to increase the number who will and to ensure the rest that they will at least be no worse off than they are now. As with the doctor's creed, the operant rule should be *primum non nocere*—"first, do no harm." American Choice provides a means to recognize and further promote the phenomenon by which many of the people who were poor twenty years ago are prosperous now. It will provide an even higher likelihood that today's poor will be able to achieve similar improvements over the next two decades.

Medicaid and Late Enrollment Penalties

What about the estimated 13,870,000 people who are eligible for Medicaid but haven't signed up for it? What happens if they also don't enroll in American Choice but later get sick and need to join? Wouldn't the late enrollment penalties result in premium rates that no state Medicaid program will be willing or able to pay?

This is a potentially big problem. An estimated 27% of Medicaid eligibles have not bothered to sign up for the coverage—though they likely would if they became sufficiently ill to require medical care. If Medicaid were an insurance program, this would become a significant problem of adverse selection; however, Medicaid, unlike

Medicare, is an entitlement program whose members pay no premiums. Adverse selection has, by definition, not been an issue.

The problem arises when Medicaid, under American Choice, shifts to becoming a funding agent that enables its beneficiaries to purchase their own insurance. If a lot of Medicaid eligibles fail to purchase health insurance until they actually need medical care, then we will have a serious adverse selection problem. Or rather, the insurers will.

Fortunately, these questions actually suggest their own answer. The fact that we can estimate the number of non-covered Medicaid eligibles means we can appropriately fund the pool for them, even without knowing specifically who they are. One way to do that would be to use what I call "John and Jane Doe" insurance policies. Each state would purchase name-to-be-determined policies based on estimates of the number of people eligible for the program but not participating.

Let's say that Colorado estimated that it had twenty-five thousand Medicaid/SCHIP eligibles whom it had not been able to identify or enroll. Colorado would fund and purchase John/Jane Doe placeholder policies for these people, paying the premium dollars to the insurers. The specific amounts would be based on estimated age/gender/location demographics of this pool and a mix of comprehensive health insurance policies to be purchased. Since there would be no actual named members to incur claims, however, none of this premium income could be earned by the insurers until they were represented by actual members. It would have to be held in restricted reserve accounts. At the point people do enroll, no matter how late, some level of past premiums paid on behalf of the Doe policies would be recognized as revenue to the insurer. Figuring out the revenue recognition formulas will doubtless provide work for a corps of actuaries and accountants. But this approach could effectively resolve the late enrollment problem.

It would also create strong incentives for both the states and the insurers to seek and find the anonymous eligibles and sign them up for coverage. The states will want to pursue them because they will have already paid for them. States will be under the gun to make sure the taxpayers get their money's worth in the form of actual services to the poor. The insurers will want to enroll them because that's the only way they can translate restricted premium reserves into actual earned premiums.

Having both sides (that is, states and insurers) actively marketing the program should minimize the adverse selection that might occur if, for example, hospital emergency rooms become the de facto sales arm of the program, funneling only the sick into membership. On the other hand, such active recruitment would also help prevent the kind of favorable selection that might occur if insurers alone were to develop selective sales techniques designed to find and sign only the healthy Medicaid/SCHIP eligibles. John/Jane Doe policies could be an effective method for encouraging universal participation by Medicaid eligibles in American Choice while protecting the actuarial soundness of the overall insurance pool.

Another approach to avoid Medicaid adverse selection could involve the use of late-enrollment options. A state could purchase options from insurers to allow Medicaid to enroll members later, as they are identified, but without any of the premium surcharges or penalties that would otherwise be due from late enrolling members. This would allow the states to avoid paying the actual premiums until each beneficiary is identified. The options prices would essentially be equivalent to the expected adverse selection cost of the late enrollees. In other words, option prices would be roughly equal to the late enrollment penalties but without the premiums. A state might thus procure such options for less money than with the fully-funded John/Jane Doe approach while preserving both late enrollment and the insurance pool against adverse selection. As with the John/Jane Doe system, any revenue from late enrollment options would not be allowable as earned revenue by the insurers until actual members enrolled.

Funding the Safety Net

Now here's the hard part. Both federal and state governments will have to be committed to providing sufficient funding to comprehensive safety-net reform to ensure that Medicare, Medicaid/SCHIP recipients *and* all low-income Americans will be able to purchase health insurance *and* purchase all needed primary and preventive care services.

Initially, this will require an increase in funding over current levels, perhaps a large one. One factor pointing to higher costs will be that these programs will no longer be able to shift provider reimbursements onto the private sector, having been stripped by American Choice of their price regulatory powers. Another factor will be the low-income people who are not in these programs but who lack the resources to participate fully in American Choice on their own.

That same elimination of cost-shifting, however, will bring down commercial insurance premiums, thus mitigating somewhat the Medicare/Medicaid/SCHIP transition to that market. So will the removal of unnecessary benefit mandates in the private insurance market. Another possibility to reduce program costs will be to establish all safety-net program HFA contributions on a sliding-scale basis, even for Medicare. The programs would gradually remove supports for progressively higher levels of recipient income. In the longer term, the health care financing and delivery system will rationalize itself under American Choice to eliminate waste, promote innovation, improve quality, effect real prevention, and drive down health care prices to an extent that will dramatically reduce costs for all government programs that support health benefits. These and other dynamics could eventually reduce such government funding below even current levels.

Many reform advocates have argued it is necessary first to reduce health care costs before providing comprehensive health care safety-net reform. They have variously argued that we must first eliminate waste, improve quality, cut hospital and doctor reimbursement rates, and exact savings from increased prevention and the use of electronic medical records. That, they argue, is the only way we'll ever be able to reform health care so that everybody can participate. Unfortunately, this is an example of yet more dependence on the failed philosophy of top-down control that helped get us into this mess in the first place—not to mention the futile reliance on the myths that increased prevention coverage and EMR will save money.

Health care purchasers—primarily employers and government—have been trying to control and reduce the cost of health care for decades, and they have failed—miserably. I have discussed in some detail why this is so and won't belabor the point here. There is no effective way (short of outright rationing and global budget restrictions) to reduce the costs of health care without revolutionizing health care purchasing and payment to incorporate a vibrant consumer market. We must shift control from government and employers to consumers under a regulated market-based system to force the system to fix itself.

To engage these market forces, we must have customers who care about quality and price and how much of their own money they are willing to spend to get the health care they require. That means turning all the money over to consumers and letting them force insurers and providers to offer transparent pricing, high-quality care, and customer service.

I know this sounds utterly radical to anyone who has bought into the concept of health care as something that exists in a different economic universe than everything else we consume. But it's really nothing more than recognition that health care is an economic good. It is fundamentally no different from food, clothing, housing, and transportation.

The first thing we need is health care financing reform. We can't wait for costs to drop first. We already have plenty of money flowing through the health care system to take care of everyone. We just need to restructure how it flows. And that flow must be routed through consumers. We have to trust that they will be as essentially rational in purchasing health care as they are in buying all their other life's necessities. They won't be perfect—many will be far from it—but they won't need to be. We just need for most of them to be pretty good at it most of the time. And there is ample evidence that they will.

With financing reform in place, the market mechanism will begin to restructure the insurance and health care delivery roles to meet consumer demands for affordable, high-quality care. Only then will prices—and costs—come down. Proponents of single payer or other forms of increased government control are wrong in arguing that we have to get costs under control first. The only way that will happen is to resort to artificial limits on who can obtain—and who can provide—which medical services—i.e., non-price rationing. Nobody wants that. And fortunately, it's not necessary.

Provider Reform

American Choice will allow consumers to demand and obtain information on who provides the best health care and which of them do it for the least amount of money.

Government reforms of taxes, insurance, and safety nets will set the stage for consumers finally to demand, receive, and act on that information. Few further legal reforms will be necessary to effect the fundamental and necessary changes in the relationships between patients and their medical providers. Instead, the financial structure created by American Choice's regulatory reforms will allow the dynamics of regulated market capitalism to reform the health care delivery system to provide improved quality and customer service at far lower cost.

The process will be that first described by economist Joseph Schumpeter as creative destruction. Providers will no longer be faced just by patients. They will be dealing with customers and consumers who will be newly empowered with control of all the money, and they will demand information and accountability. There will be no need for government regulations on provider quality, patient treatment standards, payment rules, electronic medical records subsidies, pay for performance incentives, mandatory procedure coding systems, relative value systems, or any of the other supposed desiderata commonly assumed to be within government's proper ambit for ensuring medical quality and cost. Please note that I am *not* arguing for deregulation of health insurance or health care delivery. I am calling for *reregulation* to create the boundary conditions within which a vibrant consumer health insurance and health care market can function and to get government out of businesses it has no business being in.

Ending the Monopoly of the Medical Cottage Industry

Two areas of provider reform at the legislative level will help lubricate the machinery of American Choice and make health care delivery more effective and efficient. This will be, first, to end—or at least loosen—the doctor monopoly. The other will be to enable new business models in medicine to replace the prohibitions contained in the corporate-practice-of-medicine doctrine. Both of these outmoded concepts are deeply embedded in the law books of all fifty states.

In his book *The Innovator's Prescription*[6], Clayton Christensen of the Harvard Business School emphasizes the need to disrupt what he calls the Value-Adding Process (VAP) activities of medical care. He points out that an increasing number of medical treatments have become so standard or formulaic that it is a waste of resources to have them performed by the people who do them now—primary care and specialist doctors. As he puts it, "Abilities that previously resided in the intuition of a select group of experts ultimately become so explicitly teachable that rules-based work can be performed by people with much less experience and training."

Accordingly, specialty hospitals will, to use Christensen's term, disrupt general hospitals. General hospitals will in turn focus on the undifferentiated medical problems that require a broader range of diagnostic and therapeutic resources, and they will charge appropriate prices to recover their costs and generate necessary surpluses. Nurse practitioners and other less intensively trained personnel would do many VAP activities with equal quality and far better efficiency and cost-effectiveness than doctors now achieve. Christensen calls not only for non-MDs to do much of what MDs now do, but also for primary care doctors to similarly "disrupt" specialty doctors. The more highly trained the doctor, the more she should focus on what Christensen calls "Solution Shops" to deal with the most complex patient problems that defy diagnosis or treatment by anyone else. He also emphasizes the need for flexibility and innovation in creating the new business models that will best support these changes. These will include corporate models of medical practice that enable the high levels of capital formation, organization, and integration to facilitate major innovations in the delivery of care.

American Choice will provide the economic environment to encourage these favorable disruptions. Price will suddenly matter. Hidebound traditions and legal structures that enforce the doctor monopoly and archaic business models will need to be substantially loosened for these reforms to take optimal effect. Otherwise, monopoly hospitals and doctors will not disrupt themselves.

I will leave it to better informed health care innovators than I to pursue this argument. But it is one that needs to be made.

Price Transparency

With or without reform of the medical monopoly and business models, American Choice will ensure that neither providers nor insurers will any longer be allowed to bury medical prices inside labyrinthine computer programs. Patients (and their insurers) willing and able to pay doctors and hospitals at the time of service will no longer be required to pay twice as much as insurers who pay months later. Innovative health care provider models will emerge offering low packaged prices for services and programs that help consumers control their smoking, alcohol consumption, weight, hypertension, diabetes, and cholesterol, perhaps with money-back guarantees if clients fail to earn their BAGLE insurance premium discounts.

Surgeries will be priced clearly, competitively, and publicly. Specialty hospitals and surgery centers will compete with prices that technology, innovation, and focus will continually lower, not increase. Clinical laboratories and diagnostic imaging centers will compete on price, convenience, and quality for consumers' health care dollars. Pharmacies will publicly advertise their lowest prices for prescription drugs rather than reserving and disclosing them only to PBMs and insurance companies. Hospitals will offer package prices for all manner of acute services. They will also be looking over their shoulders at international facilities, such as Bumrungrad Hospital in Bangkok, Thailand, that offer higher quality cardiac bypass procedures than many U.S. hospitals for about a fifth of the price.

Consumers demanding value will look not just at price but also at independent metrics of provider quality, much like auto buyers now look to Consumer Reports or J.D. Power for auto quality ratings. American Choice will do more than any legislative fiat to engender and enforce transparency by enabling value-savvy health care consumers to hold insurers and providers accountable for offering value, effectiveness, convenience, and customer service.

Coordination and Electronic Medical Records (EMR)

Just two of the features that savvy, prospective patients will demand from their doctors and hospitals will be coordinated care and electronic medical records. Both have been widely identified as necessary to achieve true, consistent, outcomes-based quality in health care delivery. Both are needed to improve your odds from the current fifty-fifty that your doctor will give you the correct diagnosis and best-practice treatment, and at a fair price. Both have long been seen as the wave of the future. Given the glacial pace of adoption, many of us have begun to despair that they always will be.

To understand the importance of coordination of care and electronic medical records, you need only think back to the last time you were referred to a specialist or, worse, specialists by your primary care doctor. At each doctor's office, you were required to write by hand the same information into virtually identical questionnaires on your medical history and condition, regardless of how many times you'd done it before. You were probably given many of the same expensive lab tests because each doctor didn't have access to your other doctors' records of what had been done before. The chance that your doctor followed the latest established medical guidelines to evaluate and diagnose your condition varied from a low of 20% for atrial fibrillation to a high of 85% for breast cancer. You may have been prescribed new drugs that inadvertently duplicated, negated, or, worse, complicated the effects of drugs you were already taking under different doctors' orders.

If what your specialists found and did made it back into your primary care doctor's medical record, count yourself lucky. If your primary care doctor could actually locate that information in the volumes of serially filed paper in your patient folder, count yourself even luckier. If he could make out the specialist's cryptic scribbling, *mirabile dictu!* The chances of all of your doctors conferring at once is…well, in my nearly forty years of working in health care, I've seen it happen exactly once. Overall, your chances of receiving coordinated patient care with clear, timely communication among doctors, pharmacies, laboratories, imaging centers, and hospitals are almost the same as the chances you are receiving your care at a Mayo Clinic, Cleveland Clinic, Intermountain Health Care, Virginia Mason Medical Center, or another of the integrated medical services organization that have such processes down pat. In other words, your chances are very low.

I could go into the lists of reasons why our medical delivery system is the uncoordinated, siloed, paperbound mess that it is, but I won't. Nor will I focus on the hit-or-miss attempts by federal and state governments, medical organizations, individual doctors and hospitals, medical groups, and insurers to introduce, induce, or mandate coordinated medical care, modern record keeping, and secure communications.

The fact is that under the current system of health insurance there is neither financial incentive nor customer demand for providers to change. Everybody agrees that the focus of all their activities should be the patient. Yet the patient has the least amount of say in how the system operates. That function has been taken over by the insurers, third-party administrators, pharmacy benefit managers, government payers, federal and state regulators, and the health care providers themselves. Each has its own organizational mandates and priorities. Too few of them acknowledge the patient's needs and desires as their central *raison d'être*, except in a paternalistic, trust-us-we're-here-for-you kind of way.

Expecting providers to reform without being forced to by anybody other than paying customers is, to quote Dr. Johnson, "a triumph of hope over experience." American Choice puts the health care consumer firmly in charge, with the full financial clout it takes to force real system change—by granting to the consumer the ability to grant or deny his business to any provider or insurer. Any provider that fails to measure up with consistent quality, reasonable prices, and customer service will fail to survive as a business. If consumers decide that they must receive coordinated care enabled by interoperable electronic medical records, then caregivers will provide it—or else. It's really that simple.

Doctors and hospitals that fail to adopt electronic medical records will be unable to coordinate patient care with the rest of the system or to track and report their outcome statistics. Prospective patients unable to obtain quality and value information on a provider will move on to one that can. Existing patients, discovering that other doctors offer far better coordination of care and patient outcomes than they're currently getting, will leave their established doctors for the better performing ones. Doctors, faced with the loss of patients, will finally find it worthwhile to invest the $25,000 to $45,000 for electronic records systems and to use them to make their practices more effective.[7]

Are consumers capable of making good judgments about provider quality? We certainly do not lack the ability or the intelligence. What we lack is the information, the authority, and the responsibility to do so. Much of the information we need is hardly abstruse or technical. The first thing I would like to know before going into a hospital is whether doctors and nurses wash their hands before touching a patient. The principles of antiseptic medicine were established in 1867 by Joseph Lister, so it seems obvious that all hospitals would follow them now. Yet a study reported in *The New England Journal of Medicine* on sixty-seven Michigan hospitals said otherwise.[8] It revealed that hospitals that were induced to require basic sterile precautions reduced median bloodstream infection rates from 2.7 per one thousand catheter-days to *zero* over an eighteen-month period. These changes didn't involve new technologies but were such simple precautions as hand washing, cleaning a patient's skin with antiseptic, and following full-barrier sterile precautions before inserting catheters. Michigan hospitals weren't doing these things before, and neither, by extension, are most of the nation's other 5,680 hospitals.[9] If implemented nationwide, such straightforward procedures would vastly reduce the estimated eighty thousand blood infections, twenty-eight thousand deaths, and $2.3 billion in costs to treat these hospital-caused problems every year. Yet there is currently no way to find out whether your particular hospital either measures or manages such commonsense procedures. American Choice will force them to do both and to disclose the results.

Numerous attempts are afoot by government and private watchdogs to convince or require hospitals to report various quality measures. One is the Leapfrog Group, a hospital-monitoring organization that is attempting to rally employers around demanding better hospital quality. Leapfrog asserts that improved hospital quality practices and outcomes are "unlikely to happen without the involvement of purchasers."[10] This opinion is entirely correct, but under today's health care financing system, it is deeply flawed. The problem is that the "purchaser" Leapfrog refers to is not the actual consumer but the employers who are currently writing the checks. Employers may have an economic interest in improving hospital quality, but it is not a priority that comes even close to that of the actual patient's. He is the one who risks his life, health, and livlihood whenever he enters a hospital for care.

There is no doubt that hospitals have to listen to Leapfrog's concentrated power of concerned employer groups, but who has to listen to the consumers? Until they control the money, the answer is no one. Consumers are confined to the sidelines of the quality debate because they don't have the power that comes from writing the check to pay for the care. The consumer's only recourse is to sue for malpractice when he thinks he has suffered from poor quality—a miserable, corrosive proxy for quality assurance and provider accountability. American Choice will give consumers real power by enabling them to decide how and where to spend their money on health insurance and health services.

Some might argue that insurers will end up paying for all the high-cost services unaffordable to individual consumers. Thus, consumers will still be powerless to demand provider accountability where it matters most. That argument ignores that American Choice consumers will be looking for value not just in the services they purchase directly but also those they pay for indirectly through insurers. It won't take long for savvy consumers to find out that Insurer A excludes coverage for the highest quality-rated hospitals that aren't in his residence area or that Insurer B not only includes them but makes an effort to have their policyholders treated there. The quality is higher and the cost lower.

Like the farmer and the cowman in the musical *Oklahoma*, insurers and policyholders need to turn in their adversarial relationships to become, if not friends, then co-conspirators. Their common goal? High-quality, low-cost health care. American Choice will deliver that.

Insurers that continue to pursue the old model will join the ranks of Pan Am World Airways, Packard Motor Car Company, and RCA's computer division. All got the hook for failing to adapt to the new economic realities recognized by their innovative successors, Southwest Airlines, Toyota, and Dell Computer. Joseph Schumpeter's creative destruction will find its way into health care just as it has with every other market-enabled industry—but only if there is a market to facilitate it and make it happen.

Provider Competition

With American Choice, prescription drug manufacturers will find themselves in the unaccustomed position of having to promote the price, as well as the effectiveness, of the drugs they want doctors to prescribe. Patients will demand and receive information on equally effective lower-cost alternatives. Big Pharma will no longer advertise to doctors and consumers without promoting value. Where they can now price their drugs almost as high as they like, they will be forced by consumers to price them competitively or risk losing market share against similar, lower-cost products. Even without any changes in industry pricing, consumers will discover they can immediately meet their medication needs for 35–50% less than they and their insurers are paying now. They will finally discover the already available generic and over-the-counter medications that are just as effective for a twentieth of the price.

Big Pharma will stop wasting billions of drug development money on me-too drugs that offer little or no improvement over other drugs already on the market and that sell for the much higher prices that the perverse economics of today's health care system allow. Big Pharma will become Focused Pharma, an industry with the single-minded determination to find superior pharmacological solutions to a wide array of medical problems. Some will investigate new uses for existing drugs. They will compare these drugs not just with placebos but with the drugs currently in use. Others will test new chemical and biological compounds.

Will pharmaceutical companies go out of business under American Choice? Some undoubtedly will. But they will be replaced by innovators focused on one thing: delivering better value in the form of unique products that perform better than anyone else's. The prices of *those* drugs will be very high and offer immense margins. And we (and our insurers) will be glad to pay for them. Why? Because they will provide better value and lower overall medical costs, not to mention longer and more productive lives.

Provider competition will expose the seamy underbelly of the American medical system: bad doctors and hospitals. With consumers demanding public disclosure of provider quality statistics, American Choice will shine a bright light on the best and the worst providers of care. Unlike the children in Lake Wobegon, not all of America's doctors and hospitals are above average. Exactly half are, in fact, below it (or at least the median). We will be able to find out who they are, and they will either quickly reform their ways or go out of business. Half will still be below average, but the average will improve dramatically.

Bad doctors will no longer be hidden from public view by professional courtesy and opaque disciplinary processes. Bad hospitals will no longer be able to get away with high infection rates and frequent readmissions for conditions they didn't treat properly the first time. Creative destruction will drive many of these players out of business while giving rise to entrepreneurial innovators with better solutions, better quality, better outcomes, more convenience, customer friendliness, and prices that will take your breath away with their affordability.

Health care costs could drop by as much as 75% just from quality improvements, payment simplification, and the elimination of unnecessary care while meeting all eight of American Choice's goals. But let's be conservative. Let's say they drop by only 50%. Either number may seem unimaginable now, but it was equally unimaginable in 1976 that changes in airline regulation would cut the cost of a coast-to-coast airline flight by 65% (in constant dollars) thirty years later, despite fuel prices more than doubling. Or that a three-minute transcontinental telephone call that cost the caller the equivalent of 1 hour and 44 minutes of work in 1950 would require only two minutes of labor in 1999—largely because of the simplified reregulation of the telecommunications industry and the removal of price restrictions and controls.[11]

The Cost of Insurance and Medical Care under American Choice

Under American Choice average insurance rates will initially be lower than current ones because of insurer competition, the elimination of cost-shifting, and the removal of unnecessary benefit mandates. Over time, rates will drop 50% or more as insurer and provider competition yields lower prices and reduced waste from (1) improved standards of medical care; (2) widespread adoption of those standards; (3) improved provider productivity; (4) consumer access to provider price and quality information; (5) streamlined provider reimbursement mechanisms; (6) innovative delivery models; (7) an end to cost-shifting; (8) provider competition based on quality and price; (9) reductions and elimination of preventable diseases; (10) the departure of bad providers; (11) the elimination of provider monopolies; (12) enlightened regulation; and (13) an end to provider shortages.

All this will give rise to a virtuous cycle. Consumers, controlling the money, will become the primary arbiters of value and thus price. Insurers will provide support and incentives for their members to focus on savings from price and quality (e.g., fewer complications and redos), thus driving down total claims. Insurers will offer policies that keep consumers' financial skin in the game, even for the most expensive medical procedures. Such incentives need not be negative but could offer substantial financial benefits to members who choose the highest quality *and* the lowest cost care.

All this will result in lower premiums and more market share for the insurers that best support their members. The cycle will continue with yet more consumer price consciousness, which will lead to more competitive provider pricing. Providers will reengineer their processes to eliminate waste and improve productivity to allow increased volume and lower prices.

Entrepreneurs and innovators will accelerate access to ever more effective, lower-cost diagnosis and therapy. Providers will adopt new business models and objective quality standards that focus on medical outcomes. Technology will finally drive costs down, not up. Providers will use electronic medical records to measure their own quality and to benchmark themselves against others. Doctors and hospitals that can't send this data to patients' own electronic health records will find themselves losing those patients to those who can. Patients will more often receive the correct diagnosis and the most effective treatment.

With each iteration of this cycle, quality will improve, waste will evaporate, productivity will soar, and costs will drop.

But most health care costs are incurred by the 10–20% of the population who are the sickest. Even if these people have chosen relatively high insurance deductibles under American Choice, will consumer price consciousness continue to be irrelevant when it comes to choosing health care providers? Someone needing open-heart surgery is not going to care whether it costs $50,000 or $500,000 once his $10,000 deductible is met. How will American Choice deal with this?

The big-picture answer is twofold. First, with American Choice's individual BAGLE risk-factor control incentives, we will expect a lower incidence of preventable acute disease, such as heart disease wrought by smoking, obesity, and high cholesterol.

But the question really relates to those who do suffer such serious illnesses. That is when an even more powerful effect of American Choice will kick in to reduce costs. Remember that under a consumer market approach, the insurers that are most creatively effective in meeting consumer needs for high-quality, low cost-care will become the most successful. Any presumption that insurers will simply default to the current high deductible model is a faulty one. American Choice will encourage a plethora of novel approaches, one of which is suggested in the following scenario.

A Future Scenario and Major Savings

L et's imagine one such possible and very simple variation on the high deductible model several years from now under the American Choice Health Plan.

Fifty-four-year-old Andrea Moonshine has just been told by her cardiologist, Dr. Pectus, that she needs coronary bypass surgery (CABG). Dr. Pectus emphasized that she should get the surgery soon but that it was not an emergency. He recommended a local medical center hospital and a cardiac surgeon, Dr. Carmine.

Andrea's employer contributed $15,000 per year to her HFA, and Andrea had added another $350 per month ($4,200 annually). At the time of her visit, her HFA had a balance of $16,000. Three years earlier, Andrea had chosen a health insurance policy under the American Choice program from the Aspen Insurance Company. Her policy currently had a $10,000 annual deductible and 100% insurance coverage above that. She had liked Aspen for a number of reasons, not the least for guaranteeing that her premiums would not go up by more than 2% per year for the first three years. The only condition was that Andrea had to be willing to let her deductible increase by the same percentage each year. As it turned out, her premiums had actually declined by 5% per year.

Dr. Pectus submitted his invoice to Aspen through the ComapreNet online invoicing system the same day he made his diagnosis. The bill was for Dr. Pectus's publicly quoted fee of $199.99 for the visit and was instantly adjudicated by Aspen. The Aspen computer server immediately returned a message to Dr. Pectus's billing clerk that Andrea had not spent up to her annual deductible and that she was responsible for the bill. The clerk then charged Andrea's HFA debit card for the $199.99 fee, and Dr. Pectus received the full payment twenty minutes later via bank wire transfer. He was old enough to remember when he and his colleagues had to hire squads of billing staff just to fight the daily battles with insurers for much-reduced payments, which usually didn't arrive for weeks. Now he just sets his own prices, knowing they will be paid almost immediately upon entry by his receptionist—as long as they are competitive enough to bring him patients.

In submitting his invoice, Dr. Pectus included diagnosis and treatment codes along with a link to Andrea's online electronic medical record (EMR). Dr. Pectus' automatic uploading of the new EMR data to Andrea's private electronic health record (HER) also led to immediate notification of Andrea's independent patient advocate, who called her on her phone shortly after she returned home from the doctor.

Andrea's patient advocate was a nurse named Bryan whose job was to assist his clients in getting the highest-quality health care at the lowest cost. Bryan was an independently practicing Patient Advocate-Certified (PAC) who was paid a fixed monthly fee by every consumer who chose him as her PAC. The PAC program arose shortly after the national rollout of the American Choice Health Plan. Its purpose was to assist patients in navigating their way through an often-daunting health care system to find high-quality, competitively priced health care services.

Most insurers promoted PACs because they had become so effective in helping patients. They had helped to achieve improved medical outcomes and significantly lower costs for both the patients and the insurance companies. Aspen Health Plan even included Bryan's service fee in Andrea's monthly insurance premium although Bryan had no responsibility at all to the insurer—only to Andrea.

Andrea chose Bryan after seeing him ranked highly in a Consumer Reports online article about PACs.

After confirming Bryan's identity, Andrea granted him access to her online EMR. It provided her comprehensive medical history from every doctor and health provider she had seen since adoption of the nationwide interoperable EMR coding and data storage system eight years earlier. Much of her history from before that was also viewable in PDF format. It had all been scanned into her record as searchable image files, although Andrea was considering have it updated to the more modern data format as well.

Bryan also had access to trusted online resources that confirmed Dr. Pectus had a solid professional reputation. His patient recommendations had never been successfully challenged either by independent second opinions or by third-party audits of his and his patients' electronic records. Nonetheless, Bryan ran a standard diagnostic program to check Andrea's diagnosis against the latest American College of Cardiology practice standards. He was impressed that Dr. Pectus had followed the guidelines almost to the letter, even noting the reasons for his exceptions along with hyperlinks to recent journal articles.

Bryan was also glad to see that Andrea had done her homework in choosing Dr. Pectus. He was one of the nationally recognized doctors most often recommended to render second opinions on CABG-related diagnoses. Bryan saw that Dr. Pectus had frequently found reasons to question other doctors' CABG-related diagnoses, which was particularly meaningful because of the high incidence of over-utilization of the procedure. Had Bryan found Dr. Pectus's diagnosis to be at odds with the practice standards, he could have sent the data for further review to a consulting cardiologist. He might even have recommended that Andrea seek a physical appointment and second opinion. Having confidence in the Pectus diagnosis, Bryan turned his efforts to helping Andrea find the best doctors and medical facilities for her treatment.

The advent of American Choice had generated a massive increase in consumer demand for provider quality and price information. As a result, the field of coronary bypass surgery, among others, had become highly competitive. Bryan knew that in the old days most CABG procedures were performed in local hospitals. Now there was a much smaller number of hospitals nationally and internationally that specialized in it, doing only that procedure and no other. As a result, each did thousands of them every year and had impressive, continually improving patient outcomes, all verified by independent public quality auditors with confidential access to the hospitals' and patients' electronic medical record files.

Newer procedures that obviated the need to crack a patient's chest had been quickly adopted and dramatically improved in these hospitals. These advances yielded lower mortality rates, shorter recovery times, vanishingly few infections, reduced complication rates, shorter lengths of stay, and far lower costs. Because of their specialization, advanced techniques, and high volumes, these hospitals and their surgeons were able to offer lower prices for CABG procedures while profiting mightily in the process. In medicine, higher volume frequently equates to higher quality *and* lower cost. Under American Choice, that also meant lower *prices*.

Bryan was pleased that Andrea seemed to be almost as interested in the cost of her care as she was in the quality. He remembered that during the first couple of years of American Choice, insurers weren't very sophisticated in setting their benefit levels. Their most common mistake was to place a high deductible, such as $10,000 on a health plan, and then count on that to save money. The thought was that this would motivate patients to become savvy, price-sensitive shoppers for health services. As long as a patient hadn't satisfied his deductible, it worked well.

The problem was that a high proportion of health costs were incurred by a relatively small number of people whose costs far exceeded their deductibles. Those patients no longer cared about the total cost because their insurers were paying the entire amounts above the deductibles. As a result, anyone needing a CABG, which normally cost about $60,000, would demand the highest-quality care without caring a whit about the cost. There was little consumer motivation to be price sensitive. Prices had stayed high.

One of the newer insurers, Aspen Health Plan, had a brilliant underwriter named Stewart. He had spotted this problem early on and introduced a widely copied innovation: direct-to-patient savings rebates. He knew that top-quality CABG providers were offering very competitive prices. His challenge was to figure out how to get patients to use them instead of their local hospitals.

Stewart convinced his CEO to allow Aspen Health to offer savings-based rebates to members who had their CABGs performed at these specialized hospitals. Bryan, the patient advocate, had quickly picked up on this. Whenever he received a call from an Aspen CABG patient, he would inform her that she could actually be paid as much as $13,000 to get her care at one of these hospitals. Patients' initial skepticism quickly gave way to enlightened self-interest when Bryan showed them the statistics on the hospitals' stellar outcomes.

Bryan told Andrea about Aspen's rebate program. If she decided to get a $60,000 bypass from her local hospital, Aspen would pay the entire amount above her remaining deductible. If she paid even more somewhere else, she would be responsible for the full amount above $60,000. But if she had it performed in a specialty CABG hospital in Houston for $20,000, she would receive a cash payment equal to 25% of the savings, or $10,000. There were even options for having the procedure done by American-trained cardiac surgeons in Joint Commission International accredited hospitals in Thailand and India for even less. One such hospital group was even affiliated with Harvard Medical International.

Stewart, the Aspen underwriter, had originally been concerned about offering the rebate for fear of his company being deluged by CABG patients during its annual open enrollment periods. To prevent such adverse selection, he had added a policy proviso that the rebate program was available only to those who had been Aspen members for at least three years. Since this did not in any way affect any new member's access to the full CABG treatment benefit, Stewart was able to apply this condition without violating any federal or state regulation.

Aspen was able to remove this new member time limit only two years after initiating it since virtually every insurer in the country had by then copied his idea. The rebate program had quickly become commoditized. It no longer rendered any competitive advantage to any one insurer. And with all insurers doing it, it no longer created adverse selection risk for any one insurer. But it had served to lower the average price of a CABG procedure by 60% nationwide and raised provider compliance with current standards of care to more than 95%. The loss of competitive advantage was fine with Stewart because he had a lot of other ideas to improve Aspen's marketability and bottom line—just as he had in extending similar savings rebates to a wide range of other acute and chronic care services before his competitors had copied them, too.

Faced with Andrea's diagnosis and condition, Bryan confirmed her ability to travel for care, via secure email with Dr. Pectus. After receiving confirmation, he did not hesitate to recommend several distant hospitals. Softening the stress of being away from home, Aspen had included another benefit in addition to the rebates—Andrea could be accompanied by her husband, Lars, with all expenses paid. Additionally, one of the top-ranked Indian hospitals offered to pick them up at the airport, transport them to the hospital and hotel via limousine, and then put them up at a five-star beach resort for a week of R&R after her discharge—all for $10,000. Andrea chose that option, flew to Mumbai with Lars, had the surgery, and found her care to be the best she could have imagined. Her surgeon had been trained at the Mayo Clinic in the United States, and even the hospital orderlies were all registered nurses. She enjoyed her beachside recuperation with a good book and fine food and felt that the experience had greatly enhanced her recovery.

Upon returning home, she received follow-up care arranged by Bryan and paid for by Aspen. She also collected a $12,500 rebate that went into her HFA, which left her balance at almost $23,000, even after paying for her deductible portion of the surgery. Aspen's managers were happy to have provided such great service to Andrea. They were happier still to have paid a total of only $22,500 for a procedure that five years earlier would have cost $60,000.

Andrea's case, and many others like it, had allowed Aspen to earn enviable profit margins for its investors. It had also lowered its premiums by 5% a year for the past three years. Aspen enjoyed a 98% rating of "Satisfied" or "Highly Satisfied" when its members were polled by J. D. Power and Associates. That was one of the reasons it enjoyed a high member retention rate and large growth during recent open enrollments. Many of their new members had been dissatisfied customers of other insurers that they had deserted en masse.

Andrea's surgery had also been a wake-up call that she had to take better care of herself. Addicted to cigarettes since age twelve (she had loved those old Joe Camel ads), she had a pack-a-day habit and was twenty-five pounds overweight. Her primary care doctor had been urging her to shape up.

Aspen Health had become almost annoying in reminding her of the premium reductions she would receive if she could demonstrate that she didn't smoke and had achieved a healthy body-fat percentage. She had already sent Aspen her annual test results showing healthy blood pressure, blood sugar, and cholesterol levels, and she had no DUI record or clinical evidence of alcohol abuse. Thus, she was already receiving discounts from her premiums for those factors.

She had also been concerned about Lars's health risks. They agreed during their resort stay in India to change their lifestyles. Upon returning home, both enrolled in a smoking cessation program and support group. They began to exercise and follow the dietary advice of a Culinary Institute of America-trained nutritionist. They paid for all this with funds from their respective HFAs. Once they successfully achieved their new goals, they felt better, had more stamina, and looked terrific. They also saved more than $8,000 per year in total Aspen premium reductions—a most satisfactory financial return on their investments in healthier living.

Andrea's story may be speculative fiction, but it will hardly be far-fetched under American Choice. Concepts such as independent patient advocates, premium and savings-based rebates, and the CompreNet open-source provider network barely scratch the surface of the potential for quality and cost innovations in medical care. Yet, just these three concepts have the potential to reduce health care costs by as much as half.

The Savings

Throughout this book I have suggested that health care costs under American Choice will drop by 50% or more over a period of years. I have discussed how the dynamics of a consumer market and provider competition will head us in that direction. It is useful to back up and look at the magnitude of waste in the current system that allows me to make such a seemingly rash prediction.

Just one major area in desperate need of reform is the horrendously complex dance engaged in by providers, insurers, and consumers simply to pay for services rendered by medical providers. Richard L. Clarke, president and CEO of the Healthcare Financial Management Association, has observed that the "fragmented and broken system of charging, billing and collections consumes about 31 cents out of every [health care] dollar. Medicare regulations (reported to be more voluminous than the entire IRS tax code), Byzantine payment rules, 40-plus million uninsured people, complex payment formulas…are the real problem."[1] If this estimate is accurate—and the health care financial executives I've talked to tell me it is—then a staggering $713 million is mostly wasted.

In a more rational system, this purely administrative function would cost a tiny fraction of that amount. For providers, the cost of billing and collection would be little more than the fees to process credit and debit card transactions. For insurers, claims processing based on market prices of provider services would be almost completely automated, cutting their costs by 80–90%. The net reimbursement process cost to the system would likely fall by at least an order of magnitude. (For more on this, read "Who Wants to Be a Trillionaire?" in the appendix.)

A particularly damning study released by Pricewaterhouse-Coopers' Health Research Institute estimates that a staggering $1.2 trillion of our then $2.2 trillion in annual health care expenditures (55%) is wasted. It defines waste as "costs that could have been avoided without a negative impact on quality." According to this analysis, "The top three areas of wasted spending are defensive medicine ($210 billion annually), inefficient claims processing (up to $210 billion annually), and care spent on preventable conditions related to obesity and overweight ($200 billion annually)."[2]

A study by the Milken Institute estimated potential savings of $190 billion a year in medical costs with lifestyle improvements and modest treatment advances for six diseases—cancer, diabetes, hypertension, stroke, heart disease, and pulmonary conditions.[3] Since chronic diseases account for a total of $1.5 trillion in annual expenditures, this savings estimate would seem to be, as the authors themselves suggest, conservative.

The Dartmouth Institute for Health Policy and Clinical Practice has estimated that just unnecessary hospitalizations, duplicative testing, unproven treatments, and excessive end-of-life care account for up to one-third of health care spending.[4] In her book *Overtreated*, New American Foundation senior fellow Shannon Brownlee relates a litany of waste in our health care financing and delivery system. She confirms that nearly a third of all health care spending goes for administrative "paper pushing."[5] The average hospital cost per day in the United States is four times the average in the developed world. We spend "between five hundred and seven hundred billion dollars on care that does nothing to improve our health." In three hundred enlightening but often depressing, pages, she provides as detailed an indictment as I've seen of the waste and maltreatment within the system.

These examples demonstrate that our system of health care offers a huge collective target of opportunity to reduce costs just by eliminating waste that has already been identified. What none of these studies address is the additional opportunity costs we've suffered from not having harnessed America's innovative, entrepreneurial resources to go beyond dealing with mere waste. Major opportunities exist to achieve even lower costs through innovative business models, medical process improvements, competitive pricing, and an end to the unnecessary medical monopoly.

American Choice will engage forces and resources that will eliminate most of the waste *and* unleash innovation. It will simplify billing and collection processes, promote consistent provider quality, eliminate wasteful medical practices, expand the use of formal practice guidelines, increase provider productivity, spawn innovative treatment options, reduce preventable diseases, and engage competition to reduce prices. Over time—perhaps five to fifteen years—we will see health care costs drop by half or more with dramatic improvements in the quality and quantity of necessary medical care.

I'm old enough to remember when AT&T was *the* telephone company monopoly in America. It was illegal for consumers to own their own telephone equipment or to connect any non-AT&T device to a telephone line. Long-distance telephone calls were an expensive luxury. The easiest way for a business executive to keep someone waiting outside his office was for his secretary to tell the hapless guest, "He's on long distance." It was an expensive undertaking never to be interrupted by someone's mere physical presence. Everyone complained about Ma Bell, but everyone had also come to accept its monopoly as the natural order of things. The Bell System was extremely reliable. It was also extremely slow to innovate. It never really viewed its mission as anything beyond providing reliable point-to-point voice communications.

Then came AT&T's court-ordered breakup in 1984 and the congressional telecommunication regulatory reforms in 1996. Without those, it is unlikely that we would now own fax machines; buy our own telephones; talk on ubiquitous, cheap cell phones; enjoy high-speed Internet connections (or even low-speed Internet connections); send email; access a World Wide Web; download videos; communicate via Blackberrys and iPhones; buy low-cost telephone/high-speed Internet/television packages; or make as many long-distance and local telephone calls we want for a low flat fee.

With American Choice, we will be able to see the same effect in health care. Just as almost no one in 1984 predicted today's wide-open telecommunications environment, it is difficult now to foresee how reforming health care can deliver similar benefits twenty years from now. But it will happen if we engage the power of regulated market capitalism in the cause of comprehensive health care reform.

APPENDIX

Who Wants To Be
a Trillionaire?

A ll great economic revolutions have generated opportunities for
massive accumulations of individual and institutional wealth.
Whether the innovation was railroads, the telegraph, capital markets, the telephone, automobiles, radio, television, computers, or the
Internet, visionary entrepreneurs have always emerged to harness
vast new consumer demand and to become immensely wealthy.

When it works well, America honors its great innovators and
entrepreneurs. Thomas Edison was hailed as the genius inventor
and entrepreneur of his time, much as Google founders Larry Page
and Sergey Brin have been in ours. Others like John D. Rockefeller
in the nineteenth century or Bill Gates today initially generated ac-
claim for their entrepreneurial accomplishments. Later they came to
be attacked as rapacious monopolists. Later still, they came back to
reconstitute their public images as great philanthropic benefactors.
Whether you view them as predators or heroes, it remains that each
has made significant contributions to economic growth and beneficial social change. All made vast fortunes through intelligence,
innovation, timing, toughness, and luck.

If American Choice, or anything like it, ever makes its debut on
the American economic stage, it is reasonable to expect the emergence of new titans of wealth and change to emerge as well. Is this a
good thing? Regardless of how these moguls subsequently comport
themselves and use their nouveau riches, it seems certain that the
process by which they create their fortunes will result from having

delivered orders of magnitude more value to the American public than they themselves will reap.

Many believe it is immoral for people to profit from the illness or suffering of others. To the extent this means *causing* or *perpetuating* illness and suffering, I am in complete agreement—cigarette manufacturers and certain unfortunate aspects of the current medical system come to mind. The moral high ground is held by those who alleviate the maladies with the least waste and diversion of resources from other needs of equal import. For reasons nobody fully understands, such outcomes have always flowed best from the emergent qualities of regulated market capitalism. The profit motive drives entrepreneurs to find better, more innovative, and indeed more profitable methods to achieve these good ends, even though their aims are usually more focused on their own ends of doing well.

In the realm of economic endeavor, no replacement for market forces, whether malign or well-intentioned, has been found to approach the magnificent performance of the uncoordinated, chaotic, inexplicably complex interactions of billions of situational human judgments we call a market. Attempts to design better systems have always run into the problem characterized by H.L. Mencken: "for every complex problem, there is an answer that is clear, simple, and wrong."

Today, relatively few of us begrudge Bill Gates or Steve Jobs their small shares of the relatively minor sums each of us periodically pays to Microsoft or Apple for helping us do important and trivial things with greater ease and enjoyment. I suggest the same dynamic will hold for the savvy winners in the health care revolution that will accompany American Choice. Clever entrepreneurs will figure out ways to heal us better, faster, and cheaper than anyone ever imagined possible. Some will create vast fortunes for themselves in the process.

Probably the single greatest problem with public acceptance of market capitalism is the fear that no one can predict how it will all unfold because it doesn't always unfold well for all of us all the time.

Yet history tells us that the great majority of us will end up better off, empowering us to aid those who don't do so well.

I will offer one future scenario about a specific change I think will take place as a direct result of American Choice. It would significantly benefit virtually everyone while generating massive fortunes for those who succeed in making it work.

The opportunity presents itself in the form of the hundreds of billions of dollars annually wasted on the non-productive morass of billing and collecting for health care services between providers and payers. Few of us have been spared the frustration of dealing with this aspect of our health care system, and all of us have suffered financially because of it.

The American Choice Health Plan will free doctors and hospitals to set their own prices in a competitive market, subject to consumer determinations of value, aided by their insurers. The need for us to continue throwing away so much treasure on mere billing and collection activities will go away. Here's how it might happen.

Introducing Iris Wilde and CompreNet

Shortly after the enactment of American Choice, an enterprising entrepreneur I will call Iris Wilde will successfully raise $100 million of venture capital in a series of financing rounds to form a company that she will name CompreNet.

CompreNet's mission statement is simple, if a tad megalomaniacal:

The mission of CompreNet is to revolutionize health care consumer shopping and provider pricing, billing, and collection by replacing opaque, inefficient systems with a seamless electronic network to connect every consumer in America with every health care provider, and every provider with every insurer (1) to allow consumers easily to obtain information on quality and price on every health care provider, service, and product; (2) to allow providers to prospectively determine patient insurance eligibility and ability to pay;

(3) to simplify provider submission of claims at the point of patient service; and (4) to facilitate the instantaneous adjudication and payment of these claims by consumers and their insurers. CompreNet's goal is to provide the essential information and transaction infrastructure to enable the American Choice Health Plan to achieve its full potential to improve health care quality while reducing its costs by half or more.

The idea of CompreNet came from Iris's observation in 2002 that every retail pharmacy in the United States was electronically connected to every third-party payer that insures or pays for prescription drug benefits. Whenever a pharmacy receives a patient's prescription, a pharmacist or pharmacy tech enters the client's insurance card and prescription information into a computer that transmits the data securely and instantaneously to the proper insurer's computer server. In a matter of seconds the server confirms the patient's eligibility status, calculates the allowable drug price, determines both payer and patient liability, and transmits that information back to the pharmacy. The pharmacist then fills the prescription and the pharmacy tech dispenses it to the patient after collecting the copayment as directed by the third-party payer.

As soon as the pharmacy tech enters the copayment into the system, the insurer instantly completes and adjudicates the claim. It usually pays the pharmacy by bank wire transfer within ten days. There are rarely any paper claims to deal with, so an extremely high percentage of pharmacy claims (greater than 99%) get filed, adjudicated, and paid via this electronic system. Both the payer and the patient know upfront how much they will have to pay, and the pharmacist knows how much she will collect before she ever reaches for a pill bottle or keys in computer instructions to an automated Baker Cell inventory dispenser. The system works well and costs the payer as little as $.15 per claim.

Iris realized that the pharmacy claims system was light years ahead of the dysfunctional doctor and hospital claims universe. She also saw that the pharmacy system was light years behind current technology. For example, there are no magnetic strips or microchips on customers' pharmacy benefit ID cards that allow the computer to do all the eligibility data entry on the pharmacy claims computer or to prompt the pharmacist simply to click a box for a normal re- fill of an existing prescription. Instead, almost everything has to be entered by hand by the pharmacist or a pharmacy tech. Even worse, there are frequent problems when a doctor prescribes a non-favored brand-name drug or the patient is seeking an early refill because of an upcoming vacation. When these things happen, they too often require the pharmacist to pick up the phone and call the patient's doctor and leave a message requesting a prescription change or clari- fication, which leaves the customer waiting until the doctor or his nurse returns the call and deals with the issue. Or the pharmacist has to call the insurer to correct an incorrect birth date or to explain that the patient is about to leave on vacation. Such hassles consume a high percentage of each pharmacist's day. The situation is not only galling to highly trained pharmacists, but it is also an immense drain on their professional productivity.

Iris realized that an updated system would include much more powerful computer applications to allow 99% phone-free billing and collections for pharmacies, doctors, and even hospitals. But it could only work if each patient functions as a responsible consumer with the ability to authorize the payments up to limits imposed by insur- ance coverage. Iris knew it was absurd to bill an insurance company for a $4 prescription under the current system. The labor involved in entering the data and making the phone calls often exceeded the cost of the drugs being sold.

If an insurer could be pre-notified that one of its insureds was to be hospitalized for surgery, for example, they could have already intervened with the patient prior to admission to help make sure he was making a good decision about quality and price, based on alternatives suggested by the insurer or independent third-party patient advocate. Even if the patient chose a hospital not fully covered by his insurer, he would know in advance how much he would personally be on the hook for. And he would know approximately or even exactly how much he would be paying.

It occurred to Iris that there was no technical reason why all medical claims couldn't be transmitted and processed the same way as pharmacy claims, only faster and more efficiently. In 2002 she had been stymied by the far greater complexity and labor intensity required to produce and process medical claims. Whereas a pharmacy claim consists of identifying and pricing a single standardized packaged product, a medical or hospital claim could include anywhere from several to several thousand discreet product and service items, many of which require human judgment and intervention to code properly. Much gamesmanship had arisen from the creative use of such interventions to increase provider revenues. This forced insurers to apply countervailing interventions to scrutinize claims and minimize costs—often requiring human judgment and dueling computers.

The problem in fully automating such a process was not its constantly escalating complexity. Any high-volume activity that can be defined algorithmically can be more efficiently processed by computers than by humans. The problem was that computers don't do judgment—they only do if-then-else rules. Iris also came to understand the perverse economics of health care that allow insurers to pay the lowest provider reimbursement rates and to pay them late. That left the uninsured, cash-paying consumers to pay higher prices—often two-and-a-half times as much.

Another problem contributed to the need for such a combination of mindless and mindful complexity. There was no widely accepted standard for what constituted a fair price for anything delivered by doctors or hospitals. That is not so in the rest of our economy because both the prices and quantities of things to be paid for *are agreed to in advance* between buyers/consumers and sellers. Billing and collection is then a simple, inexpensive process for both sides.

In medical care, there is rarely any such pre-agreement between buyer/consumer and seller. Why? The major reason is that the buyer and the consumer are almost never the same person. The insurer is the buyer, and the patient is the consumer. Thus, consumers don't pay, and payers don't consume. Neither has sufficient information to determine the true value of the product or service being delivered.

The consumer may be convinced he needs the service, but he knows nothing of its price. The insurer normally doesn't even know that the service has been consumed until it receives a bill. Even then it doesn't know whether the service was needed. In fact, it doesn't know for sure, even after receiving the bill, whether the service has actually been provided! Assuming a service has been both provided and needed, the insurers have only rough proxies for its value. Mostly these are arbitrary standards, like the Resource Based Relative Value System (RBRVS) created by the federal government, which puts a dollar value on everything a doctor could charge for. "Value" may have been in the name of the system, but it was nowhere to be found in its contents, which are based on very rough estimates of cost.

Iris's insight in 2002 was that there could be a solution to all this. Medical care could be made as simple to price and bill as any other good or service. All it required was for the buyer of the service and the consumer of the service to be the same person—the patient. If someone could figure out how to do that, then medical care could be priced and sold just like cars and bananas.

Unfortunately, Iris had been in no position to make this happen. The medical billing problem was a huge systemic one dominated on top by the Centers for Medicare and Medicaid Services (CMS), which set virtually all of the non-prescription-drug pricing rules used by virtually all doctors and hospitals in the private sector. Instead, Iris had to remain happy as the owner/CEO of a physician billing and collection service. She assuaged her disappointment with her Lamborghini, a summer house in the Hamptons, and frequent trips to the Cote d'Azur with her poodle Leona.

The debut of American Choice changed all that. Its consumer focus suddenly made simplified, transparent provider pricing not just possible but absolutely necessary. Iris dug further into the pricing issue. She learned more about CPT, HCPCS, DRG, ICD, and other coding standards for medical diagnoses, products, and services. It dawned on her that the previously opaque complexity of provider pricing had arisen not because of the use of such codes but because of the government's standardization of their relative values and the resulting cloud of prices allowed for providers by different insurers. Moreover, even with American Choice's removal of government price regulation, there was still a need for widely accepted health care product and service coding standards. Just as every product in a supermarket carries a Universal Product Code to facilitate inventory control and checkout, so must every health care product and service be identifiable by a unique code if there is to be efficient claims and payment processing.

Iris's inspiration was that it is possible to combine multiple codes into simple service-specific baskets—she dubbed them UberCodes—to enable doctors, hospitals, and other providers to price and market their services as easily labeled bundles of services that were readily understood by consumers while affording identifiability to computers in the form of the underlying component codes. For example, under the old system, providing a patient with cardiac bypass surgery would have generated detailed individual provider claims by the hospital, the surgeon, the assistant surgeon, the anesthesiologist, and the pathologist, with a total of hundreds or even thousands of distinct service codes, each priced at a rate that no one ever expected to be paid. It was like buying a car based on the total prices of its thousands of different parts. If the hapless patient-to-be happened to ask someone—anyone—how much this episode of care was going to cost, there was no way to know or find out the answer until after the fact.

Iris's innovation was to show hospitals and doctors how they could standardize their pricing for complete bundles of services and then combine them into all-inclusive global service pricing that any patient, hospital billing clerk, or insurance claims administrator could understand. There was some precedent for this idea going back at least to the diagnosis related groups (DRGs) implemented by Medicare in the 1980s for hospital reimbursement, but Iris's concept was to extend the idea to virtually all medical services everywhere with the use of UberCodes. A single cardiac bypass surgery could be publicly priced by a hospital on Iris's CompreNet website at $25,000, for example, inclusive of all doctor and hospital fees and charges. Only late payers would be subject to financing charges, late payment fees, and collection surcharges imposed by providers forced to carry accounts receivable and to chase payment from slow-paying insurers or consumers. Otherwise, the actual price paid would be the same price originally quoted by the hospital—to the penny—as long as the payment was made on a fast, timely basis.

Iris's second epiphany was that UberCoding would allow providers to set their own prices for all their services and to make those prices applicable to all their patients, whether insured or not. She reasoned that, just as Wal-Mart and Bloomingdales set different prices for identical products, doctors and hospitals could do the same thing as long as consumers have strong incentives to seek and purchase the services with the lowest prices and highest quality. Consumers, with the aid of the insurers and other resources, could become their own pricing police for medical services, just as they have always been for almost everything else they buy. No longer would it be necessary or even desirable for insurers and government agencies to negotiate prices because a far more self-interested and effective system would be enforced by the consumers themselves. The insurers would just have to make damn sure that their insurance policies provided sufficient incentives for their members to pay a lot of attention to price (see Andrea Moonshine scenario in the conclusions section above for an example of this.) To protect themselves against price gouging, however, American Choice Health Plan-participating insurers would also need to set publicly disclosed maximum price limits on how much they would pay for specific high cost services.

With the advent of independent provider quality-rating services, Iris realized she could enable consumers to shop online for health care providers based on the quality and the prices of their services. There even emerged a third category of independent rankings for doctors' and hospitals' levels of customer service, based on such factors as the friendliness and helpfulness of staff, whether the doctor actually apologized for delays, and whether his nurse made a follow-up call to see how the patient was doing.

CompreNet immediately became a must-have service for every insurer, provider, and consumer in America. It dramatically accelerated by years the achievement of all of American Choice's ambitious goals.

Excerpts from CompreNet's Business Plan[1]

What Is CompreNet?

CompreNet is an innovative health service information and payments facilitator formed by a group of experienced entrepreneurs and investors led by CEO Iris Wilde.

CompreNet offers a secure, Internet-based information and payment network to connect America's physicians, hospitals, and ancillary providers to consumers and insurers to provide seamless consumer information on providers, products, and services and to facilitate the resulting financial transactions when services are rendered. With CompreNet, health care providers are able to post their prices publicly for all their health care products and services, much as a supermarket posts its prices online. Any provider's posted prices are subject to one simple rule: These are the prices offered by the provider to any patient for whom full payment is made within one business day of the date of service. Only patients or insurers paying later than that can be required to pay more. CompreNet is available to any insurer that agrees to process and pay claims instantly subject to this rule.

The mission of CompreNet is to provide patients and insurers with a price-based incentive to pay for health care services in full at the time of service and to give providers an incentive to post their best, most competitive prices for consumers and insurers willing to eliminate provider accounts receivable and all the incident costs.

What Are CompreNet's Core Principles?

1. *To Slash Transaction Costs*: We at CompreNet believe that 31% is too high a cost for billing and collection for medical care. It should cost less than a tenth as much.

2. *To Enhance the Doctor-Patient Relationship*: We believe that health insurers do not belong in the middle of the physician/patient relationship. The insurer is an underwriter of risk, not a manager of care.

3. *Transparent Fair Market Value*: We believe that health care providers and patients, participating in a competitive marketplace with access to transparent information on quality and price, are capable of establishing the fair market value of the medical services they alone respectively produce and consume.

4. *Timely Payment*: We believe that patients and their insurers should pay for services at, or immediately following, the time of care and that all parties benefit when they do.

5. *A Universal Need*: We believe that the insurance market needs to move swiftly in this direction. CompreNet wants to be part of the solution by providing easy-to-use tools for all the parties.

The Need for CompreNet

1. *The Current System Subtracts Value*: The Healthcare Financial Management Association (HFMA) has estimated that health care charging, billing, and collecting consume 31 cents out of

every health care dollar. These costs add little value and are a significant barrier to the provision of quality, affordable medical care.

2. *Price Opacity Hurts Patients*: Health insurers have become so enmeshed in the complexity of their own claims processing and payment systems that provider fee schedules have become, at best, irrelevant and, at worst, misleading. This situation interferes with the physician/patient relationship in ways that prevent either party from knowing the cost of care or the source of payments before services are rendered. The net effect is that everybody loses under this system.

3. *Patients Need Price Transparency*: Patients need to know doctor and hospital prices and rates *before* they purchase services. Under the current system, there is no way for this to happen.

4. *Providers Need Payment Certainty*: Providers need to know how much and when they will be paid *before* they agree to render services. Under the current system, they have little or no idea.

5. *Providers Must Price Competitively*: Providers need a means to deal with patients who are becoming increasingly price sensitive. This started with the advent of MSAs, HRAs, and HSAs but has accelerated greatly as a result of the American Choice Health Plan, which now allows all patients to pay directly for much of their own medical care from their own health funding accounts.

6. *Righting a Capsized System*: All patients, payers, and providers need a system in which those who pay first also pay the least. Under the current system, insurers pay later *and* less than anyone who is willing to pay cash at the time of service. This is completely backward.

7. *Price Deregulation*: Under the American Choice Health Plan, consumer purchasing of all health insurance and services, combined with CMS's abdication to the market of all responsibility

for system-wide pricing, has eliminated any need to continue the current, wasteful, dueling-computers system of billing and collection.

8. *Slashing Transaction Costs*: With the elimination of the current system, we have an opportunity to adapt successful pharmacy and debit/credit card transaction-processing models for medical care delivery at a tiny fraction of current costs.

9. *A Standardized Process*: The health insurance industry needs a streamlined, low-cost, commoditized health care payment system that will allow insurers to focus their competitive energies on providing high levels of financial protection; customer-pleasing service; encouragement to seek cost-effective care; and incentives for personal responsibility for disease prevention.

10. *Consumer Value Pricing*: Consumers and insurers need to pay the lowest available prices for the best, most effective services.

11. *Fast, Assured Payments*: Providers need to be paid quickly and assuredly.

12. *Aiding Providers' Competitive Advantage*: Efficient, high-quality providers need better methods to market their services to existing and prospective patients.

CompreNet's Value Proposition

1. *Clear Prices, Simple Rules*: All health care providers should be able to post fair, non-negotiable prices for their services to patients and insurers who are willing and able to pay within one business day of the time of service. Anyone who pays later must pay more to cover the incremental costs of invoicing, financing, and collection.

2. *Market Pricing*: Providers should be able to decide what those prices will be and to change them at any time, as their own circumstances and competitive judgments dictate.

3. *A Rational System*: Health service prices available to patients and insurers who pay at the time of service should be:

   a. Simple for all parties to understand and execute.

   b. The best prices available from that provider.

      i. If the patient pays at the time of care, the price should initially reflect the provider's improvement in cash flow and the elimination of associated costs of claims submission, patient invoicing, financing, frustration, uncertainty, and risk. Longer term, provider prices will be based on the value to consumers.

      ii. Patients and insurers who pay cash immediately should pay the lowest price of any other payer, instead of an uncertain amount paid at a much later time.

4. *Provider Utility*: Providers will be able to use the CompreNet site to:

   a. Post their best cash prices on the public CompreNet website at no cost to prospective patients.

   b. Simplify their pricing, based on UberCoded bundled packages of services to be provided to patients.

   c. Hyperlink or Widget their CompreNet listings to their own websites, appointment scheduling, and to independent quality rating services.

   d. Instantly confirm patient insurance eligibility and coverage prior to service delivery, as well as patient ability to pay charges not covered by insurance.

   e. Based on a patient's insurance coverage, estimate the patient's liability prior to service and place a hold on patient's credit card or HFA debit card account for that amount. The provider is thus assured of payment upon patient certification once the service has been provided.

   f. Integrate their own electronic charge-capture systems with CompreNet for seamless insurance claim filing before the patient has left the doctor's exam room, ER, OR, or other facility.

g. Determine patient approval of service and payment authorization via electronic patient signature or private PIN entry.

h. Electronically submit patient claims to insurers immediately upon delivery of service, based on patient approval—all before patient has left the building.

i. Immediately receive from insurer the final claim adjudication information, funds transfer advice, and notice of amount to collect from patient before he/she leaves the provider facility.

j. Collect patient portion of charges directly from the patient via HFA debit card, credit card, cash, or check.

k. Receive all necessary claims and collection data to populate provider's journal and general ledger entries.

5. *Consumer Utility*: Consumers and prospective patients will be able to use the CompreNet site to:

a. Compare providers and services according to independent quality rankings.

b. Segregate information on any providers that the consumer's insurance company will not reimburse.

c. Search for the highest quality, lowest cost providers for any needed health care service or product.

d. Determine exact or approximate prices for services before they are rendered by any provider.

e. Pay provider charges for which consumers are liable, utilizing an HFA debit card, any major credit card, or bank wire transfer. Patients may also pay via check or cash at the time of service for later reimbursement by their HFAs and/or insurers.

f. Receive all necessary claims and payment data to support any required consumer tax filing or audit.

g. Manage HFA deposits, transfers, investment options, and payments.

6. *Insurer Utility*: Insurers will use the CompreNet site to:

   a. Receive provider queries and immediately confirm or confute member eligibility and coverage information.

   b. Receive and immediately adjudicate provider-submitted, patient-approved claims upon a member's receipt of services.

   c. Electronically transfer insurer payments to the provider within one business day.

   d. Immediately advise a provider of any residual claims liability by the patient and electronically transmit a detailed explanation of benefits (EOB) statement to the patient.

   e. Invoice member premiums.

   f. Accept member premium payments.

   g. Provide complete member premium, claims, and payment histories.

7. *Turnkey MD Practice and Hospital Management Systems*: CompreNet additionally offers providers complete turnkey systems that incorporate the following:

   a. Appointment-desk online verification of patient's insurance eligibility and coverage information.

   b. Remote (Internet) and local online patient registration.

   c. Check-in desk patient ID card readers/RF transponders and immediate link to CompreNet-enabled insurance revalidation and debit card funds hold.

   d. Electronic point-of-service charge capture, including integration with provider's accounting and electronic medical record systems.

   e. Checkout-desk patient signature or PIN-entry electronics, verification of service and price, authorization for insurance adjudication, and patient authorization for charges to HFA debit card, credit card, or other bank account.

   f. Printed or electronic patient receipt generation and transmission.

g. Invoice printing or electronic transmission for delayed payments.

h. Comprehensive provider financial, utilization, and productivity reporting.

i. Full turnkey accounting system, with generation of all journal and general ledger entries.

j. Full EMR integration and support.

8. *Turnkey Insurer/TPA Back Office Systems*: CompreNet offers insurers complete turnkey eligibility, claims, and patient liability accounting and processing systems that incorporate the following:

a. Production and distribution of member coverage cards that include:

   i. Member identification

   ii. Electronic provider and CompreNet recognition via standard and RF card readers

   iii. Integrated HFA debit card

   iv. Optional integrated credit card

   v. Card-swipe or RF emergency facility access to patient EMR or PHR

b. Receive and respond to CompreNet-mediated provider requests for member eligibility and coverage information.

c. Calculate pre-service estimates of insurer and member liability based on provider or member query via CompreNet.

d. System to receive and instantly adjudicate all CompreNet-mediated provider claims submissions, returning instant payment advices and patient EOBs to providers and members.

e. Update accounting for member deductibles and out-of-pocket payments.

f. Provide complete, secure access to appropriate provider and member payment histories, including pending status.

    g. Complete insurer payment and claims payable accounting and reporting.

    h. Complete integration with insurer's or TPA's accounting systems.

    i. Other features too numerous to summarize (see CompreNet client service agreement for complete recitation of services and fees).

CompreNet's Revenue Model

CompreNet has five integrated sources of revenue:

1. Fees for claims transaction services.

2. License fees for turnkey provider and service bureau front-end systems and services.

3. License fees for turnkey insurer and TPA back-end systems and services.

4. Consulting and advisory fees from providers and insurers.

5. Advertising fees from providers and insurers.

Epilogue

CompreNet's rollout was an immediate success, with the firm's annual revenue quickly reaching $5 billion and net income of $1.8 billion. CompreNet's IPO was historic, placing Iris's net worth at the end of the first day of trading well north of $100 billion. CompreNet's constant innovation was widely credited as a significant factor in the subsequent fifteen-year decline in inflation-adjusted health care costs that leveled off at only 41% of health care expenditures (constant dollars) incurred during the last full year before American Choice's debut. CompreNet's innovations spread to a worldwide market that revolutionized consumer health care markets virtually everywhere. At CompreNet's peak stock price, Iris became the world's first trillionaire.

CompreNet was subsequently broken into multiple pieces by the combined efforts of the European Competition Commission and the U.S. Justice Department's Antitrust Division. As a result, Iris became even wealthier. CompreNet was able to reassemble itself from its dispersed components twenty years later, after the death of European Commissioner for Competition Neelie Kroes and the first American election of a Republican president in decades.

About the Author

STEPHEN HYDE is the author of *Prescription Drugs for Half Price or Less* (Bantam-Dell, 2006). The former federal chief HMO financial regulator and a certified actuary, he started and grew Peak Health Care, Inc., into a highly successful public managed-care company, recognized by *Business Week* as one of "America's Best Small Companies." He has extensive experience in managed-care operations and strategy, health insurance, managed-care regulation, consumer-driven health care, pharmacy benefits, disease management, medical information technology, medical group management, medical network and PPO operations, health benefit design and pricing, health insurance underwriting, community rating, and health service product development and marketing.

He has an MBA from Harvard Business School and a BA in financial administration "with high honor" from Michigan State University. He currently lives in Colorado Springs where he is CEO of Hyde Rx Services Corp., a health care management consultancy. He may be contacted at sshyde@q.com and welcomes your compliments and criticisms, preferably in Pareto proportions.

Acknowledgments

IN APPROACHING a subject as intimidating as health care reform, I feel like a gnat standing on the shoulders of giants. There are few, if any, truly new ideas embodied in The American Choice Health Plan. If I have added any originality, it derives from the way I've reengineered, extended, and arranged existing ideas and concepts—mostly well proven elsewhere—into what I hope to be a comprehensive structure for viewing, analyzing, and solving the health care crisis.

My mentors and intellectual forebears are numerous, and I am grateful to them all. I apologize to those who may feel I've taken their perfectly good ideas and stitched them into something that only Victor Frankenstein could love.

My early mentors included my mother, who set me up in my first business, a Kool Aid stand to compete with the neighbor kids who didn't know to put sugar in theirs. In college, Professor Roland Robinson taught me how to take apart a balance sheet. He gave me a textbook editing job that allowed me to stay in school and out of rice paddies. I also suspect he wrote the recommendation letter that got me into Harvard Business School. At Harvard, entrepreneurial studies Professor Pat Liles taught me that the business comes before the deal. And never, ever run out of cash. Over a single beer in 1970 Kaiser's late Carl Berner had one of those once-in-a-lifetime pivotal roles that led me into the career I've followed ever since. Professor Brandt Allen taught me never to make a decision until I have to. I'm sure I learned other things at HBS, but I can't remember them just now. Professor Earl Sasser has endured me and helped me for forty years.

At my first insurance company job, Security Industrial C.E.O. E.J. Ourso taught me the power of audacity backed by solid analysis, preparation, and pre-negotiation role playing. My first business partner, David Whelan, taught me the value of extroversion. He, along with the Center for Creative Leadership, helped me to move from I to E on the Meyers Briggs.

Christopher Stanley Cross and Gar Puryear taught me that bank presidents are human too. Darrel and Hazel Smith were there for me when I hit bottom after an early business failure. Joe Ryan hired me out of my Ozark log cabin into Arthur Young and Company in Washington, D.C., to help create the HMO industry on a cost-plus-fixed-fee basis. There, Jack Wirnowski protected me from the bureaucracy. Later, in Chicago, Jim Deason tolerated my undisciplined floundering in a job for which I was ill-suited. Bill McLeod rescued me from that and other mires, becoming my boss, protector, mentor, and great friend. I still mourn his passing.

Without Keith Ketelsen, Chuck Bowles, John Smith, Larry Silver, and Jim Harding to provide the canvas, paints, easel, and painting lessons, my tenure at Peak Health Care would not have been nearly as revolutionary, satisfying, or fun as it turned out to be. Investment bankers Paul Felton and Charlie Murphy did the heavy lifting to take us public. I am grateful to you all and look forward to our continuing friendships.

There are a lot of endnotes in this book. My being able to learn from and build on the ideas, facts, opinions, and hard, scholarly work of the authors I cite has often been exhilarating. You all have my unbounded respect and gratitude.

There are three people who, more than any others, helped me shift my focus from working to make more money from health care to making health care work for more people. All would be surprised to hear me say this. In 1992, Bill Niskanen, now Chairman Emeritus of the Cato Institute held my feet to the fire to produce and present a paper on one of my more radical ideas for provider reform. It had never occurred to me that anyone would care to hear anything I had to say on matters of policy. The favorable response I received from (most of) the people in the audience kindled my interest in paying more attention to health policy.

Then my friend, fellow wine aficionado, and American Enterprise Institute scholar Charles Murray encouraged me to put my health reform ideas into book form. When I failed to respond, he nudged me along by asking my opinions on the health care commentary in his draft of "What It Means to Be a Libertarian." He honored me even further by acknowledging me in the same paragraph as Milton Friedman. I still have the notes from my conversation with Charles on how to write a book. He could write a book about that.

Then Regi Herzlinger invited me to write a piece on health insurance reform, which she published in her encyclopedic *Consumer-Driven Health Care*. That was the first time I had ever written even a summary of what was to become The American Choice Health Plan, which had been forming in my mind for many years. Regi additionally asked me to review the draft of her authored portion of the book. Over the years she has taught me more than I can acknowledge. Her respect for my contrary opinions has given me the confidence to think them through better and then to abandon or stick with them. Thanks to you all, Bill, Charles, and Regi.

I have had occasion to discuss health reform with many people more informed than I am about a lot of it. They have uniformly been generous with their time and gentle in correcting my howlers. My thanks to the following friends and respected colleagues:

- Martha Barton for knowing everyone and for helping me to understand end-of-life care and hospice.

- Mike Huotari for introducing me to the Colorado health reform process and for knowing everyone Martha may have missed.

- Peter Miterko for his expertise on ERISA and other legal aspects of health benefits.

- Rob Ruiz-Moss and John Herbers for contributing to and encouraging my further development of the business plan upon which the appendix is based. Most of what I know about individual health insurance is because of them.

- Charlie Zinn, MD, for his support, ideas, insights on cancer treatment, and for connecting me to the Mayo folks.

- Eric Sipf for his input on many aspects of health care cost and fraud control, not to mention our nearly thirty-year friendship.

- John Legere for triangulating Robert Heinlein's long out-of-print *Life-Line*.

- Peter Carman and Sharon Erikson for reviewing and commenting on key chunks of the manuscript.

- Linda Gorman, a real economist, for her insights on market-driven health care.

- Bill Kendall, another professional economist, for taking the time to review and comment on key elements of the American Choice Health Plan.

- Beth McGlynn of RAND Corporation and Shannon Brownlee of the New American Foundation for providing eye-opening insights and data on health care quality.

- George Tracy for teaching me about retail pharmacy operations those many years ago.

- Harvard and Columbia Professor Marta Wosinska for reviewing and commenting on various manuscript excerpts, including an early introductory chapter that, thanks to her, will never see the light of day.

- Former health care executive and California HMO regulator Mike Henry for a third of a century of insight, support, deep friendship, and, more recently, access to his encyclopedic knowledge on the early days of California HMOs.

- Milliman actuary Bruce Pyenson for reviewing my musings on adverse selection and for our continuing dialogue on various aspects of health insurance reform.

- Dayton Ault for his incisive insights on managed care underwriting.
- Greg Scandlen for continually reminding me how commonsensical the idea of consumer markets in health care really is.
- My editor Allan Burns for saving me from myself on numerous occasions.
- HobNob publisher Rob Simon for, well, everything.
- Jeff Millburn for keeping me abreast of the continuing challenges and rewards of helming a large multispecialty medical group over the past 25 years.
- Jackie Driscoll for her insights into hospital financial operations and economics.
- For those of you who have gotten this far down the list only to find I've not included you, please don't be shy about reminding me of your contributions in case I'm fortunate enough to include them in subsequent editions. It's negligence, not ingratitude that has caused me to leave you out.

More than anyone, my wife and closest friend, Loren George has been unfailingly supportive throughout the year-and-a-half effort to produce this book. Much of it was during odd, late-night hours when we could have otherwise been enjoying each other's company. Thank you, my love. I'm back. Likewise, my children Evan and Erin have encouraged me and reminded me why it is so important that we pass on a better health care system to future generations than the one we've created for ourselves.

Finally, my thanks to Mrs. McConathy for teaching me how to diagram sentences (and my apologies for my love of hyphens and dashes) and to Mr. Byars for teaching me how to type. It remains my only real skill.

Notes

Introduction: The Upside-Down Economics and Persistent Myths of American Health Care

1. Paul Krugman, "The Age of the Anti-Cassandra," http://krugman.blogs. nytimes.com/2008/03/25/the-age-of-the-anti-cassandra/ (accessed June 2, 2008).

2. Thomas Sowell, *Economic Facts and Fallacies* (New York: Basic Books, 2008).

Chapter 1: The Fundamental Problem with American Health Care and a Proposal to Remedy It

1. Benjamin Brewer, "Even Doctors Guess At Health Charges," *The Wall Street Journal*, May 21, 2008.

2. Herbert S. Levine, "Why Soviet Central Planning Failed," address to AAASS, February 1995, http://www.ssc.upenn.edu/east/spring95/levin.html (accessed December 28, 2007).

3. Michael Rothschild, *Bionomics* (New York: Henry Holt, 1990).

4. Eric D. Beinhocker, *The Origin of Wealth* (Watertown, MA: Harvard Business School Press, 2006).

5. Andrew H. Beck, "The Flexner Report and the Standardization of American Medical Education," JAMA (2004), http://jama.ama-assn.org/cgi/content/full/291/17/2139 (accessed January 10, 2009).

Chapter 2: Health Care Delivery: The Key Problems and Issues

1. J.A. Poisal, et al., "Health Spending Projections Through 2016: Modest Changes Obscure Part D's Impact," *Health Affairs* 26.2 (2007), http://content.healthaffairs.org/cgi/content/abstract/26/2/w242 (accessed April 30, 2009). Reed Abelson and Milt Freudenheim, "Even the Insured Feel Strain of Health Costs," *The New York Times*, May 4, 2008, http://www.nytimes. com/2008/05/04/business/04insure.html?_r=1&oref=slogin (accessed May 17, 2008). Angie C. Marek, "Under the Knife: Cutting Medical Bills," *Smart-*

Money Magazine, March 28, 2008, http://www.smartmoney.com/mag/index.
cfm?story=april2008-cut-medical-bills (accessed April 11, 2008). Kathleen
Blanchard, RN, "Employees Paying More For Health Insurance, Trend
Continues," *Emax Health*, November 28, 2008, http://www.emaxhealth.
com/1020/72/26914/employees-paying-more-health-insurance-trend-
continues.html (accessed December 3, 2008). The Henry J. Kaiser Family
Foundation, "Employee Health Benefits: 2007 Annual Survey,"
September 11, 2006, http://www.kff.org/insurance/7672/index.cfm
(accessed April 30, 2009).

2. C. Borger et al., "Health Spending Projections through 2015: Changes on the
   Horizon," *Health Affairs Web Exclusive, March/April 2006.* "Health Insur-
   ance Costs," The National Coalition on Health Care, 2008, http://www.
   nchc.org/facts/cost.shtml (accessed May 17, 2008). Uwe E. Reinhardt, Peter
   S. Hussey and Gerard F. Anderson, "U.S. Health Care Spending In An
   International Context," *Health Affairs* 23.3 (2004), http://content.healthaf-
   fairs.org/cgi/content/full/23/3/10 (accessed April 30, 2009). (R. Pear, "U.S.
   Health Care Spending Reaches All-Time High: 15% of GDP," *The New York
   Times*, January 9, 2004). Scott Gottlieb, MD, "Organ Transplants Within the
   U.S. & Abroad," American Enterprise Institute for Public Policy Research,
   ReachMD Interview, http://www.reachmd.com/xmsegment.aspx?sid=2602
   (accessed May 28, 2008).

3. "Table 46. Income before taxes: Shares of average annual expenditures and
   sources of income, Consumer Expenditure Survey, 2006," U. S. Bureau of
   Labor Statistics, http://www.bls.gov/cex/2006/share/income.pdf (accessed
   April 30, 2009). "Table 2301: Higher income before taxes: Shares of average
   annual expenditures and sources of income, Consumer Expenditure Survey,
   2006," http://www.bls.gov/cex/2006/share/higherincome.pdf (accessed May
   18, 2008).

4. Mark Kantrowitz, "FinAid—The Smart Student Guide to Financial Aid,"
   http://www.finaid.org/savings/tuition-inflation.phtml (accessed May 28,
   2008).

5. "National Income and Product Accounts Table 2.5.5. Personal Consumption
   Expenditures by Type of Expenditure," U.S. Bureau of Economic Analysis,
   2006 data, http://www.bea.gov/national/nipaweb/TableView.asp?SelectedTab
   le=73&FirstYear=2005&LastYear=2006&Freq=Year (accessed May 19, 2008).

6. Uwe E. Reinhardt, Peter S. Hussey and Gerard F. Anderson, "U.S. Health
   Care Spending In An International Context," *Health Affairs* 23.3 (2004),
   http://content.healthaffairs.org/cgi/content/full/23/3/10 (accessed April 30,
   2009).

7. The Henry J. Kaiser Family Foundation, "Employee Health Benefits: 2007 Annual Survey," September 11, 2006, http://www.kff.org/insurance/7672/index.cfm (accessed April 30, 2009).

8. "Overview of Employer Mandate Policy Options," Rand Compare, http://www.randcompare.org/options/mechanism/employer_mandate (accessed February 15, 2009). "Plan for a Healthy America—Barack Obama and Joe Biden's Plan," http://usliberals.about.com/gi/dynamic/offsite.htm?zi=1/XJ&sdn=usliberals&cdn=newsissues&tm=14&f=00&tt=2&bt=0&bts=0&st=16&zu=http%3A//www.barackobama.com/issues/healthcare/ (accessed February 15, 2009).

9. J. Le Grand, "Methods of Cost Containment: Some Lessons from Europe" (paper presented at the Fourth International Health Economics Association World Congress, San Francisco, June 2003), 6. N. Devlin, J. Appleby, and D. Parkin, "Patients' Views of Explicit Rationing: What Are the Implications for Health Service Decision-Making?" *Journal of Health Services Research and Policy* 8.3 (2003): 183–186.

10. Gardiner Harris, "British Balance Benefit vs. Cost of Latest Drugs," *The New York Times* December 2, 2008, http://www.nytimes.com/2008/12/03/health/03nice.html?em (accessed December 3, 2008).

11. Greg D'Angelo, "The 2007 Medicare Trustees Report: A Trigger for Reform?" The Heritage Foundation, May 3, 2007, http://www.heritage.org/Research/HealthCare/wm1442.cfm (accessed May 21, 2008). "How Much Do We Spend on End-of-Life Care?" PBS Online/Thirteen WNET New York, http://www.thirteen.org/bid/sb-howmuch.html (accessed May 21, 2008).

12. Jane Gross, "For the Elderly, Being Heard About Life's End," *The New York Times*, May 5, 2008, http://www.nytimes.com/2008/05/05/health/05slow.html?th&emc=th (accessed May 12, 2008).

13. Theo Francis, "More Choices Drive Cost of Health Care," *Wall Street Journal*, April 7, 2008, pB8, http://online.wsj.com/article/SB120752201349093441.html?mod=home_health_right&apl=y&r=340312 (accessed March 11, 2008).

14. Martin Sipkoff, "9 Ways To Reduce Unwarranted Variation," *Managed Care*, November 2003, http://www.managedcaremag.com/archives/0311/0311.variation.html (accessed February 23, 2008).

15. Martin Sipkoff, "9 Ways To Reduce Unwarranted Variation," Managed Care, November 2003, http://www.managedcaremag.com/archives/0311/0311.variation.html (accessed February 23, 2008).

16. Matthew DoBias, "AMA, AHA Wary of CMS Nonpayment Proposals," ModernHealthcare.com, December 3, 2008, http://www.modernhealthcare.com/apps/pbcs.dll/article?AID=/20081203/REG/312039971 (accessed December 3, 2008).

17. John E. Wennberg, MD, MPH, et al, "The Care of Patients With Severe Chronic Illness (2006), An Online Report on the Medicare Program by the Dartmouth Atlas Project," Center for the Evaluative Clinical Sciences, 65, http://www.dartmouthatlas.org/atlases/2006_Chronic_Care_Atlas.pdf (accessed February 24, 2008).

18. Robert L. Barclay, MD, et al, "Colonoscopic Withdrawal Times and Adenoma Detection during Screening Colonoscopy," *The New England Journal of Medicine*, December 14, 2006, http://content.nejm.org/cgi/content/abstract/355/24/2533 (accessed March 5, 2008).

19. Gina Kolata, "Study Questions Colonoscopy Effectiveness," *The New York Times*, Decemeber 14, 2006, http://www.nytimes.com/2006/12/14/health/14colon.html (accessed March 5, 2008).

20. Martin Sipkoff, "9 Ways To Reduce Unwarranted Variation," *Managed Care*, November 2003, http://www.managedcaremag.com/archives/0311/0311.variation.html (accessed February 23, 2008).

21. (1) Martin Sipkoff, "9 Ways To Reduce Unwarranted Variation," *Managed Care*, November 2003, http://www.managedcaremag.com/archives/0311/0311.variation.html (accessed February 23, 2008; D. Solomon et al., "Adherence with osteoporosis practice guidelines: A multilevel analysis of patient, physician, and practice setting characteristics," *The American Journal of Medicine*, 117.12 (2004): 919–924, http://patient-research.elsevier.com/patientresearch/displayAbs?key=S0002934304005728&referrer=www.google.com%252Fsearch%253Fhl%253Den%2526rlz%253D1B3GGGL_en US237US237%2526q%253Dfrequency%252Bof%252Bpatients%252Brecei ving%252Bmedical%252Bpractice%252Bguideline%252Bstandard%252Bo f%252Bcare%252Bfrom%252Btheir%252Bdoctor%2526btnG%253DSearch (accessed February 23, 2008); (2) Alan M. Muney, MD, MHA; "Evidence-Based Medicine Needs To Be Promoted More Vigorously," *Managed Care*, February 2002, http://www.managedcaremag.com/archives/0202/0202.muney.html (accessed February 23, 2008). (3) B Romanowski, Y M Zdanowicz, and S T Owens; "In search of optimal genital herpes management and standard of care (INSIGHTS): doctors' and patients' perceptions of genital herpes," *Sexually Transmitted Infections*, 84 (2008): 51–56, http://sti.bmj.com/cgi/content/full/84/1/51 (accessed February 23, 2008); (4) Elizabeth A. McGlynn, Ph.D., et al., "The Quality of Health Care Delivered to Adults in the United States," *The New England Journal of Medicine*, 346.26 (2003):

2635–2645, http://content.nejm.org/cgi/content/abstract/348/26/2635 (accessed April 11, 2008).

22. Glenn S. Takata, MD et al., "Development, Testing, and Findings of a Pediatric-Focused Trigger Tool to Identify Medication-Related Harm in US Children's Hospitals," *Pediatrics* 121.4 (2008): e927–e935, http://pediatrics.aappublications.org/cgi/content/full/121/4/e927 (accessed April 11, 2008).

23. Elizabeth A. McGlynn, Ph.D. et al., "The Quality of Health Care Delivered to Adults in the United States," *The New England Journal of Medicine*, 346.26 (2003): 2635–2645, http://content.nejm.org/cgi/content/abstract/348/26/2635 (accessed April 11, 2008).

24. Stephen S. Hyde, "The Last Priesthood: The Coming Revolution in Medical Care Delivery," Cato Institute, *Regulation Magazine*, Fall 1992, http://www.cato.org/pubs/regulation/reg15n4h.html (accessed February 24, 2008).

25. Stephen S. Hyde, "The Last Priesthood: The Coming Revolution in Medical Care Delivery," Cato Institute, *Regulation Magazine*, Fall 1992, http://www.cato.org/pubs/regulation/reg15n4h.html (accessed February 24, 2008).

26. (1) John E. Wennberg, MD, MPH, et al., "The Care of Patients With Severe Chronic Illness (2006), An Online Report on the Medicare Program by the Dartmouth Atlas Project," Center for the Evaluative Clinical Sciences, 65, http://www.dartmouthatlas.org/atlases/2006_Chronic_Care_Atlas.pdf (accessed February 24, 2008). (2) Shannon Brownlee, *Overtreated: Why Too Much Medicine Is Making Us Sicker and Poorer* (New York: Bloomsbury USA, 2007).

27. Marilyn J. Field and Kathleen N. Lohr, eds., *Guidelines for Clinical Practice: From Development to Use* (Washington DC: National Academies Press, 1992).

28. Jenny Doust, "Why Do Doctors Use Treatments That Do Not Work?" *BMJ* 328 (2004): 474–475, http://www.bmj.com/cgi/content/full/328/7438/474#REF6 (accessed March 4, 2008). Steve Connor, "Glaxo Chief: Our Drugs Do Not Work on Most Patients," *The Independent/UK*, December 8, 2003, http://www.commondreams.org/headlines03/1208-02.htm (accessed March 4, 2008).

29. Jenny Doust, "Why Do Doctors Use Treatments That Do Not Work?" *BMJ* 328 (2004): 474–475, http://www.bmj.com/cgi/content/full/328/7438/474#REF6 (accessed March 4, 2008).

30. Rita Rubin, "Drug Warnings Outline Danger," *USA Today*, March 25, 2005, http://www.usatoday.com/news/health/2005-04-25-black-box-cover_x.htm (accessed March 4, 2008).

31. Maggie Mahar, "Making Use of Comparative Effectiveness Research," Taking Note, December 5, 2008, http://takingnote.tcf.org/2008/12/making-use-of-comparative-effectiveness-research.html (accessed January 21, 2009).

32. Ceci Connolly, "Comparison Shopping for Medicine," *Washington Post*, March 17, 2009, http://www.washingtonpost.com/wp-dyn/content/article/2009/03/16/AR2009031602913.html (accessed March 10, 2009).

33. Tom Daschle, with Scott S. Greenberger and Jeanne M. Lambrew, *Critical: What We Can Do about the Health-Care Crisis* (New York: Thomas Dunne Books, 2008).

34. Eric D. Beinhocker, *The Origin of Wealth* (Watertown, MA: Harvard Business School Press, 2006).

35. Michael F. Cannon, "A Better Way to Generate and Use Comparative-Effectiveness Research," Cato Institute, *Policy Analysis*, February 6, 2009, http://www.cato.org/pub_display.php?pub_id=9940 (accessed April 30, 2009).

36. Christopher Murray et al., "Eight Americas: Investigating Mortality Disparities across Races, Counties, and Race-Counties in the United States" *PLoS Medicine* 3.9 (2006), http://medicine.plosjournals.org/perlserv/?request=getdocument&doi=10.1371/journal.pmed.0030260 (accessed April 30, 2009).

37. Kurt Ullman, "Linking Doctors' Pay to Performance Has Little Effect on Diabetes Outcomes," Health Behavior News Service, November 1, 2007, http://hbns.org/getDocument.cfm?documentID=1611 (accessed February 22, 2008).

38. "Keeping Up with Medication Dosage and Frequency is Vital to Your Health," Group Insurance Commission, Commonwealth of Massachusetts, Winter 2005, http://www.mass.gov/gic/healthartdrugcompliance.htm (accessed February 26, 2008).

39. Laura Landro, "Incentives Push More Doctors to E-Prescribe," *The Wall Street Journal*, January 21, 2009, http://online.wsj.com/article/SB123249533946000191.html?mod=djemHL (accessed January 21, 2009).

40. Nicola Howell et al., "Compliance With Statins in Primary Care," *The Pharmaceutical Journal* 272 (2004), http://www.pjonline.com/pdf/papers/pj_20040110_compliance.pdf (accessed February 23, 2008).

41. "Keeping Up with Medication Dosage and Frequency is Vital to Your Health," Group Insurance Commission, Commonwealth of Massachusetts, Winter 2005, http://www.mass.gov/gic/healthartdrugcompliance.htm (accessed February 26, 2008).

42. Jay Crosson, MD, "Dr Garfield's Enduring Legacy—Challenges and Op-portunities," http://xnet.kp.org/permanentejournal/summer06/legacy.html (accessed January 25, 2009).

43. "Is Preventive Medical Care Cost Effective?" National Center for Policy Analysis, November 9, 1995, http://www.ncpa.org/ba/ba188.html (accessed April 6, 2008).

44. "Is Preventive Medical Care Cost Effective?" National Center for Policy Analysis, November 9, 1995, http://www.ncpa.org/ba/ba188.html (accessed April 6, 2008).

45. Joshua T. Cohen, Peter J. Neumann, and Milton C. Weinstein, "Does Preventive Care Save Money? Health Economics and the Presidential Candidates," *NEJM* 358.7 (2008): 661–663, http://content.nejm.org/cgi/content/full/358/7/661#R3 (accessed May 7, 2008).

46. Louise B. Russell, "Preventing Chronic Disease: An Important Investment, But Don't Count On Cost Savings," *Health Affairs* 28.1 (2009), http://content.healthaffairs.org/cgi/content/abstract/28/1/42 (accessed April 3, 2009).

47. "The Health Insurance Experiment—A Classic RAND Study Speaks to the Current Health Care Reform Debate," RAND Corporation, 2006, http://www.rand.org/pubs/research_briefs/2006/RAND_RB9174.pdf (accessed April 30, 2009).

48. Hodan Farah Wells and Jean C. Buzby "Dietary Assessment of Major Trends in U.S. Food Consumption, 1970–2005," USDA, March 2008, http://www.ers.usda.gov/Publications/EIB33/EIB33.pdf (accessed April 6, 2008).

49. "Trends and Indicators in the Changing Health Care Marketplace: Exhibit 2.13: Number: Number and Distribution of HMO Enrollment, by Model Type, 1984–2004," Kaiser Family Foundation, http://www.kff.org/insurance/7031/print-sec2.cfm (accessed April 6, 2008).

50. Laura Landro, "Submitting to the Science of Prevention," *The Wall Street Journal*, November 26, 2008, http://online.wsj.com/article/SB122765661371658079.html?mod=djempersonal (accessed December 5, 2008).

51. "Report Cites Major Reduction in Teenage Smoking," New York State Department of Health, August 30, 2007, http://www.health.state.ny.us/press/releases/2007/2007-08-30_teenage_smoking_reduction.htm (accessed April 7, 2008).

52. "AIDS Transmission Rate Falls," *The Wall Street Journal*, December 10, 2008, pA16. "Trends in HIV/AIDS Diagnoses—33 States, 2001—2004," CDC, *MMWR Weekly*, November 18, 2005, http://www.cdc.gov/MMWR/preview/mmwrhtml/mm5445a1.htm (accessed April 7, 2008).

53. Nicholas A. Christakis and James H. Fowler, "The Spread of Obesity in a Large Social Network over 32 Years," *The New England Journal of Medicine* 357.4 (2007): 370–379, http://content.nejm.org/cgi/content/full/357/4/370 (accessed December 5, 2008). Nicholas A. Christakis and James H. Fowler, "The Collective Dynamics of Smoking in a Large Social Network," *The New England Journal of Medicine* 358.21(2008): 2249–2258, http://content.nejm.org/cgi/content/full/358/21/2249 (accessed December 8, 2008).

54. "Report of the Council on Medical Service," CMS Report 7-A-00, June 2000, www.ama-assn.org/ama/upload/mm/372/a00cms7doc.doc (accessed April 7, 2008).

55. "Heart and Stroke Death Rates Steadily Decline; Risks Still Too High," *AHA News*, January 22, 2008, http://www.americanheart.org/presenter.jhtml?identifier=3053235 (accessed April 7, 2008).

56. PHM van Baal et al., "Lifetime Medical Costs of Obesity: Prevention No Cure for Increasing Health Expenditure," 2008, *PLoS Medicine* 5.2 (2008), http://www.plosmedicine.org/article/info%3Adoi%2F10.1371%2Fjournal.pmed.0050029 (accessed May 24, 2008).

57. Jacob Goldstein, "Health Reform and the High Cost of Healthy Living," *The Wall Street Journal—Health Blog*, February 15, 2008, http://blogs.wsj.com/health/2008/02/05/health-reform-and-the-high-cost-of-healthy-living/ (accessed May 24, 2008).

58. Graphic at http://talkingtails.files.wordpress.com/2007/07/800px-maslows_hierarchy_of_needssvg.png?w=399&h=266 (accessed December 8, 2008).

Chapter 3: Consumer Roles and Rights

1. "Fallacy of Composition," NationMaster.com Encyclopedia, http://www.nationmaster.com/encyclopedia/Fallacy-of-composition (accessed February 1, 2009).

2. "HealthGrades Study Finds Patient Outcomes at Lenox Hill Hospital Among Nation's Best For Cardiac Services and Coronary Interventional Procedures," LenoxHill Hospital, http://www.lenoxhillhospital.org/press_releases.aspx?id=624 (accessed February 1, 2009). HealthGrades, http://www.healthgrades.com/hospital-directory/new-york-ny-manhattan/hospital-awards-HGST750A7B36330101/user_agreement (accessed February 1, 2009).

3. Kathleen Blanchard, RN, "Employees Paying More For Health Insurance, Trend Continues," *Emax Health*, November 28, 2008, http://www.emaxhealth.com/1020/72/26914/employees-paying-more-health-insurance-trend-continues.html (accessed December 3, 2008). "Treasury, IRS Issue 2009 Indexed Amounts for Health Savings Accounts," U.S. Treasury, May 13, 2008, http://www.ustreas.gov/press/releases/hp975.htm (accessed January 21, 2009). Robin A Cohen, Michael Martinez and Heather Free, "Health Insurance Coverage: Early Release of Estimates from the National Health Interview Survey," Centers for Disease Control and Prevention, January 13, 2009, http://www.cdc.gov/nchs/data/nhis/earlyrelease/insur200809.htm#F3 (accessed January 19, 2009).

4. Vanessa Fuhrmans, "Insurer Jumps Into Web," *The Wall Street Journal*, December 1, 2008, http://online.wsj.com/article/SB122809638906868099.html?mod=djemHL (accessed December 1, 2008). Laura Landro, "What's New (Or Improved) in Health Sites," *The Wall Street Journal*, January 7, 2009, http://online.wsj.com/article/SB123128697040459161.html?mod=djempersonal (accessed January 19, 2009),

5. Laura Landro, "What's New (Or Improved) in Health Sites," *The Wall Street Journal*, January 7, 2009, http://online.wsj.com/article/SB123128697040459161.html?mod=djempersonal (accessed January 19, 2009).

6. Laurie Goering, "Medical Tourism Soars as Americans Seek Major Savings on Health Care," *Chicago Tribune*, April 1, 2008, http://www.ahiphiwire.org/News/Default.aspx?doc_id=158092 (accessed April 11, 2008).

7. Joel Millman, "How the Amish Drive Down Medical Costs," *The Wall Street Journal*, February 21, 2006, http://online.wsj.com/article/SB114048909124578710.html (accessed March 24, 2008).

8. Laurie Goering, "Medical Tourism Soars as Americans Seek Major Savings on Health Care," *Chicago Tribune*, April 1, 2008 http://www.ahiphiwire.org/News/Default.aspx?doc_id=158092 (accessed April 11, 2008).

9. Tilman Ehrbeck, Ceani Guevara, and Paul D. Mango, "Mapping the Market for Medical Travel," *The McKinsey Quarterly*, May 2008, http://www.mckinseyquarterly.com/Health_Care/Strategy_Analysis/Mapping_the_market_for_travel_2134 (accessed April 25, 2009).

10. Uday Khandeparkar, "Outsourcing Health Care to India," *The Wall Street Journal*, December 15, 2008, http://online.wsj.com/article/SB122933146963306435.html (accessed December 15, 2008).

11. "Galichia Heart Hospital Launches Medical Tourism Program," http://www.ghhospital.com/pr_washpost.php (accessed April 3, 2009).

12. Dinah Wisenberg Brin, "Pharmacies Fight Tough Battle on Generic Prices," *The Wall Street Journal*, December 22, 2008, http://online.wsj.com/article/ SB122990612110525373.html?mod=djemHL (accessed December 22, 2008).

13. Stephen S. S. Hyde, *Prescription Drugs For Half Price or Less* (New York: Bantam Dell Division of Random House, Inc., 2006).

14. Patricia Barnes, Barbara Bloom, and Richard Nahin, "Complementary and Alternative Medicine Use Among Adults and Children: United States, 2007," National Health Statistics Report, no. 12, National Center for Health Statistics, December 10, 2008, http://nccam.nih.gov/news/2008/nhsr12.pdf (accessed December 26, 2008).

15. David M. Eisenberg, et al., "Trends in Alternative Medicine Use in the United States, 1990–1997: Results of a Follow-up National Survey," *JAMA*, 280.18 (2008): 1569–1575.

16. "1997 National Health Expenditures Survey," Centers for Medicare & Medicaid Services.

17. Steve Salerno, "The Touch That Doesn't Heal," *The Wall Street Journal*, December 26, 2008, W11.

18. Abby Ellin, "Lasik Surgery: When The Fine Print Applies To You," *The New York Times*, March 13, 2008, http://www.nytimes.com/2008/03/13/fashion/ 13SKIN.html?_r=1&scp=1&sq=lasik&st=nyt&oref=slogin (accessed March 18, 2008).

19. "LCA-Vison Reports Quarterly Performance of LasikPlus Vision Centers," *Lasik Surgery News*, December 2, 2007, http://lasiksurgerynews.com/news/ LCAV-LasikPlus-20071203.shtml (accessed March 18, 2008).

20. Steve Forbes, "Fact and Comment," *Forbes Magazine*, October 29, 2008, http://www.forbes.com/opinions/forbes/2008/1117/017.html (accessed November 3, 2008).

21. Abby Ellin, "Lasik Surgery: When The Fine Print Applies To You," *The New York Times*, March 13, 2008, http://www.nytimes.com/2008/03/13/fashion/ 13SKIN.html?_r=1&scp=1&sq=lasik&st=nyt&oref=slogin (accessed March 18, 2008). Sabine Vollmer, "Eyeing the Risks of LASIK Eye Surgery," October 11, 2007, http://seattletimes.nwsource.com/html/health/2003941235_ lasik11.html (accessed March 18, 2008).

22. Rhonda L. Rundle, "Competitive Squeeze—Industry Giants Push Obesity Surgery," *The Wall Street Journal*, March 31, 2008, http://online.wsj.com/ article/SB120692909065176045.html (accessed March 31, 2008).

23. John B. Dixon, MBBS, PhD, et al., "Adjustable Gastric Banding and Conventional Therapy for Type 2 Diabetes—A Randomized Controlled Trial," *JAMA*, January 23, 2008, http://jama.ama-assn.org/cgi/content/abstract/299/3/316?maxtoshow=&HITS=10&hits=10&RESULTFORMAT=&fulltext=gastric+banding+diabetes&searchid=1&FIRSTINDEX=0&resourcetype=HWCIT (accessed March 31, 2008).

24. Rhonda L. Rundle, "Obesity Surgery Is Called Cost-Effective," *The Wall Street Journal*, September 8, 2008, http://online.wsj.com/article/SB122082794026608293.html?mod=djemHL (accessed April 25, 2009).

25. John Kasprak, "Backgrounder: Retail-Based Medical Clinics," September 10, 2008, http://www.cga.ct.gov/2008/rpt/2008-R-0457.htm (accessed January 15, 2009).

26. Milt Freudenheim, "Wal-Mart Will Expand In-Store Medical Clinics," *The New York Times*, February 7, 2008, http://www.nytimes.com/2008/02/07/business/07clinic.html?_r=2 (accessed January 15, 2009).

27. Amy Merrick, "Walgreen Broadens Its Health-Care Reach," *The Wall Street Journal*, January 14, 2009, http://online.wsj.com/article/SB123189349214879393.html?mod=djemHL (accessed January 15, 2009).

28. Milt Freudenheim, "Wal-Mart Will Expand In-Store Medical Clinics," *The New York Times*, February 7, 2008, http://www.nytimes.com/2008/02/07/business/07clinic.html?_r=2 (accessed January 15, 2009).

29. Milt Freudenheim, "Wal-Mart Will Expand In-Store Medical Clinics," *The New York Times*, February 7, 2008, http://www.nytimes.com/2008/02/07/business/07clinic.html?_r=2 (accessed January 15, 2009).

30. Clayton Christensen, Jerome Grossman, and Jason Hwang, *The Innovator's Prescription: A Disruptive Solution for Health Care* (New York: McGraw Hill, 2009).

31. Milt Freudenheim, "Wal-Mart Will Expand In-Store Medical Clinics," *The New York Times*, February 7, 2008, http://www.nytimes.com/2008/02/07/business/07clinic.html?_r=2 (accessed January 15, 2009).

32. Joel Millman, "How the Amish Drive Down Medical Costs," *The Wall Street Journal*, February 21, 2006, http://online.wsj.com/article/SB114048909124578710.html (accessed March 24, 2008).

33. Barbara Martinez, "Generic Drugs By Mail Can Be a Raw Deal," *The Wall Street Journal*, February 15, 2005, B1.

34. "Health Plan Initiatives, Trends and Research in Consumer-Driven Care," Blue Cross Blue Shield Association, October 20, 2008, http://www.bcbs.com/about/search.jsp?query=consumer+driven (accessed November 3, 2008).

35. Emily Berry, "Taking It to the Bank: A New Strategy for Health Plans," *AMNews*, December 22, 2008, http://www.ama-assn.org/amednews/2008/12/22/bisa1222.htm (accessed December 26, 2008).

36. "Making the Leap from 'Monopoly Money,'" Harvard Pilgrim Health Care, https://www.harvardpilgrim.org/pls/portal/docs/PAGE/BROKER/HSA-WP-FINAL-10-12-07.PDF (accessed April 11, 2009).

37. AP, "AMA Joins Suit Against Aetna, Cigna Over Payment Data," *The Wall Street Journal*, February 10, 2009, http://online.wsj.com/article/SB123431749077271205.html?mod=djemHL (accessed February 11, 2009).

38. Richard L. Clarke, "Healthcare Complexities Work Against All of Us," Letter to *The Wall Street Journal*, November 28, 2003, http://www.hfma.org/about/positions/pa_healthcare_comlexities.htm (accessed March 11, 2008).

39. "Federal Employee Health Benefits Program Premiums for 2009," National Treasury Employees Union Chapter 293, http://www.secunion.org/HealthPlan9292008 (accessed November 15, 2008).

40. Frank Diamond, "Blueprint for the Future? Or Trapped in a Lockbox?" *Managed Care*, January 2001, http://www.managedcaremag.com/archives/0101/0101.fehbp.html (accessed November 17, 2008).

41. "Federal Employee Health Benefits Program Premiums for 2009," National Treasury Employees Union Chapter 293, http://www.secunion.org/HealthPlan9292008 (accessed November 15, 2008).

42. "FEHBP Premium Rise for 2009 Extremely Troubling," National Treasury Employees Union Chapter 293, http://www.secunion.org/FEHBRise92008 (accessed November 17, 2008).

43. "How Much Do I Pay for Coverage?" U.S. Office of Personnel Management, http://www.opm.gov/insure/federal_employ/index.asp?AnswerId=70 (accessed November 15, 2008).

44. Brittany Ballenstedt, "Federal Health Premiums to Rise 7% in 2009," September 25, 2008, http://www.govexec.com/story_page.cfm?articleid=41054&printerfriendlyvers=1 (accessed November 17, 2008).

45. "Non-Postal Premium Rates for the Federal Employees Health Benefits Program," http://www.opm.gov/insure/health/rates/nonpostalffs2009.pdf (accessed November 17, 2008).

46. CMS Office of Public Affairs, "Lower Medicare Part D Costs Than Expected in 2009—Beneficiary Satisfaction Remains High," August 14, 2008, http://www.cms.hhs.gov/apps/media/press/release.asp?Counter=3240&intNumPerPage=10&checkDate=&checkKey=&srchType=1&numDays=3500&srchOpt=0&srchData=&keywordType=All&chkNewsType=1%2C+2%2C+3%2

C+4%2C+5&intPage=&showAll=&pYear=&year=&desc=&cboOrder=date (accessed April 25, 2009).

47. Tyler Cowen, "Public Goods," Library of Economics and Liberty, http://www.econlib.org/library/Enc/PublicGoods.html (accessed January 20, 2009).

48. About.com:Economics, http://economics.about.com/library/glossary/bldef-economic-good.htm (accessed January 20, 2009).

49. In his book, *What It Means To Be A Libertarian*,"(Broadway, 1997, p. xii), Charles Murray coined the term "lower-case libertarian" to connote a classical liberal who is "too fond of tradition and the nonrational aspects of the human spirit" to adopt the pure, uncompromising tenets of "the leading thinkers of the libertarian movement—Libertarians with a capital L."

50. Charles P. Kindleberger and Robert Aliber, *Manias, Panics, and Crashes—A History of Financial Crises*, Fifth Edition (Hoboken, NJ: John Wiley & Sons, Inc., 2005).

Chapter 4: Health Insurance: What's Wrong with It and What Needs to Be Done About It?

1. "CNN Poll: Americans Say Health Care Too Expensive," CNN, March 19, 2009, http://politicalticker.blogs.cnn.com/2009/03/19/cnn-poll-americans-say-health-care-too-expensive/ (accessed April 13, 2009).

2. Carmen DeNavas-Walt, Bernadette D. Proctor, and Jessica C. Smith, "Income, Poverty, and Health Insurance Coverage in the United States: 2008," U.S. Census Bureau, August 2008, http://www.census.gov/prod/2008pubs/p60-235.pdf (accessed January 8, 2009).

3. "Overview of the Uninsured in the United States: An Analysis of the 2005 Current Population Survey," U.S. Department of Health and Human Services Office of the Assistant Secretary for Planning and Evaluation, September 22, 2005, http://aspe.hhs.gov/health/reports/05/uninsured-cps/index.htm#fig4 (accessed March 27, 2008).

4. "Annual Population Estimates 2000 to 2007; Table 1: Annual Estimates of the Population for the United States, etc.," U.S. Census Bureau, http://www.census.gov/popest/states/NST-ann-est.html (accessed March 28, 2008).

5. Amy J. Davidoff, Bowen Garrett, and Alshadye Yemane, "Medicaid-Eligible Adults Who Are Not Enrolled—Who Are They and Do They Get the Care They Need?" October 1, 2001, http://www.urban.org/url.cfm?ID=310378 (accessed March 28, 2008).

6. Matthew Collier and Lisa Walsh, "The New Insurance Frontier," *The Wall Street Journal*, January 7, 2008, http://online.wsj.com/article_print/SB119966521932671081.html (accessed April 25, 2009).

7. Thomas P. Miller, "What DO We Know About the Uninsured?" *The American*, July/August 2008, http://american.com/archive/2008/july-august-magazine-contents/what-do-we-know-about-the-uninsured (accessed January 8, 2009).

8. Victoria Craig Bunce and JP Wieske, "Health Insurance Mandates in the States 2008," Council for Affordable Health Insurance, http://www.cahi.org/cahi_contents/resources/pdf/HealthInsuranceMandates2008.pdf (accessed February 10, 2008).

9. Scott Gottlieb, "Obama's Health Care Record," *The Wall Street Journal*, May 5, 2008, A15, http://online.wsj.com/article/SB120995014765166523.html?mod=opinion_main_commentaries (accessed April 25, 2009).

10. Ezekiel Emanuel and Ron Wyden, "Why Tie Health Insurance to a Job," *The Wall Street Journal*, December 10, 2008, A19.

11. Spineline, http://www.medtronicsofamordanek.com/spineline/hospital/definitions.html (accessed November 28, 2008).

12. Bruce Pyenson, "Health Care Reform 2008," Milliman Interview, June 2008.

13. "Employer-Sponsored Health Insurance: Trends in Cost and Access," Agency for Health Care Research and Quality, U.S. DHHS, http://www.ahrq.gov/research/empspria/empspria.htm (accessed January 24, 2008).

14. "Employer Health Benefits—2007 Annual Survey," The Kaiser Family Foundation and Health Research and Educational Trust, http://www.kff.org/insurance/7672/upload/Summary-of-Findings-EHBS-2007.pdf (accessed January 24, 2008).

15. University of Missouri-St. Louis, Continuing Education, Human Resource Management Program, http://www.umsl.edu/divisions/conted/business/noncredit/cert_hrm_topics.htm (accessed January 12, 2009).

16. Phil Primack, "Small Employers and Expanded Health Insurance Coverage," Policy Brief 07-5, New England Public Policy Center at the Federal Reserve Bank of Boston, July 2007, http://www.bos.frb.org/economic/neppc/briefs/2007/briefs075.pdf (accessed February 16, 2009).

17. Jamie Peck and Nik Theodore, "Flexible Recession: The Temporary Staffing Industry and Mediated Work in the United States," *Cambridge Journal of Economics*, January 2007, http://cje.oxfordjournals.org/cgi/content/abstract/31/2/171?HITS=10&sortspec=relevance&hits=10&maxtoshow=&FIRSTINDEX=0&resourcetype=HWCIT&fulltext=acyclical&searchid=1&RESULTFORMAT= (accessed February 16, 2009).

18. "Futurework," *Occupational Outlook Quarterly*, US Bureau of Labor Statistics, Summer 2000, 36, http://www.bls.gov/opub/ooq/2000/Summer/art04.pdf (accessed February 16, 2009).

19. Ezekiel Emanuel, and Ron Wyden, "Why Tie Health Insurance to a Job," *The Wall Street Journal*, December 10, 2008, A19.

20. Lydell C. Bridgeford, "Public-Sector Employers Still Wary of CDHPs," *Employee Benefit News*, January 20, 2009, http://ebn.benefitnews.com/asset/article/2658541/public-sector-employers-still-wary-cdhps.html (accessed January 20, 2009).

21. Ezekiel Emanuel and Ron Wyden, "Why Tie Health Insurance to a Job," *The Wall Street Journal*, December 10, 2008, A19.

22. Andrew Stern, "Employment-Based Health Insurance: A Prominent Past, but Does it Have a Future?" The Brookings Institution, June 16, 2006, http://www.brookings.edu/events/2006/0616health-care.aspx (accessed April 25, 2009).

23. Sarah Rubenstein, "How to Fix Your Life in 2009," *The Wall Street Journal*, December 31, 2008, D2.

24. Robin A Cohen, et al., "Health Insurance Coverage: Early Release of Estimates from the National Health Interview Survey," Centers for Disease Control and Prevention, January 13, 2009, http://www.cdc.gov/nchs/data/nhis/earlyrelease/insur200809.htm#F3 (accessed January 19, 2009).

25. Burton T. Beam, Jr. and John J. McFadden, *Employee Benefits*, 6th Edition (Chicago: Dearborn Trade Publishing, 2004) 228–229, http://books.google.com/books?id=yN9vHhgi5lQC&pg=PA228&lpg=PA228&dq=blue+cross+community+rating&source=web&ots=ASHWZMPOqK&sig=3i4MG_int7hLb7-fDr7PW5luIbQ&hl=en&sa=X&oi=book_result&resnum=8&ct=result#PPA229,M1 (accessed January 20, 2009).

26. Jonathan Gruber and Ebonya Washington, "Subsidies to Employee Health Insurance Premiums and the Health Insurance Market," February 2003, http://www.jcpr.org/conferences/health_policy/gruber.pdf; "First, roughly one-quarter of the uninsured are individuals who are offered health insurance through their job or the job of a family member, but do not take it up. These are individuals who have access to the employer provided insurance system, and for whom employers are already paying a sizeable share of their insurance costs. Thus, it seems that these are the 'low hanging fruit' of the uninsured population, the cheapest group to bring into the ranks of the insured. Second, the decline in insurance coverage over the past two decades has been almost exclusively through reduced takeup of insurance among those offered, not reduced offering."

27. "Overview of the Uninsured in the United States: An analysis of the 2005 Current Population Survey," U.S. Department of Health and Human Services Office of the Assistant Secretary for Planning and Evaluation, September 22, 2005, http://aspe.hhs.gov/health/reports/05/uninsured-cps/index.htm#fig4 (accessed March 27, 2008).

28. "2007 Employer Health Benefits Survey," The Kaiser Family Foundation and Health Research Educational Trust, http://www.kff.org/insurance/7672/upload/76723.pdf (accessed April 25, 2009).

29. Robert Pear, "Women Buying Health Policies Pay a Penalty," *The New York Times*, October 29, 2008, http://www.nytimes.com/2008/10/30/us/30insure.html?_r=2&pagewanted=2&th&emc=th&oref=login (accessed November 3, 2008).

30. Paul Krugman, *The Conscience of a Liberal* (New York: W.W. Norton & Company, Inc., 2007) 239.

31. "Licensed Drivers, Vehicle Registrations and Resident Population," Highway Statistics 2004, Federal Highway Administration, http://www.fhwa.dot.gov/policy/ohim/hs04/htm/dlchrt.htm (accessed April 25, 2009).

32. Paul Krugman, *The Conscience of a Liberal* (New York: W.W. Norton & Company, Inc., 2007) 239.

33. Ben Pimentel, "Who Is Paying For Uninsured Medical Patients?" *Stanford GSB News*, June 2007, http://www.gsb.stanford.edu/news/research/kessler_uninsured.html (accessed March 3, 2008).

34. Joanne Wojcik, "AHIP Proposes Universal Coverage Mandate," *Business Insurance*, November 19, 2008, http://www.businessinsurance.com/cgi-bin/news.pl?id=14553 (accessed April 25, 2009).

35. Michael E. Porter and Elizabeth Olmsted Teisberg, *Redefining Health Care—Creating Value-Based Competition on Results* (Watertown, MA: Harvard Business School Press, 2006).

36. Michael Porter, Comments made during the Mayo Clinic Health Reform Symposium, Leesburg, VA, March 10, 2008.

37. Regina Herzlinger, *Who Killed Health Care? America's $2 Trillion Medical Problem—and the Consumer-Driven Cure* (New York: McGraw Hill, 2007) 257, 253.

38. Charles Murray, *In Our Hands—A Plan to Replace the Welfare State* (Washington, DC: The AEI Press, 2006) 45.

39. Newt Gingrich, *Real Change* (Washington, DC: Regnery Publishing, Inc, 2008) 227.

40. Michael F. Cannon and Michael D. Tanner, *Healthy Competition—What's Holding Back Health Care and How to Free It*, Second Edition (Washington, DC : Cato Institute, 2007) 43–47.

41. Greg Scandlen, "Consumer Power Report #82," June 1, 2007, www.chcchoices.org. (accessed April 28, 2009).

42. Robert Hartman and Paul van de Water, "The Budgetary Treatment of an Individual Mandate to Buy Health Insurance," Congressional Budget Office Memorandum, August 1994, http://www.cbo.gov/doc.cfm?index=4816&type=0 (accessed April 28, 2009).

43. "Overview of the Uninsured in the United States: An Analysis of the 2005 Current Population Survey," U.S. Department of Health and Human Services Office of the Assistant Secretary for Planning and Evaluation, September 22, 2005, http://aspe.hhs.gov/health/reports/05/uninsured-cps/index.htm#fig4 (accessed March 27, 2008).

44. Karl Manheim and Jamie Court, "Not So Fast on the Insurance Mandates," *Los Angeles Times*, March 24, 2008, http://www.latimes.com/news/opinion/la-oe-court24mar24,0,204686.story (accessed April 11, 2008).

45. Elisha Maldonado, "Mass. Consumers Pay $1.3 Billion a Year for Mandated Insurance Benefits," Health Care News, September 2008, 7.

46. Kevin Sack, "Massachusetts Faces a Test on Health Care," *The New York Times*, November 25, 2007, http://www.nytimes.com/2007/11/25/us/politics/25mass.html?_r=1&oref=slogin (accessed April 28, 2009).

47. John Goodman, "John Goodman's Health Policy Blog," September 17, 2007, http://www.john-goodman-blog.com/advice-for-hillary-bravo-for-stossel/ (accessed April 4, 2009).

48. David Cutler, interview by Richard Eskow, Grasping Reality with Both Hands: Economist Brad DeLong's Fair, Balanced, and Reality-Based Semi-Daily Journal, February 7, 2008, http://delong.typepad.com/sdj/2008/02/richard-eskow-t.html (accessed April 7, 2008).

Chapter 5: Medicare, Medicaid, and SCHIP

1. Greg D'Angelo, "The 2007 Medicare Trustees Report: A Trigger for Reform?" The Heritage Foundation, May 3, 2007, http://www.heritage.org/Research/HealthCare/wm1442.cfm (accessed May 21, 2008).

2. Robert R. Kulesher, "Medicare's Operational History and Impact on Health Care," *Health Care Manager*, January/March 2006, http://www.accessmylibrary.com/coms2/summary_0286-13793090_ITM (accessed December 27, 2007).

3. Gregory J. Przybylski, M.D., "Understanding and Applying a Resource-Based Relative Value System to Your Neurosurgical Practice," Posted May 21, 2002 at http://www.medscape.com/viewarticle/433288_2 (accessed December 30, 2007). "History of the RBRVS," *AMA*, http://www.ama-assn.org/ama/pub/category/16393.html (accessed December 30, 2007).

4. "CMS Financial Data," Centers for Medicare and Medicaid Services, http://www.cms.hhs.gov/CapMarketUpdates/downloads/2005walletcard.pdf (accessed April 28, 2009).

5. Jane Zhang, "Medicare Spending to Surge," *The Wall Street Journal*, February 26, 2008, http://online.wsj.com/article/SB120399640594392887.html (accessed March 3, 2008).

6. Julie Rovner, "Trustees: Medicare Funds Will Be Depleted By 2017," NPR, 3/13/9, http://www.npr.org/templates/story/story.php?storyId=104079588 (accessed May 16, 2009).

7. Jagadeesh Gokhale, "Medicaid's Soaring Costs: Time to Step on the Brakes," Cato Institute Policy Analysis no. 597, 7/19/7.

8. Michael Cannon, "Hey Buddy, Can You Spare $86 Trillion," Cato @ Liberty, May 1, 2006, http://www.cato-at-liberty.org/category/health-care/page/24/ (accessed April 24, 2009).

9. William M. Welch, "Medicare: The Next Riddle for the Ages," *USA Today*, March 13, 2006, http://www.usatoday.com/news/washington/2005-03-16-medicare-riddle_x.htm (accessed March 3, 2008).

10. Jane Zhang, "Why We Need 1,170 Codes for Angioplasty," *The Wall Street Journal*, November 11, 2008, http://online.wsj.com/article/SB122636897819516185.html (accessed November 17, 2008).

11. MargaretAnn Cross, "Confronting The Medicare Cost Shift," *Managed Care*, December 2006, http://www.managedcaremag.com/archives/0612/0612.costshift.html (accessed April 28, 2009).

12. Gregory J. Przybylski, M.D., "Understanding and Applying a Resource-Based Relative Value System to Your Neurosurgical Practice," Posted May 21, 2002 at http://www.medscape.com/viewarticle/433288_2 (accessed December 30, 2007).

13. Miguel A. Faria, Jr., MD, "The AMA, Ethics and Gun Control," Newsmax.com, May 3, 2001, http://archive.newsmax.com/archives/articles/2001/5/3/23021.shtml (accessed May 5, 2008).

14. Gregory J. Przybylski, M.D., "Understanding and Applying a Resource-Based Relative Value System to Your Neurosurgical Practice," Posted May 21, 2002 at http://www.medscape.com/viewarticle/433288_2 (accessed December 30, 2007).

15. Benjamin Brewer, MD, "Planned Medicare Cuts Weigh on Primary Care," *The Wall Street Journal*, December 11, 2007, http://online.wsj.com/article_print/SB119732809319620055.html (accessed December 11, 2007).

16. Richard Stengel and Adi Ignatius, "A Bible, But No E-mail," *Time*, http://www.time.com/time/specials/2007/personoftheyear/article/ 0,28804,1690753_1690757_1691279,00.html (accessed April 11, 2008).

17. Jane Zhang, "Why We Need 1,170 Codes for Angioplasty," *The Wall Street Journal*, November 11, 2008, http://online.wsj.com/article/ SB122636897819516185.html (accessed November 17, 2008).

18. Benjamin Brewer, MD, "Planned Medicare Cuts Weigh on Primary Care," *The Wall Street Journal*, December 11, 2007, http://online.wsj.com/article_ print/SB119732809319620055.html (accessed March 3, 2008).

19. James Arvantes, "Congress Provides Six-Month Reprieve From Medicare Payment Cuts—AAFP Decries Temporary Fix," *AAFP News Now*, December 19, 2007, http://www.aafp.org/online/en/home/publications/news/ news-now/government-medicine/20071219medicarebill.printerview.html (accessed April 28, 2009).

20. "Doctor Salaries," The-Travel-Nurse.com, http://www.the-travel-nurse. com/doctor_best_salaries.html (accessed April 12, 2009).

21. Associated Press, "Shortage of Family Doctors Predicted by 2020," September 27, 2006, http://www.msnbc.msn.com/id/15020430 (accessed April 28, 2009).

22. Diane Levick, "Fewer Primary Care Physicians Take Medicare Patients," *Hartford Courant*, April 9, 2008, http://www.courant.com/news/health/ hc-docfind0409.artapr09,0,178348.story (accessed April 11, 2008). Krystle Russin, "Fewer Doctors Are Accepting Medicare Cases," *Health Care News*, September 2008, 1.

23. Theo Francis and Vanessa Fuhrmans, "Report Finds Health Work Force Is Unprepared for Elderly Boomers," *The Wall Street Journal*, April 15, 2008, http://online.wsj.com/article/SB120818216377212673.html (accessed April 15, 2008).

24. Vanessa Fuhrmans, "Medical Specialties Hit By a Growing Pay Gap," *The Wall Street Journal*, May 5, 2008, A1, http://online.wsj.com/article/ SB120995022062766515.html?mod=djemHL (accessed May 5, 2008).

25. Benjamin M. Friedman, *The Moral Consequences of Economic Growth* (New York: Vintage Books, 2005).

26. "Medicaid and Managed Care," Kaiser Commission on Medicaid and the Uninsured, December 2001, http://www.kff.org/medicaid/upload/Medicaid- and-Managed-Care-Fact-Sheet.pdf (accessed April 28, 2009).

27. "Overview of the Uninsured in the United States: An Analysis of the 2005 Current Population Survey," U.S. Department of Health and Human Services Office of the Assistant Secretary for Planning and Evaluation, September 22, 2005, http://aspe.hhs.gov/health/reports/05/uninsured-cps/index.htm#fig4 (accessed March 27, 2008).

28. "Provider Reimbursement Rates Fiscal Year 2003–2004: Proviso 8.34, A Report to the Governor (SC), the Ways and Means Committee, and the Senate Finance Committee," Submitted by the Department of Health and Human Services, January 31, 2003, http://www.scstatehouse.net/archives/HealthHumanServices/prov8-34rpt03.doc.

29. Ben Pimentel, "Who Is Paying For Uninsured Medical Patients?" *Stanford GSB News*, June 2007, http://www.gsb.stanford.edu/news/research/kessler_uninsured.html (accessed March 3, 2008).

30. Heather Won Tesoriero, "Aetna, Cigna Rank Highest in Efficiency," *The Wall Street Journal*, May 29, 2008, http://online.wsj.com/article/SB121203008624228397.html (accessed June 2, 2008).

31. Alex Wayne, "Congress Unlikely to Avert Medicaid Cost Shift," *CQ Today*, February 11, 2008, http://public.cq.com/docs/cqt/news110-000002669279.html (accessed April 28, 2009).

32. "Total SCHIP Expenditures, FY2006," The Henry J Kaiser Foundation, http://www.statehealthfacts.org/comparetable.jsp?ind=235&cat=4 (accessed April 28, 2009).

33. Michael F. Cannon and Michael D. Tanner, *Healthy Competition—What's Holding Back Health Care and How to Free It*, Second Edition (Washington, DC: Cato Institute, 2007) 94, 97–101.

34. "The Health Insurance Experiment—A Classic RAND Study Speaks to the Current Health Care Reform Debate," RAND Corporation, 2006, http://www.rand.org/pubs/research_briefs/2006/RAND_RB9174.pdf (accessed April 28, 2009). Leighton Ku, "Charging the Poor More for Health Care: Cost-Sharing in Medicaid," Center on Budget and Policy Priorities, May 7, 2003, http://www.cbpp.org/5-7-03health.htm (accessed April 28, 2009).

35. Dennis Cauchon, "Medicaid insures historic number," *USA Today*, August 1, 2005, http://www.usatoday.com/news/washington/2005-08-01-medicaid_x.htm (accessed April 28, 2009).

36. Clifford J. Levy and Michael Luo, "New York Medicaid Fraud May Reach Into Billions," *The New York Times*, July 18, 2005, http://www.nytimes.com/2005/07/18/nyregion/18medicaid.html?ex=1279339200&en=b7bf75d8d29b6c0b&ei=5088&partner=rssnyt&emc=rss (accessed April 28, 2009).

37. Steven Malanga, "How to Stop Medicaid Fraud," *City Journal*, Spring 2006, http://www.city-journal.org/html/16_2_medicaid_fraud.html (accessed April 28, 2009).

38. "2008 Actuarial Report on the Financial Outlook for Medicaid," U.S. Department of Health and Human Services, 2008, http://www.cms.hhs.gov/ActuarialStudies/downloads/MedicaidReport2008.pdf (accessed April 12, 2009).

39. Carmen DeNavas-Walt, Bernadette D. Proctor, and Jessica Smith," Income, Poverty, and Health Insurance Coverage in the United States: 2006," U.S. Census Bureau, August 2007, http://www.census.gov/prod/2007pubs/p60-233.pdf (accessed April 28, 2009). Bernadette D. Proctor and Joseph Dalaker, "Poverty Status of People by Family Relationship, Race, and Hispanic Origin: 1959 to 2002," U.S. Census Bureau, September 2003, http://www.census.gov/prod/2003pubs/p60-222.pdf (accessed April 28, 2009).

40. Vernon Smith, Ph.D. et al., "As Tough Times Wane, States Act to Improve Medicaid Coverage and Quality: Results from a 50-State Medicaid Budget Survey for State Fiscal Years 2007 and 2008," Kaiser Commission on Medicaid and the Uninsured, October 2007, http://www.kff.org/medicaid/upload/7699.pdf (accessed April 28, 2009).

Chapter 6: HMOs, ERISA, and CDHC

1. John Barnes, "Failure of Government Central Planning Washington's Medical Certificate of Need Program," January 2006, http://www.washingtonpolicy.org/Centers/healthcare/policybrief/06_barnes_constudy.html (accessed April 28, 2009).

2. Charles B. Dew, *Ironmaker to the Confederacy—Joseph R. Anderson and the Tredegar Iron Works*, Second Edition (Richmond: Library of Virginia, 1999) 315–316.

3. Marc J. Perry and Paul J. Mackun, "Population Change and Distribution," U.S. Census Bureau, April 2001, www.census.gov/prod/2001pubs/c2kbr01-2.pdf (accessed April 28, 2009). "Comparative International Statistics," U.S. Census Bureau, Statistical Abstract of the United States: 2004–2005, http://www.census.gov/prod/2004pubs/04statab/intlstat.pdf (accessed April 28, 2009).

4. "Hospitals, Vertically Integrated Health Systems and Other Personal Health Service Organizations," Slide 49, University of Michigan, based on AHA Hospital Statistics 2005, twww.med.umich.edu/csp/Course%20materials/Summer%202005/Lichtenstein_Hospitals05.ppt (accessed April 6, 2008).

5. "Employer Health Benefits Survey 2007," Kaiser Family Foundation and Health Research Educational Trust, http://www.kff.org/insurance/7672/upload/76723.pdf (accessed April 28, 2009).

6. "ERISA," American College of Emergency Physicians, http://www.acep.org/patients.aspx?id=25934 (accessed January 13, 2008).

7. "Employment Size of Firms, Table 2a. Employment Size of Employer and Nonemployer Firms, 2004," U. S. Census Bureau, http://www.census.gov/epcd/www/smallbus.html (accessed January 25, 2009). "Employer Firm Births and Deaths by Employment Size of Firm, 1989–2005," Small Business Administration, http://www.sba.gov/advo/research/dyn_b_d8905.pdf (accessed January 25, 2009).

8. John C. Goodman, "A Brief History of Health Savings Accounts," National Center for Policy Analysis, http://cdhc.ncpa.org/about/brief-history-of-health-savings-accounts (accessed March 8, 2008). "Health Saving Accounts: How They Work," Medical Savings Health Plan, http://www.medicalsavings.com/Pages/otherQA.htm (accessed December 8, 2008).

9. Merrill Matthews Jr. and Jack Strayer, "Real Patient Protection: Expanding Medical Savings Accounts," National Center for Policy Analysis, July 16, 1998, http://www.ncpa.org/pub/ba/ba275/ (accessed March 8, 2008).

10. Alvin R. Tarlov, "HMO Enrollment Growth and Physicians: The Third Compartment," *Health Affairs*, Spring 1986, http://content.healthaffairs.org/cgi/reprint/5/1/23.pdf (accessed May 1, 2008).

11. "Lets Talk Health Care Quick Guide: Massachusetts Health Care Reform—Updated December 2007," http://www.letstalkhealthcare.org/wp-content/uploads/2007/12/ma-health-care-reform-guide-rev-december-07.pdf (accessed January 26, 2008).

12. Greg Scandlen, "Consumer Power Report #128," Consumers For Health Care Choices at The Heartland Institute, http://www.heartland.org/CHCC/ (accessed May 21, 2008).

Chapter 7: The Quieter Complications

1. Andrew H. Beck, "The Flexner Report and the Standardization of American Medical Education," JAMA, May 5, 2004, http://jama.ama-assn.org/cgi/content/full/291/17/2139 (accessed January 10, 2009).

2. George J. Stigler, "The Theory of Economic Regulation," *The Political Economy: Readings in the Politics and Economics of American Public Policy*, Ed. Thomas Ferguson and Joel Rogers (Armonk, NY: M.E. Sharpe, Inc., 1984) 68, http://books.google.com/books?id=94G2VY_lLHMC&pg=PA68&lpg=PA68&dq=As+a+rule,+regulation+is+acquired+by+the+industry+and+is+

designed+and+operated+primarily+for+its+benefit&source=web&ots=
Y1yepLs4rS&sig=F3qi7AljQX1X80_CY9Ov_snHpGU&hl=en
(accessed May 16, 2008).

3. Clayton Christensen, Jerome Grossman, and Jason Hwang, *The Innovator's Prescription: A Disruptive Solution for Health Care* (New York: McGraw Hill, 2009).

4. Shannon Brownlee, *Overtreated—Why Too Much Medicine is Making Us Sicker and Poorer* (New York: Bloomsbury USA, 2007).

5. Paul Kinnersley, et al., "Randomised Controlled Trial of Nurse Practitioner Versus General Practitioner Care for Patients Requesting 'Same Day' Consultations in Primary Care," *BMJ*, April 15, 2000, http://www.bmj.com/cgi/content/full/320/7241/1043 (accessed March 8, 2008); Mary O. Mundinger, et al., "Primary Care Outcomes in Patients Treated by Nurse Practitioners or Physicians: A Randomized Trial. JAMA 283.1 (2000): 59–68. Sharon A. Brown and Deanna E. Grimes, *Nurse Practitioners and Certified Nurse-Midwives: A Meta-Analysis of Studies on Nurses in Primary Care Roles* (Washington, DC: American Nurse Publishing, 1993). A. Bessman, "Comparison of Medical Care in Nurse Clinician and Physician Clinics in Medical Affiliated Hospitals," *Journal of Chronic Diseases*, 27 (1974): 115–25. H. Sox, "Quality of Patient Care by Nurse Practitioners and Physician Assistants: A Ten-year Perspective," *Annals of Internal Medicine*, 91 (1979): 459–68.

6. George J. Stigler, "The Theory of Economic Regulation," *The Political Economy: Readings in the Politics and Economics of American Public Policy*, Ed. Thomas Ferguson and Joel Rogers (Armonk, NY: M.E. Sharpe, Inc., 1984) 68, http://books.google.com/books?id=94G2VY_lLHMC&pg=PA68&lpg=P A68&dq=As+a+rule,+regulation+is+acquired+by+the+industry+and+is +designed+and+operated+primarily+for+its+benefit&source=web&ots =Y1yepLs4rS&sig=F3qi7AljQX1X80_CY9Ov_snHpGU&hl=en (accessed May 16, 2008).

7. Robert M. Huston, M.D., *Medical Examiner and Record of Medical Science* (Philadelphia: Lindsay and Blakiston, 1847) 487, http://books.google.com/ books?id=WBcCAAAAYAAJ&pg=PA487&dq=merest+pittance+in+the+wa y+of+remuneration+is+scantily+doled+out (accessed May 16, 2008).

8. Richard Lichtenstein, Lecture on US Hospitals in HMP 600 at the University of Michigan School of Public Health, Department of Health Management and Policy. Cited with permission of Dr. Lichtenstein.

9. Patrick John McGinley, "Beyond Health Care Reform: Reconsidering Certificate of Need Laws in a Managed Competition System," *Florida State University Law Review*, 1995, http://www.law.fsu.edu/journals/lawreview/ issues/231/mcginley.html#heading4_2 (accessed April 28, 2009).

10. Patrick John McGinley, "Beyond Health Care Reform: Reconsidering Certificate of Need Laws in a Managed Competition System," *Florida State University Law Review*, 1995, http://www.law.fsu.edu/journals/lawreview/issues/231/mcginley.html#heading4_2 (accessed April 28, 2009).

11. Patrick John McGinley, "Beyond Health Care Reform: Reconsidering Certificate of Need Laws in a Managed Competition System," *Florida State University Law Review*, 1995, http://www.law.fsu.edu/journals/lawreview/issues/231/mcginley.html#heading4_2 (accessed April 28, 2009).

12. D. Grabowski, M. Morrisey, and R. Ohsfeldt, "The Effects of Certificate-of-Need Repeal on Medicaid Long-Term Care Expenditures," *Academy for Health Services Research and Health Policy*, 18 (2001): 99, http://gateway.nlm.nih.gov/MeetingAbstracts/102273348.html (accessed April 28, 2009). Mark E. Kaplan, "An Economic Analysis of Florida's Hospital Certificate of Need Program and Recommendations for Change," *Florida State University Law Review*, 1991: 475, 478.

13. "Certificate of Need," American Health Planning Association, http://www.ahpanet.org/copn.html (accessed December 21, 2007).

14. Victoria Craig Bunce and JP Wieske, "Health Insurance Mandates in the States 2008," Council for Affordable Health Insurance, http://www.cahi.org/cahi_contents/resources/pdf/HealthInsuranceMandates2008.pdf (accessed February 10, 2008).

15. Laura Meckler and Anna Wilde Mathews, "McCain's Regulated-market Health Plan Would Boost Role of High-Risk Pools," *The Wall Street Journal*, June 2, 2008, http://online.wsj.com/article/SB121236916701936663.html?mod=djemHL (accessed June 2, 2008).

16. "Massachusetts' Health Care Reform Plan: Too Many Sticks; Not Enough Carrots," The Council for Affordable Health Insurance, May 2006, http://www.cahi.org/cahi_contents/resources/pdf/massachusetts.pdf (accessed January 26, 2008).

17. Robert Steinbrook, M.D., "Health Care Reform in Massachusetts—Expanding Coverage, Escalating Costs," *The New England Journal of Medicine*, June 26, 2008, http://content.nejm.org/cgi/content/full/358/26/2757?query=TOC (June 26, 2008).

18. *Rupp's Insurance and Risk Management Glossary* (Chatsworth,CA: NILS Publishing, 2002), http://insurance.cch.com/rupps/any-willing-provider-law.htm (accessed May 14, 2008).

19. Todd J. Zywicki, Susan A. Creighton, Luke M. Froeb, and David Hyman, "Letter to Patrick C. Lynch, Attorney General, State of Rhode Island and Providence Plantations," April 8, 2004, http://www.ftc.gov/os/2004/04/ribills.pdf (accessed May 15, 2008).

20. Michael G. Vita, "Regulatory Restrictions on Selective Contracting: An Empirical Analysis of 'Any Willing Provider' Regulations," *Journal of Health Economics*, 20 (2001): 955–966. This study controls for differences in the states' populations, including factors such as age, ethnicity, educational background, employment background (government, agriculture, manufacturing, etc.), income, population density, and the population growth rate.

21. Charles F. Kaiser III and Marvin Friedlander, "Corporate Practice of Medicine," http://www.irs.gov/pub/irs-tege/eotopicf00.pdf (accessed May 15, 2008).

22. Stephen Hyde, "The Last Priesthood—The Coming Revolution In Medical Care Delivery," CATO Regulation, Fall 1992, http://www.cato.org/pubs/regulation/regv15n4/reg15n4h.html (accessed May 16, 2008).

23. Nicole Huberfeld, "Be Not Afraid of Change: Time to Eliminate the Corporate Practice of Medicine Doctrine," *Health Matrix: Journal of Law-Medicine*, 14. 2 (2004), http://papers.ssrn.com/sol3/papers.cfm?abstract_id=498664#PaperDownload (accessed May 16, 2008).

24. Clayton Christensen, Jerome Grossman, and Jason Hwang, *The Innovator's Prescription: A Disruptive Solution for Health Care* (New York: McGraw Hill, 2009).

25. Brigitte C. Madrian, "Health Insurance Portability—The Consequences of COBRA," *Regulation: The Cato Review of Business and Government*, 21.1 (1998), Cato Institute, http://www.cato.org/pubs/regulation/regv21n1/21-1f2.pdf (accessed May 16, 2008).

26. Anna Wilde Mathews, "Newly Out of a Job? Here's How To Replace the Health Benefits," *The Wall Street Journal*, November 20, 2008, http://online.wsj.com/article/SB122704352826838437.html?mod=djempersonal (accessed November 20, 2008).

27. "Employer Health Benefits—2008 Annual Survey," The Kaiser Family Foundation and Health Research and Educational Trust, http://ehbs.kff.org/pdf/7790.pdf (accessed November 20, 2008).

28. M.P. McQueen, "Stimulus Makes Cobra Coverage a Better Bet," *The Wall Street Journal*, March 19, 2009, http://online.wsj.com/article/SB123500263888517825.html (accessed April 3, 2009).

29. Barbara Martinez, "Doctor-Owned Hospitals Fare Poorly in Child Health Bill," *The Wall Street Journal*, January 22, 2009, http://online.wsj.com/article/SB123258770557404699.html?mod=djemHL (accessed February 26, 2009).

30. David Whelan, "Bad Medicine," *Forbes*, March 10, 2008, http://www.forbes.com/forbes/2008/0310/086.html (accessed May 24, 2008).

31. "Specialty Hospitals—Geographic Location, Services Provided, and Financial Performance," United States General Accounting Office, October 2003, http://www.gao.gov/new.items/d04167.pdf (accessed April 28, 2009).

32. David P. Hamilton, "Insurers Take On Botched Medical Work—With Their Checkbooks," BNET Health Care Industry, April 4, 2008, http://industry.bnet.com/healthcare/2008/04/04/insurers-take-on-botched-medical-work-with-their-checkbooks (accessed April 28, 2009).

33. David Whelan, "Bad Medicine," *Forbes*, March 10, 2008, http://www.forbes.com/forbes/2008/0310/086.html (accessed May 24, 2008).

34. U.S. Senators Chuck Grassley and Max Baucus Letter to Michael O. Leavitt, Secretary, Department of Health and Human Services, February 14, 2006, http://www.americashospitals.com/issues/congressional_communications/Grassley,%20Baucus%20letter%20re%20specialty%20hospital%20safety%2002.14.06.pdf (accessed May 23, 2008).

35. "Nonprofit Hospitals and Tax Arbitrage," Congressional Budget Office, December 2006, http://www.cbo.gov/ftpdocs/76xx/doc7696/12-06-Hospital-Tax.pdf (accessed May 23, 2008).

36. John Carreyrou, "Nonprofit Hospitals, Once for the Poor, Strike It Rich," April 4, 2008, http://www.wsbt.com/news/consumer/17296354.html (accessed April 28, 2009).

37. Barbara Martinez & John Carreyrou, "Minority of Tax-Exempt Hospitals Provide Most Charity Care," *The Wall Street Journal*, February 13, 2009, http://online.wsj.com/article/SB123446379679978451.html?mod=djemHL (accessed February 18, 2009).

38. Regina Herzlinger, *Market-driven Health Care: Who Wins, Who Loses in the Transformation of America's Largest Service Industry* (Reading, MA: Addison-Wesley Publishing Company, Inc., 1997).

39. Clayton Christensen, Jerome Grossman, and Jason Hwang, *The Innovator's Prescription: A Disruptive Solution for Health Care* (New York: McGraw Hill, 2009).

40. Christopher J. Conover and Emily P. Zeitler, "Costs and Benefits of EMTALA," (Draft), Duke University Center for Health Policy, Law and Management, May 2004, http://www.hpolicy.duke.edu/cyberexchange/Regulate/CHSR/HTMLs/F1-EMTALA.htm (accessed April 28, 2009).

41. Hippocrates, *Of the Epidemics*, Book 1 translated by Francis Adams, http://classics.mit.edu/Hippocrates/epidemics.1.i.html (accessed May 27, 2008).

42. Robert Pear, "Fed Chief Addresses Health Care and Its Costs," *The New York Times*, June 17, 2008, http://www.nytimes.com/2008/06/17/health/policy/17health.html?_r=4&oref&oref=slogin&oref=slogin (accessed June 23, 2008).

43. Michael F. Cannon, "A Better Way to Generate and Use Comparative-Effectiveness Research," Cato Institute, February 6, 2009, http://www.cato.org/pub_display.php?pub_id=9940 (accessed April 28, 2009).

Part III—The Cure

1. Uwe E. Reinhardt, Peter S. Hussey, and Gerard F. Anderson, "U.S. Health Care Spending In An International Context," *Health Affairs*, 23. 3 (2004): 10–25, http://content.healthaffairs.org/cgi/content/full/23/3/10 (accessed April 28, 2009).

2. "2008 Annual Report of the Boards of Trustees of the Federal Hospital Insurance and Federal Supplementary Medical Insurance Trust Funds," March 25, 2008, http://www.cms.hhs.gov/ReportsTrustFunds/downloads/tr2008.pdf (accessed January 24, 2009).

3. Eric D. Beinhocker, *The Origin of Wealth* (Boston: Harvard Business School Press, 2006) 19 and 458 quoting Brian Arthur (1999) in *Science*: "Complexity economics is not a temporary adjunct to static economic theory, but theory at a more general, out-of-equilibrium level."

4. Bryan Caplan, "Singapore's Health Care System: A Free Lunch You Can Sink Your Teeth Into," Library of Economics and Liberty, January 13, 2008, http://econlog.econlib.org/archives/2008/01/singapores_heal.html (accessed April 13, 2009).

Chapter 8: Why Not Single Payer?

1. Pete Stark, "Medicare For All," *The Nation*, February 6, 2006, http://www.thenation.com/doc/20060206/stark (accessed April 28, 2009).

2. John Conyers, H. R. 676, "'The United States National Health Insurance Act,' Or 'Expanded & Improved Medicare For All,'" http://www.house.gov/conyers/news_hr676.shtml (accessed May 24, 2008).

3. Paul Krugman, *The Conscience of a Liberal* (New York: W.W. Norton & Company, Inc., 2007) 238.

4. Richard L. Clarke, "Healthcare Complexities Work Against All of Us," Letter to *The Wall Street Journal*, November 28, 2003, http://www.hfma.org/about/positions/pa_healthcare_comlexities.htm (accessed April 11, 2008).

5. Merrill Matthews, Ph.D., "Medicare's Hidden Administrative Costs: A Comparison of Medicare and the Private Sector (Based in Part on a Technical Paper by Mark Litow of Milliman, Inc.)," Council For Affordable Health Insurance, January 10, 2006, http://cahi.org/cahi_contents/.../CAHI_Medicare_Admin_Final_Publication.pdf (accessed April 28, 2009).

6. "Summary of Reform Task Force Meetings," National Bipartisan Commission on the Future of Medicare, http://medicare.commission. gov/medicare/summary.htm (accessed January 25, 2008).

7. Richard A. Sherer, "Are They Honest Mistakes or Medicare Fraud? Complicated Rules Lure Doctors and Government Into an Endless Loop," *Psychiatric Times*, September 2000, http://www.psychiatrictimes.com/ p000901a.html (accessed January 25, 2008).

8. Merrill Matthews, Ph.D., "Medicare's Hidden Administrative Costs: A Comparison of Medicare and the Private Sector (Based in Part on a Technical Paper by Mark Litow of Milliman, Inc.)," Council For Affordable Health Insurance, January 10, 2006, http://cahi.org/cahi_contents/.../CAHI_ Medicare_Admin_Final_Publication.pdf (accessed April 28, 2009).

9. "Fraud in Medicare," National Center for Policy Analysis, www.ncpa. org/~ncpa/health/pdh5.html (accessed January 3, 2008).

10. "Insurance Fraud," November 2007, Insurance Information Institute, http:// www.iii.org/media/hottopics/insurance/fraud/ (accessed April 28, 2009).

11. "Presidential Candidates and Health Care Information Technology: Where Do They Stand?" 12/16/7, http://www.electronic-medical-record.blogspot. com/ (accessed May 24, 2008).

12. Anna Wilde Mathews, "CBO Questions Savings From Digital Health-Care Records," *The Wall Street Journal*, May 22, 2008, http://online.wsj.com/ article/SB121142088466812947.html?mod=djemHL (accessed May 24, 2008).

13. Robert Solow, Review of *Manufacturing Matters*, by Stephen Cohen and John Zysman, *New York Review of Books*, July 12, 1987.

14. U.S. Department of Labor, 1998, cited by Jack E. Triplett, http://www.csls. ca/journals/sisspp/v32n2_04.pdf (accessed December 3, 2008).

15. Michael T. Kiley, "Computers and Growth with Frictions: Aggregate and Disaggregate Evidence," http://www.sciencedirect.com/science?_ob= ArticleURL&_udi=B6V8D-454738H-8&_user=10&_rdoc=1&_fmt=& _orig=search&_sort=d&view=c&_acct=C000050221&_version=1&_ urlVersion=0&_userid=10&md5=09f3ab81e922310a626de118fd1cd738 (accessed December 3, 2008).

16. Vitaliy Katsenelson, "The Profit Margin Paradigm," *The Motley Fool*, March 1, 2006, http://www.fool.com/investing/value/2006/03/01/the-profit-margin-paradigm.aspx (accessed April 28, 2009).

17. "Net Profit Margins—The Top Ten," The Online Investor, www. theonlineinvestor.com/margin_topten.phtml (accessed January 2, 2008).

18. "Net Profit Margins—The Top Ten," The Online Investor, www.theonlineinvestor.com/margin_topten.phtml (accessed January 2, 2008).

19. "2002 Drug Industry Profits: Hefty Pharmaceutical Company Margins Dwarf Other Industries," Public Citizen, www.citizen.org/documents/Pharma_Report.pdf (accessed April 28, 2009).

20. http://www.nytimes.com/2006/02/10/business/10aetna.html?_r=1&oref=slogin (accessed April 28, 2009).

21. http://www.fool.com/investing/value/2006/03/01/the-profit-margin-paradigm.aspx.

22. Julie Rovner, "Trustees: Medicare Funds Will Be Depleted By 2017," NPR, 3/13/9, http://www.npr.org/templates/story/story.php?storyId=104079588 (accessed May 16, 2009).

23. Jagadeesh Gokhale, "Medicaid's Soaring Costs: Time to Step on the Brakes," Cato Institute Policy Analysis no. 597, July 19, 2007, http://www.cato.org/pubs/pas/pa-597.pdf (accessed April 28, 2009).

24. P.J. O'Rourke, "The Problem Is Politics," *Cato's Letter*, 6 (Spring 2008), Cato Institute, www.cato.org/pubs/catosletter/catosletterv6n2.pdf (accessed April 28, 2009).

25. David Gratzer, MD, "The Ugly Truth About Canadian Health Care," *City Journal*, Summer 2007, http://www.city-journal.org/html/17_3_canadian_healthcare.html (accessed April 28, 2009).

26. "Is Preventive Medical Care Cost Effective?" National Center for Policy Analysis, November 9, 2005, http://www.ncpa.org/ba/ba188.html (accessed April 6, 2008).

27. "Defining Overweight and Obesity," Centers for Disease Control and Prevention, http://www.cdc.gov/nccdphp/dnpa/obesity/defining.htm (accessed March 13, 2009).

28. N. Gregory Mankiw, "Beyond Those Health Care Numbers," *The New York Times*, November 4, 2007, http://www.nytimes.com/2007/11/04/business/04view.html?_r=1&oref=slogin&pagewanted=print (accessed April 28, 2009).

29. Robert L. Ohsfeldt and John E. Schneider, *The Business of Health—The Role of Competition, Markets, and Regulation* (Washington, DC: The AEI Press, 2006) 19–20.

30. Robert L. Ohsfeldt and John E. Schneider, *The Business of Health—The Role of Competition, Markets, and Regulation* (Washington, DC: The AEI Press, 2006) 21.

31. N. Gregory Mankiw, "Beyond Those Health Care Numbers," *The New York Times*, November 4, 2007, http://www.nytimes.com/2007/11/04/business/04view.html?_r=1&oref=slogin&pagewanted=print (accessed April 28, 2009).

32. Robert L. Ohsfeldt and John E. Schneider, *The Business of Health—The Role of Competition, Markets, and Regulation* (Washington, DC: The AEI Press, 2006) 18.

33. Dr. David Gratzer, *The Cure: How Capitalism Can Save American Health Care* (New York: Encounter Books, 2006) 167.

34. "Canada Health Act Overview—What is the Canada Health Act?" Health Canada, November 25, 2002, http://www.hc-sc.gc.ca/ahc-asc/media/nr-cp/2002/2002_care-soinsbk4_e.html (accessed March 30, 2008).

35. David Gratzer, MD, "The Ugly Truth About Canadian Health Care," *City Journal*, Summer 2007, http://www.city-journal.org/html/17_3_canadian_healthcare.html (accessed April 28, 2009).

36. "Wait Times Power Point Presentation," Canadian Institute for Health Information, http://secure.cihi.ca/cihiweb/dispPage.jsp?cw_page=PG_549_E&cw_topic=549&cw_rel=AR_1385_E (accessed March 29, 2008).

37. Interview with David Gratzer posted 7/30/7 at http://www.qando.net/details.aspx?Entry=6555 (accessed March 30, 2008).

38. Scott Gottlieb, MD, "Organ Transplants Within the U.S. and Abroad," American Enterprise Institute for Public Policy Research, ReachMD Interview, http://www.reachmd.com/xmsegment.aspx?sid=2602 (accessed May 28, 2008).

39. Jeanne Whalen, "Europe's Drug Insurers Try Pay-for-Performance," *The Wall Street Journal*, October 12, 2007, http://online.wsj.com/article/SB119214458748556634.html (accessed April 28, 2009).

40. Jeanne Whalen, "British Agency Impugns Value Of Four Costly Cancer Drugs," *The Wall Street Journal*, August 8, 2008, http://online.wsj.com/article/SB121812494680320949.html?mod=djemHL (accessed April 28, 2009).

41. "Brits Resort to Pulling Own Teeth," CNN.com, October 15, 2007, http://www.cnn.com/2007/WORLD/europe/10/15/england.dentists/index.html (accessed March 29, 2008).

42. Dr. David Gratzer, *The Cure: How Capitalism Can Save American Health Care* (New York: Encounter Books, 2006) 177.

43. David Gratzer, MD, "The Ugly Truth About Canadian Health Care," *City Journal*, Summer 2007, http://www.city-journal.org/html/17_3_canadian_healthcare.html (accessed April 28, 2009).

44. Dr. David Gratzer, *The Cure: How Capitalism Can Save American Health Care* (New York: Encounter Books, 2006) 176.

45. Dr. David Gratzer, *The Cure: How Capitalism Can Save American Health Care* (New York: Encounter Books, 2006) 172.

46. Milton Friedman, "How to Cure Health Care," *Public Interest*, Winter 2001: 32.

47. David Hogberg, Ph.D., "Sweden's Single-Payer Health System Provides a Warning to Other Nations," *National Policy Analysis*, The National Center for Public Policy Research, May 2007, http://www.nationalcenter.org/NPA555_Sweden_Health_Care.html (accessed March 30, 2008).

48. Michael Tanner, "The Grass Is Not Always Greener—A Look at National Health Care Systems Around the World," Cato Institute, March 18, 2008, http://www.cato.org/pub_display.php?pub_id=9272 (accessed April 28, 2009).

49. "The Michael Moore Chronicles," National Center for Policy Research, http://sicko.ncpa.org/french-system-more-responsive-to-patient-needs (accessed March 30, 2008).

50. Helen Disney et al., "Impatient for Change—European Attitudes To Health Care Reform," http://209.85.173.104/search?q=cache:FUTJ3eqGS1cJ:www.healthpowerhouse.com/files/Impatient%2520for%2520change.pdf+disney+impatient+for+change&hl=en&ct=clnk&cd=1&gl=us (accessed March 30, 2008).

51. David Gratzer, "The Ugly Truth About Canadian Health Care," *City Journal*, Summer 2007, http://www.city-journal.org/html/17_3_canadian_healthcare.html (accessed April 28, 2009).

Chapter 9: The American Choice Health Plan

1. Gary Marcus, "Forget About Survival of the 'Fittest,'" *The Wall Street Journal*, February 11, 2009, A17.

2. "Retiree Accounting: More Than Meets The Eye," *Business Week*, January 30, 2006, http://www.businessweek.com/magazine/content/06_05/b3969080.htm (accessed April 28, 2009).

3. Dennis Cauchon, "Benefits Neglected for Civil Retirees—Governments Face a Steep Medical Tab," *USA Today*, February 16, 2009, http://www.usatoday.com/printedition/news/20090216/1aretiree16_st.art.htm (accessed April 28, 2009).

4. Jason Zweig, "Pay Collars Won't Hold Back Wall Street's Big Dogs," *The Wall Street Journal*, February 7, 2009, B1.

5. Wayne T. Brough, "New Federal Insurance Regulations Will Harm Consumers," March 22, 2007, http://www.freedomworks.org/informed/issues_template.php?issue_id=2811 (accessed April 10, 2008).

Chapter 10: Free Rider Prevention and Insurance Company Regulation

1. Linda Gorman, "Medical Bankruptcy Myths," John Goodman's Health Policy Blog, April 2, 2008, http://www.john-goodman-blog.com/medical-bankruptcy-myths/#more-189 (accessed April 28, 2009).

2. J. Newhouse, "Reimbursing Health Plans and Health Providers: Selection Versus Efficiency in Production," *Journal of Economic Literature*, 43.3 (1996): 1236–63. Jay Crosson, MD, "Dr Garfield's Enduring Legacy—Challenges and Opportunities," *Permanente Journal*, 10.2 (2006), http://xnet.kp.org/permanentejournal/summer06/legacy.html (accessed January 25, 2009).

3. Merrill Mathews, "A Health-Insurance Solution," *The Wall Street Journal*, Commentary, December 12, 2007, http://online.wsj.com/article/SB119742880091722751.html?mod=relevancy (accessed February 2, 2009).

4. Benjamin Brewer, MD, "The Doctor's Office—Finding a Medical Home May Be Just What the Doctor Ordered," February 12, 2008, *The Wall Street Journal*, http://online.wsj.com/article/SB120277184155560513.html (accessed April 28, 2009).

Chapter 11: Premium Reform

1. Christopher J. Murray, et al., "Eight Americas: Investigating Mortality Disparities across Races, Counties, and Race-Counties in the United States," September 2006, http://medicine.plosjournals.org/perlserv/?request=get-document&doi=10.1371/journal.pmed.0030260 (accessed April 28, 2009).

2. "Keeping Up with Medication Dosage and Frequency is Vital to Your Health," Winter 2005, Group Insurance Commission, Commonwealth of Massachusetts, http://www.mass.gov/gic/healthartdrugcompliance.htm (accessed February 26, 2008).

3. Premium discount based on estimated annual smoking-attributable medical costs per smoker from "Annual Smoking-Attributable Mortality, Years of Potential Life Lost, and Economic Costs—United States 1995–1999," United States Centers for Disease Control and Prevention, http://iier.isciii.es/mmwr/preview/mmwrhtml/mm5114a2.htm (accessed February 20, 2008). Cigarette costs based on nationwide average of $4.63/pack; "State Cigarette Prices, Taxes, and Costs per Pack," Campaign for Tobacco-Free Kids," http://www.tobaccofreekids.org/research/factsheets/pdf/0207.pdf (accessed February 20, 2008).

4. J. Newhouse, "Reimbursing Health Plans and Health Providers: Selection Versus Efficiency in Production," *Journal of Economic Literature*, 43.3 (1996): 1236–63. Jay Crosson, MD, "Dr Garfield's Enduring Legacy—Challenges and Opportunities," *Permanente Journal*, 10.2 (2006), http://xnet.kp.org/ permanentejournal/summer06/legacy.html (accessed January 25, 2009).

5. Joshua T. Cohen, et al., "Does Preventive Care Save Money? Health Economics and the Presidential Candidates," *NEJM*, February 14, 2008, http://content.nejm.org/cgi/content/full/358/7/661#R3 (accessed May 7, 2008).

Chapter 12: Toward Universal Participation, Provider Reforms, and Lower Costs

1. Matthew Collier and Lisa Walsh, "The New Insurance Frontier," *The Wall Street Journal*, January 7, 2008, http://online.wsj.com/article/ SB119966521932671081.html (accessed April 28, 2009).

2. Sandy Szwarc, BSN, RN, CCP; "Uninsured—Making a Diagnosis," July 2, 2007, http://junkfoodscience.blogspot.com/2007/07/uninsured-making-diagnosis.html (accessed January 9, 2008).

3. Stan Dorn, J.D., and Genevieve M. Kenney, Ph.D., "Automatically Enrolling Eligible Children and Families Into Medicaid and SCHIP: Opportunities, Obstacles, and Options for Federal Policymakers," June 16, 2006, The Commonwealth Fund, http://www.commonwealthfund.org/publications/ publications_show.htm?doc id=376814 (accessed February 29, 2008).

4. Diane Rowland, "Poverty and Health," *Gale Encyclopedia of Public Health* (New York: Macmillan Reference, 2002), http://www.healthline.com/ galecontent/poverty-and-health (accessed January 27, 2009).

5. "Chart 22—Distribution of Persons Served Through Medicaid and Payments by Basis of Eligibility, Fiscal Year 2000," *Program Information on Medicaid & State Children's Health on Insurance Program (SCHIP)*, Centers for Medicare and Medicaid Services, 2004, http://aspe.hhs.gov/medicaid/jul/ InfoMedicaid_schip.pdf (accessed January 30, 2008).

6. Clayton Christensen, Jerome Grossman, and Jason Hwang, *The Innovator's Prescription: A Disruptive Solution for Health Care* (New York: McGraw Hill, 2009).

7. Laura Landro, "Incentives Push More Doctors to E-Prescribe," *The Wall Street Journal*, January 21, 2009, http://online.wsj.com/article/ SB123249533946000191.html?mod=djemHL (accessed January 21, 2009).

8. Peter Pronovost, M.D., Ph.D., et al., "An Intervention to Decrease Catheter-Related Bloodstream Infections in the ICU," *The New England Journal of Medicine*, December 28, 2006, https://content.nejm.org/cgi/reprint/355/26/2725.pdf?ck=nck (accessed January 27, 2008).

9. "Fast Facts on American Hospitals, American Hospital Association," http://www.aha.org/aha/resource-center/Statistics-and-Studies/fast-facts.html (accessed January 27, 2008).

10. "Fact Sheet: Evidence-based Hospital Referral (EBHR)," The Leapfrog Group, http://www.leapfroggroup.org/media/file/Leapfrog-Evidence-Based_Hospital_Referral_Fact_Sheet.pdf (accessed January 28, 2008).

11. Thomas J. DiLorenzo, *How Capitalism Saved America: The Untold History of Our Country, From the Pilgrims to the Present* (New York: Crown Publishing, 2004) 98.

Conclusion: A Future Scenario and Major Savings

1. Richard L. Clarke, "Healthcare Complexities Work Against All of Us," Letter to *The Wall Street Journal*, November 28, 2003, http://www.hfma.org/about/positions/pa_healthcare_comlexities.htm (accessed April 11, 2008).

2. "The Price of Excess, Identifying Waste in Healthcare Spending," PricewaterhouseCoopers' Health Research Institute, http://blogs.wsj.com/health/files/2008/04/price-of-excess-paper-final.pdf (accessed April 11, 2008).

3. Ross DeVol and Armen Bedroussian, "An Unhealthy America: The Economic Burden of Chronic Disease," Milken Institute, http://www.milkeninstitute.org/pdf/chronic_disease_report.pdf (accessed February 21, 2008).

4. Maggie Mahar, "The State of the Nation's Health," *Dartmouth Medicine*, Spring 2007, http://dartmed.dartmouth.edu/spring07/pdf/atlas.pdf (accessed April 11, 2008).

5. Shannon Brownlee, *Overtreated—Why Too Much Medicine is Making Us Sicker and Poorer* (New York: Bloomsbury USA, 2007).

Appendix: Who Wants to Be a Trillionaire?

1. Adapted and expanded from an unpublished 2007 business plan by the author, based on his 2002 concepts.

Index

Schneider, John
  The Business of Health, 273–74
Schumpeter, Joseph, 24, 87, 207, 376, 384
self-destructive behaviors, 3, 17, 28, 35,
  59–62, 67, 72–73, 111–12, 125, 129,
  140, 144, 195–96, 289–90, 350, 354–55,
  359, 367, 369, 387, 397
Service Employees International Union,
  142
70/20 rule, 130, 330
Shaw, George Bernard, 56
Sicko, 262, 275
Singapore, 258
single-payer system, 9, 79, 177, 234, 285,
  330
    arguments for, 259–62
    creeping, 152, 329
    critique of, 262–82
    definition, 257
    in other countries, 272–81
    not necessary, 281–82
    opposition to, 258
    problems with, 84
    two-tier, 282
Sipkoff, Martin, 47
60 Minutes, 91
small business, 4–5, 138–39, 214–15,
  239–40, 299
Smith, Adam, 2, 30, 33
smoking, 66–67, 69–70, 72–73, 331–32,
  356, 361–63, 395
Social Security, 161, 175
Solow, Robert, 267
"Solution Shops," 378
South Carolina
    Medicaid program, 186
Soviet Union, 20, 257
    Gosplan, 179, 228
Sowell, Thomas, 9
Sparrow, Malcolm, 265
special interests, 145, 166–67, 169, 179,
  215, 227, 253, 264, 337, 344
standards of living, 39, 152, 183, 256
Stark, Pete, 259–60, 269
Stark II law, 248
state
    benefit mandates, 145–46, 149, 214

corporate practice of medicine
  (CPOM) laws, 237–38
fraudulent schemes, 186–87
guaranteed-issue requirements,
  233–34
medical practice laws, 224
minimum insurance benefit laws,
  230–32
regulators, 289
states'-rights advocates, 309
Stern, Andrew, 142
Stigler, George J., 226
stomach ulcers, 52, 56
strokes, 66
supply and demand, 2, 15, 25, 154, 228–30
Sweden, 257, 280
Switzerland, 31, 128, 258
Symptom Analyst Plus, 50

take-home pay, 40, 141, 142, 195
Tanner, Michael, 166, 280
tax
    benefits and group coverage, 131, 133
    code, 308
    credits, 304–307
    equity, 30
    exclusion, 307–308
    exemptions, 249, 304
    neutrality, 295
    out-of-pocket benefits, 149
    payers, 151–52, 164
    payroll, 40, 131, 146, 218, 275, 291,
      295, 300, 305
    penalty, 146, 295
    policy, 42, 223, 307, 308
    reform, 29, 293, 294–308
    refundable credits, 303
    returns, 166, 170, 305–306
    unlegislated, 176
    without representation, 167–69
technology, 4, 24, 93, 387
Texas Medical Association, 182
Thailand, 379, 393
third-party administrators (TPAs), 99, 137
third-party payers, 22, 229, 245, 404
Thoreau, Henry David, 30
ToxTown, 81
transition period, 153

Breinigsville, PA USA
07 April 2011
259361BV00004B/18/P